Nursing Care and the Activities of Living

Dedication

This book is dedicated to all the student nurses who do make a difference.

Nursing Care and the Activities of Living

Second Edition

Edited by

Ian Peate

EN(G), RGN, DipN (Lond), RNT, BEd (Hons), MA (Lond), LLM
Head of the School of Nursing and Midwifery
Faculty of Health and Human Sciences
Thames Valley University
Middlesex, UK

WILEY-BLACKWELL
A John Wiley & Sons, Ltd., Publication

This edition first published 2010

Blackwell Publishing was acquired by John Wiley & Sons in February 2007. Blackwell's publishing programme has been merged with Wiley's global Scientific, Technical, and Medical business to form Wiley-Blackwell.

Registered office
John Wiley & Sons, Ltd., The Atrium, Southern Gate, Chichester, West Sussex, PO19 8SQ, United Kingdom

Editorial office
9600 Garsington Road, Oxford, OX4 2DQ, United Kingdom
2121 State Avenue, Ames, Iowa 50014-8300, USA

For details of our global editorial offices, for customer services and for information about how to apply for permission to reuse the copyright material in this book please see our website at www.wiley.com/wiley-blackwell.

Library of Congress Cataloging-in-Publication Data

Nursing Care and the Activities of Living / edited by Ian Peate. 2nd ed.
p. ; cm.
Rev. ed. of: Compendium of clinical skills for student nurses / edited by Ian Peate. 2005.
Includes bibliographical references and index.
ISBN 978-1-4051-9458-7 (pbk. : alk. paper)
1. Nursing–Textbooks. I. Peate, Ian. II. Compendium of clinical skills for student nurses.
[DNLM: 1. Nursing Care–Great Britain. WY 100 C737 2010]
RT41.C7445 2010
610.73–dc22

2009021836

A catalogue record for this book is available from the British Library.

Set in 9/12.5 pt Interstate Light by Aptara® Inc., New Delhi, India
Printed and bound in Malaysia by KHL Printing Co Sdn Bhd

1 2010

Contents

Contributors

David Briggs, *RN, DN (Cert), CPT, DPSN, BA (HONS), PGCE (NMC recorded), MSc, FHEA*
David began his career in 1980 at the North Middlesex Hospital, becoming a Staff Nurse and working on a medical ward. He progressed his career within District Nursing and became a District Nursing Charge Nurse in 1985. He mentored and assessed many pre-registration nurses within a community environment and also delivered the practical element of the district nurse training to several district nurses. He joined the University of Hertfordshire in 2000. His portfolio consists of teaching many practical nursing skills, for example moving and handling, nutrition and communication. He is a fellow of the Higher Education Academy.

Victoria Darby, *RGN, BSc (Hons) MA (Education)*
Victoria trained for 4 years at City University and qualified in 1996 to work as a Staff Nurse in pancreatic surgery. She worked as a Placement Support Nurse from 2000 and then within the University setting from 2003. Victoria's areas of interests are interprofessional education, study skills and social policy. She is currently a Senior Lecturer at the University of Hertfordshire.

Debbie Davies, *RN, DipN (Lond), RNT, PGCE(HE), BSc(OU), MSc*
Debbie began her nursing career in 1977 at The Middlesex Hospital, Mortimer Street, London W1. As a Registered Nurse, she worked in a variety of clinical areas including surgery and intensive care. She became a Ward Sister in cardiovascular surgery and undertook a clinical teaching role in the intensive care unit at St Mary's Hospital, Praed Street, London W2. She has worked in nurse education since 1987. Her key areas of interest are clinical nursing practice and theory and psychosocial aspects of nursing. She is currently Pre-Registration Nursing Admissions Coordinator whose portfolio centres on recruitment and marketing.

Guy Dean
Guy qualified in 1981 and specialised in intensive care nursing, coronary care as a Charge Nurse. He then became a clinical nurse manager, for a short time, and decided to enter nurse education. He completed his teacher training and degree in nursing and became a Registered Clinical Nurse Teacher and Registered Nurse Tutor. He subsequently, since 1998, became a lecturer at the University of Herefordshire. He developed the first degrees in Paramedic Sciences and Physician Assistants in the UK. His key areas of interest are patient assessment. He is currently Programme Leader for the BSC (Hons) Emergency Nursing.

Mary Greeno, *MA, BSc (Hons), PGCE, RN, SCM, RCNT, RNT, FLTHE*
Mary did her general nursing and midwifery training in University College Hospital, Galway. She undertook an ENB theatre course in Edgware General Hospital, where she worked as a Staff Nurse and Sister for a number of years. She then worked as an Accident and Emergency Sister in Edgware General Hospital. She did her clinical teaching course at the Royal College of Nursing, followed by the PGCE at Harrow Polytechnic College. Following a number of years teaching as both a Clinical Teacher and Nurse Tutor at Barnet College of Nursing and Midwifery, she undertook a BSc (Hons) in nursing at the University of Hertfordshire, followed by an MA at Middlesex University. She is currently working as Senior Lecturer at the University of Hertfordshire. Her interests are in dignified patient care, theatre nursing and palliative care.

Laureen Hemming, *RGN, DipN (Lond), RCNT, BA (Open), PGCEA, BPhil Complementary Health Care*
Laureen is currently Programme Tutor for Oncology Nursing and Palliative Care Degree pathways; two degrees that she authored as well as manages and has been teaching in this field since 1990. Her nursing career commenced in the 1960s at Addenbrookes Hospital, Cambridge, and she had various posts in medical and surgical nursing, elderly care and orthopaedics before settling in St Albans and focussing on end-of-life care. Her interests include complementary therapies, psychosocial end-of-life care, bereavement and nurse education. Laureen has published in journals and written a chapter on personal care in the Compendium of Clinical Skills for Student Nurses and has presented at National and International Conferences on various aspects of cancer, palliative care and nurse education.

Jackie Hulse, *BA (Hons), RGN, MSc, PGCE, RNT, PGDip (TESOL)*
Jackie Hulse worked in cardiac care and critical care settings in London for 12 years before becoming a Nurse Teacher. In addition to pre-registration and post-registration teaching, Jackie now works predominantly with students on the Overseas Nurses Programme and the International Nursing programme at UH and she has also trained as an English Language Teacher to gain expertise in supporting these students.

Sean Mallon, *RN, BA (Lond), PGDip (Lond), MSc (Lond)*
Sean began his nursing in 1990 at Mount Vernon Hospital by working in an acute medical ward. He later worked in coronary care and studied both his BA and his MSc in that specialist area. Having been a Charge Nurse in CCU for 5 years, he then moved into a Lecturer Practitioner role and continues now to work in nurse education. He is currently a Senior Lecturer in Adult Nursing and his portfolio centres on foundation skills and clinical skills for nurses.

Janet G. Migliozzi, *RGN, BSc (Hons), MSc (Lond), PGDEd, FHEA*
Janet commenced her nursing career in London, becoming a Staff Nurse in 1988. She has worked at a variety of hospitals across London, predominately in vascular, orthopaedic and high dependency surgery before specialising in infection prevention and control and has worked in nurse education since 1999. Her key interests include microbiology particularly in relation to health care associated infections, vascular/surgical nursing, health informatics and nurse education. Janet is currently

programme leader for the Infection Prevention and Control degree pathways and has published in journals and written a chapter on minimising risk in relation to health care-associated infection and is a member of the Infection Prevention Society.

Muralitharan Nair, *SRN, RMN, DipN (Lond) RNT, Cert Ed., BSc (Hons) MSc (Surrey), Cert in Counselling, FHEA*
Muralitharan commenced his nursing career in 1971 at Edgware General Hospital becoming a Staff Nurse. In 1975 he commenced his mental health nurse training at Springfield Hospital and worked as a Staff Nurse for approximately 1 year. He has worked at St Mary's Hospital Paddington and Northwick Park Hospital returning to Edgware General Hospital to take up the post of Senior Staff Nurse and then Charge Nurse. He has worked in nurse education since 1989. His key interests include physiology, diabetes, surgical nursing and nurse education. Muralitharan has published in journals and written a chapter on elimination and published a textbook on Pathophysiology. He is a fellow of the Higher Education Academy.

Ian Peate, EN(G), *RN, DipN (Lond), RNT, BEd (Hons), MA (Lond), LLM*
Ian began his nursing career in 1981 at Central Middlesex Hospital, becoming an Enrolled Nurse working in an intensive care unit. He later undertook a 3-year student nurse training at Central Middlesex and Northwick Park Hospitals, becoming a Staff Nurse and then a Charge Nurse. He has worked in nurse education since 1989. His key areas of interest are nursing practice and theory, sexual health and HIV/AIDS. He is Head of the School of Nursing and Midwifery in the Faculty of Health and Human Sciences.

Lynn Quinlivan, *RN(G), DipT&L, BSc (Hons) OU*
Lynn began her nursing career in 1978 at the Royal Isle of Wight School of Nursing, becoming a State Registered Nurse working in acute care. Lynn undertook the Intensive Care Course at Charing Cross Hospital 1982 and continued to work in Acute Care over the next 20 years as a Staff Nurse and then a Sister. She has worked in nurse education since 2003. Currently, Lynn is a Senior Lecturer; her key areas of interest are clinical practice and management skills.

Jane Say, *RN, RNT, BSc (Hons), PGDE, MSc*
Originally, Jane trained at the Royal Liverpool University Hospital and studied biochemistry at Liverpool University. Before entering nurse education, Jane worked in a variety of acute medical areas including, renal, cardiology and respiratory care. Her key areas of interest include nutritional care and assessment, the biosciences as applied to nursing practice and the development of teaching and learning in nurse education. Currently, Jane is a Programme Tutor within the Pre-Registration Nursing Programme at the University of Hertfordshire.

Lynda Sibson, *MSc, RGN, RSCN, CTHE, Independent Nurse Consultant*
Lynda began her nursing career in 1983 at Epsom District Hospital, later trained at Great Ormond Street Hospital as a paediatric nurse. She later worked as a Practice Nurse in a GP surgery and later following qualifying as a Nurse Practitioner, worked in a nurse-led Minor Treatment Centre in Central London. Following the use of telemedicine to support this clinical role, Lynda then worked for a telemedicine organisation, completing her Master's dissertation on patient satisfaction with teledermatology.

Lynda was Principal Lecturer at the University of Hertfordshire and was also a nurse consultant. She has set up her consulting company, Sibson Consulting Ltd. (www.sibsonconsulting.com). She is currently working with West Midlands Ambulance Service NHS Trust in a senior management position and project managing a postgraduate programme for air ambulance paramedics.
Lynda is also one of the Consultant Editors of the *Journal of Paramedic Practice* and Honorary Fellow, University of Warwick.

Kim Walter, *RN, DipN, RNT, BSc, MA*
Kim began her nursing career in 1983 as a Staff Nurse at the Lister Hospital, Stevenage. She initially worked as a theatre/anaesthetic nurse until moving into chronic neuro-disability nursing in 1990 working for the Sue Ryder Foundation, where she became a ward Sister. She then moved to the Leonard Cheshire Foundation in 1998, where she became a training coordinator for the service she was based in. In 2002, she moved to the Royal Hospital for Neuro-disability in Putney, becoming a full-time teacher as part of the staff development team. She joined the University of Hertfordshire as a lecturer in 2004. Her areas of special interest are chronic neurology and manual handling. She is also currently acting as the Branch Programme Tutor for the Diploma of Nursing in Higher Education.

Acknowledgements

I would like to express my gratitude to a number of people for all their encouragement. I thank Mrs Frances Cohen for her continued help and assistance. I also thank my partner Jussi Lahtinen for his unyielding support and my brother Anthony Peate who contributed to a number of the illustrations.

Introduction

There has been much change in the spheres of health and social care provision as well as nurse education since the first edition of this text was published. Lord Darzi, the author of a government publication, sets a new foundation for a health service that empowers staff and provides patients with choice in England (Department of Health [DH], 2008). The initiative ensures that health care will be provided on a personalised basis, and that it will be fair, will include the most effective treatments provided within a safe system and will help patients to stay healthy.

All four chief nursing officers of the UK have provided nurses with their vision that is based on the report *Modernising Nursing Careers* (DH, 2006), which sets the direction for modernising nursing careers. The priorities contained within the report centre on the careers of registered nurses; however, it is noted in this publication that nurses do not work in isolation and nursing teams often include more than registered nurses. As well as the proposed changes in nursing careers, it must be acknowledged that there will be changes in the careers of other professional groups. This report accepts that careers can and do take different forms: there are some nurses who will choose to climb an upward ladder of increasing responsibility and as such reap higher rewards; others will choose a more lateral career trajectory, moving within and between care groups and settings. This book takes into account the changes and proposals made in the two key initiatives described above.

The text has been written for students in order to help them find their way through the many clinical issues they may face on a daily basis when nursing adults on wards, in clinics and in the community setting. The overarching aim of this text is to reflect the central tenet that underpins the Code of Professional Conduct (Nursing and Midwifery Council, 2008) – that is, to provide safe and effective care in order to protect the public.

The book encourages students to provide care that is safe and effective; it will also help them assimilate knowledge gained and apply it to the skills needed by the nurse when providing patient care. The information in the book is offered in order to assist students whilst on clinical placement and also takes into account the fact that they have academic work to produce for their educational institution; therefore, it is laid out in a format that is easy to use. We do not intend that the reader reads the text from cover to cover but envisage that students will dip in and out of it when clinical issues or concerns emerge.

The text embraces the concepts associated with the Roper, Logan and Tierney's Activities of Living Model for Nursing Roper et al.'s (1996) with the intention of guiding and steering students through their learning and caring when they work with and for their patients. This model of nursing is used in a number of clinical areas in the UK, Republic of

Ireland, Australia and some European countries; we believe the framework that it uses is a valuable framework for the delivery of care.

The chapters will examine and focus upon an activity of living; however, it must be noted that each activity will impinge on another and that they are all interrelated. Many of the chapters will explore various nursing skills associated with the particular activity of living that the student will encounter when in clinical practice. We hope that the information offered here will encourage the student to explore further, to delve deeper into the issues discussed and to reflect on their practice.

The chapters will provide the reader with a practical focus underpinning the theory of nursing – the art and science of caring. Throughout the text the reader is reminded that the nurse is accountable for his or her actions and omissions at all times, and because of this, care must be delivered in such a way that it is evidence based.

In this edition we have made a number of other changes; for example, every chapter explicitly states what its aims are; we have called these learning opportunities and have done this in an attempt to encourage learning. There are also pre- and post-chapter quizzes for each chapter.

A glossary of terms regarding the terminology used in each chapter will be provided; this will help students find their way through the intricacies related to nursing and medical terminology. An appendix called 'Normal Values' is also supplied to help students understand 'abnormal/altered' blood and biochemical results.

The chapters

Chapter 1 places the text into context, providing the reader with an insight into the opportunities and challenges that nurses face in the twenty-first century. The roles and responsibilities of the nurse are outlined in this chapter. The Nursing and Midwifery Council is cited and reference is made to its core function of setting standards and ensuring that they are maintained in order to safeguard the health and well-being of the public. Professional nurse regulation, the nursing register and the nurse's duty of care are discussed. The chapter concludes by reminding the reader that the best interests of the patient must always come first.

In an enlightened progressive society there must be an awareness of the vulnerability of some adults to abuse or neglect. Chapter 2 provides the reader with an understanding of the complex term 'vulnerability' and the issues associated with safeguarding vulnerable adults; a definition of 'vulnerable adult' is also provided. Four important ethical concepts related to the practice setting are described and discussed. There are many ways in which the violation of an individual's human and civil rights can occur, and this chapter discusses a number of them. The nurse needs to know about the ways in which an adult may be abused as well as understand who can perpetrate abuse.

Chapter 3 introduces the complexities associated with assessing individual needs and presents the reader with some of the building blocks that underpin a safe, effective nursing practice. Here the nursing process and an introduction to nursing models are discussed. Practical examples are given that will help the reader begin to assess, plan, implement and evaluate care. The chapter explains how the complex activity of assessment is carried out and how to then plan care by setting goals that are patient-centred and realistic. Having provided care in association with care plans or care pathways, the important aspect of measuring and evaluating interventions is discussed. The chapter encourages the reader to adapt and adopt assessment strategies to a variety of care settings.

When patients access and use care or are the recipients of care provision, they should be assured it is carried out in a safe and effective manner. Chapter 4 considers the important issue of safety and draws on current thinking on risk management. Key specific areas are highlighted, which include drug administration, prevention of falls, infection prevention and control. The important issue of hand washing is described, and it is reiterated how important this simple yet often overlooked activity is to protect patients and staff. Ways in which to minimise risks related to these areas are explored. Maintaining a safe environment does not only depend on the infrastructure, but also on the equipment and materials used as well as the nurse's understanding of crucial issues. This chapter notes that all health care personnel, irrespective of the setting, are responsible for maintaining a safe environment.

Chapter 5 provides much practical advice to those who are new to nursing practice. This chapter is key to all other chapters; it points out that if the nurse is unable to communicate effectively with his or her patient then the patient is at risk of substandard, if not dangerous, care interventions. The art and science of nursing depends on nurses communicating in an effective manner with all patients, families and co-workers; nurses communicate continually in a variety of ways. This chapter also acknowledges the fact that in this age of increased technology and high-level skills, communication (verbal and non-verbal) is just as important and should be given careful consideration.

Eating and drinking are complex activities of living. Chapter 6 is dedicated to these very important fundamental activities. Contemporary thinking related to nutrition and nutritional assessment is described in detail, giving the reader a thorough insight into these activities of living that are responsible for sustaining life.

By understanding the complex principles discussed in this chapter, the reader will be able to deliver the care required for those patients who have particular care needs in order to maintain their eating and drinking needs as well as preventing any potential problems from becoming actual problems. The roles of the nurse and the multidisciplinary team are explained in detail. Chapter 6 specifically describes some of the practical aspects associated with eating and drinking.

Urinary and faecal elimination are discussed in Chapter 7. An overview of the gastrointestinal and renal tracts is offered, with the aim of explaining how eliminatory needs can be addressed and met. There are a number of common conditions discussed in this chapter; these are conditions that the nurse may come across on a regular basis. This chapter also draws on the assessment aspect of nursing and, in particular, provides the reader with advice concerning practical nursing interventions.

Stoma care and urinary catheterisation are described, with hints and tips provided to help the novice nurse begin to manage these aspects of essential care. The chapter encourages the reader to consider the patient in a holistic way and, as such, reflects on the physical, psychological and social elements of care.

Chapter 8 considers the activity of breathing and begins by guiding the reader through the essential anatomy and physiology of the respiratory system and an understanding of what is vital if the nurse is to assist and support those who may have actual or potential breathing problems. The chapter draws on the content of other chapters to explain how to communicate with a breathless patient and how to assess the complex activity of breathing.

Common respiratory diseases are described, and the nursing care needed to help the patient is outlined. There are also practical examples regarding specimen collection and the importance of documenting findings.

Chapter 9 details the needs of the patient from a personal cleansing and dressing perspective. The chapter will take the reader through this important activity in detail and focuses on helping patients maintain their personal hygiene according to their own personal preferences and practices. Important cultural perspectives are discussed. Maintaining hygiene is crucially important for the physical, psychological, emotional and social well-being of the individual. Many people refer to this activity as an element of 'basic' care provision; however, it undermines the importance of the activity and the significance that it has for patients who may be unable to meet their own hygiene needs. The chapter concludes with a plea for this aspect of nursing to receive the recognition it rightly deserves, as it is an important component of essential patient care.

All activities of living are linked with mobility. Chapter 10 explains the association of movement and mobility with health and well-being of the patient and the nurse. The chapter draws upon ergonomics to explain how it is the musculoskeletal system that provides movement and how mobility is an intrinsic aspect of living.

An evidence-based approach is used to help the reader understand the principles of safe manual handling and encourages the nurse to appreciate the fundamental aspects associated with the musculoskeletal system and how it operates in order to assist and promote the activity of mobility. The chapter provides a fundamental understanding of spinal anatomy and then describes how back injury can occur. It goes on to explore how ergonomics are used to promote safe systems at work, promoting effective mobility. The chapter clearly explains the dangers to both the nurse and the patient if unsafe practice is adopted.

Maintaining body temperature is the theme of Chapter 11. The chapter begins by explaining the dynamics associated with thermoregulation and the role of the nurse in ensuring that the patient's body temperature is maintained as is appropriate. For all forms of life, this chapter explains, temperature is a fundamental issue and human beings are no exception to this. If a patient has too high a temperature then it will place the patient in danger, and on the other hand, if the patient has too low a temperature then it can be just as detrimental to the patient's health and well-being.

In order to help the nurse assess a patient's temperature effectively so that appropriate actions are taken if there is an anomaly in the findings, the various body temperature sites and different techniques associated with assessing temperature at these sites are detailed.

Chapter 12 considers working patterns and leisure interests and the importance of these when admitting or assessing a patient. It then goes on to explain that a holistic assessment must include an assessment of working and leisure activities, encouraging the reader to address such issues as they are vital if due consideration is to be given to the 'whole' patient. A number of important issues are acknowledged and discussed in this chapter, which will help the nurse offer a holistic approach to care giving. A socio-economic approach is used, but the chapter also includes the psychological and social implications that work, leisure and unemployment can have on an individual's health and well-being.

In Chapter 13 the complex issue of sexuality is considered. Sexuality as an activity of living can often be neglected by nurses as it can have the potential to cause embarrassment and anxiety for both the nurse and the patient. Sex and sexuality are central to what humans are, and because of this, nurses are in danger of disregarding a major aspect of the patient's being if they ignore the patient's sexuality and any issues surrounding their sexual health needs. Chapter 13 provides an insight into this complex activity of living.

Sleeping and resting are discussed in Chapter 14, which provides the reader with an understanding of the pathophysiology related to sleep. There are pointers offered that will enable the nurse to help a patient sleep and rest. This activity of living is often neglected by health care professionals, and the important issue about sleep deprivation and the effects it will have on an individual's quality of life is raised.

Finally, the last chapter, Chapter 15, considers death and dying. The chapter provides practical advice to the nurse who may be facing for the first time the death of a patient to whom he or she was providing care. Death and dying can be an upsetting event for all concerned - patient, family and nurse - as this chapter points out. The chapter considers the care of a person facing death and loss. The psychological, physical, spiritual, religious needs and social support are also considered; there is a discussion concerning religious and cultural needs after death. After reading this informative chapter the nurse should have gained more insight into this sometimes a 'taboo' subject and may be able to offer closer, more effective support to the patient and those near to him or her.

Terms used in the text

There are a number of different terms used in this text and it is important from the outset to define some of these terms. Different terms can mean a number of different things to different people. There are, for example, a number of terms that can be used to describe people who come into contact with health and social care providers. Using any term can lead to labeling and stereotyping.

A term used often in the NHS is 'patient', and on a number of occasions this has been used in this text. It has to be acknowledged that not everyone embraces the use of the passive concept associated with this term, and there are a number of reasons for this; for example, it can highlight the medical focus of the relationship between the person and the service.

The term 'client' has also been used. Some may suggest that the use of this term can have the potential to emphasise the professional nature of the relationship. 'Client' along with 'consumer' has its genesis in health care provision during the 1980s and 1990s when market forces and consumerism were at the fore.

Recently the term 'expert' has often been used; the stress when using this term is on a participative approach, respecting a person's capacity to work towards his or her own rehabilitation. Experts are seen to be the equivalent to those experts who provide care, for example, a nurse or doctor. The term 'expert' values the views and experiences of the expert - the service user.

Some people do not like the term 'service user' or 'user'; it could lead to the grouping together of an otherwise diverse community of individuals with very individual needs. The term 'user' may bring to mind some negative connotations connected with it. It could, for example, be used to identify those who are involved in the use of illicit substances.

The Nursing and Midwifery Council (2008) has chosen to use the word *person* for those who are recipients of the services of nurses, midwives or health visitors. Previously the term 'client' or 'patient' was used.

This text uses a number of terms and aims to promote the care and support of those with health care needs. The terms that have been used here are used to address a diverse range of experiences that may affect any person at any time.

The term 'carer' has been used on a number of occasions in this book. This term is used to describe those who look after others, be they ill, healthy or have a disability. 'Carer' has many interpretations and may refer to an employed health care provider or someone who provides care that is unpaid. Carers include parents, grandparents and, in a number of instances, siblings who are looking after sick children.

We want this text to whet your appetite and in so doing encourage you to delve deeper. We hope that the text will encourage, motivate and excite you as well as instil in you the yearning, confidence and capability to practise to the best of your ability. What you need to bring is your desire to care with compassion and understanding for those whom you have the privilege to care for.

References

Department of Health (2006) *Modernising Nursing Careers: Setting the Direction*. London: DH.

Department of Health (2008) *High Quality Care for All: NHS Next Stage Review Final Report*. London: DH.

Nursing and Midwifery Council (2008) *The NMC Code, Standards of Conduct, Performance and Ethics for Nurses and Midwives*. London: NMC.

Roper, N., Logan, W.W. and Tierney, A.J. (1996) *The Elements of Nursing: A Model for Nursing Based on A Model of Living*, 4th ed. Edinburgh: Churchill Livingstone.

Chapter 1
The Nature of Nursing

Lynn Quinlivan

Learning opportunities

This chapter will help you to:

1. Understand the key functions of the Nursing and Midwifery Council
2. Define key roles associated with nurses as they progress from newly qualified staff nurses to modern matrons
3. Begin to appreciate the importance of professional regulation
4. Describe key themes associated with 'fitness to practise'
5. Understand terminology associated with the phrase 'Agenda for Change'
6. Discuss the importance of the Knowledge and Skills Framework

Pre-chapter quiz

1. The Nursing and Midwifery Council has five key functions. What are they?
2. Define 'fitness to practise'
3. What is the role of a health care assistant?
4. Describe the usual nursing hierarchy for a ward
5. Why is confidentiality important?
6. What does the acronym KSF stand for?
7. What is the significance of the Bolam test?
8. What is the definition of 'reasonable care'?
9. To whom is the nurse accountable?
10. Describe the difference between responsibility and accountability

Introduction

The central role of a nurse is to deliver high-quality, appropriate care to patients within a variety of care settings. The role of a nurse is dynamic; it is continually evolving in all aspects of health care. This chapter will introduce the reader to the role of the Nursing and Midwifery Council (NMC) and the impact of current UK government policies upon the delivery of clinical care within the community, hospitals and the independent sector. It will also outline the hierarchical structure often associated with nursing and the roles and responsibilities of specific nursing posts.

'The National Health Service is not just a great institution but a unique and very British expression of an ideal that health care is not a privilege to be purchased but a moral right secured for all' (Department of Health [DH], 2008a).

The Nursing and Midwifery Council

The NMC was established in 2002. It has taken over the responsibility for professional regulation of nurses, midwives and health visitors from the United Kingdom Central Council (UKCC) and the associated four national boards that had been established in 1979.

The NMC's function is that of a regulatory body. The NMC sets standards of conduct and performance (NMC, 2008a); it also maintains a live register of qualified nurses and midwives.

The NMC acts as a resource available to registered and non-registered nurses, their employers and the general public, offering advice and guidance on matters pertaining to nursing practice, such as delegation, advocacy and autonomy (NMC, 2008b). In addition to the above, the NMC provides advice and guidance on professional standards and considers allegations relating to an individual's fitness to practise, which could be a result of lack of competency, professional misconduct or illness.

Registration and professional accountability

The NMC validates programmes of study provided by schools of nursing and departments of nurse education throughout the UK. With regard to pre-registration nursing, the aim is to ensure that the theoretical and practical components of a programme fulfil set criteria for the admission of graduates to the professional register. The NMC's representatives periodically visit clinical care areas to which student nurses are allocated in order to ensure that the learning experience is appropriate and meaningful and that practice assessors and mentors adequately support student nurses within the clinical care environments (NMC, 2006a).

Following the completion of a period of undergraduate study, such as Diploma of Higher Education in Nursing, the higher education institution formally notifies the NMC that an individual has followed a recognised undergraduate programme of study and is thus eligible to register as a registered nurse. The higher education institution and the registrant complete and sign a declaration that the registrant is of good heath and good character. Students who have commenced their pre-registration education after September 2007 are allocated a sign-off mentor for their final clinical placement (NMC, 2006b). The sign-off mentor, who has met additional criteria, must make the final assessment of practice and confirm to the NMC that the required proficiencies for entry to the register have been achieved.

Standards of conduct and performance

The Code (NMC, 2008a) states that the 'people in your care must be able to trust you with their health and well being'. To justify that trust, you, the nurse, must:

- Make the care of people your first concern, treating them as individuals and respecting their dignity
- Work with others to protect and promote the health and well-being of those in your care, their families and carers, and the wider community
- Provide a high standard of practice and care at all times
- Be open and honest, act with integrity and uphold the reputation of your profession

As a registered nurse you are individually accountable for actions and omissions when practising and must always be able to justify your decisions. Furthermore, you must always act lawfully, whether those laws relate to your professional practice or personal life. If a registered nurse fails to comply with the tenets of the code, it may bring his or her fitness to practise into question and endanger his or her registration.

Maintenance of a register of nurses and midwives

Another key function (defined in law) is to maintain the professional register. The register is central with respect to the NMC's function in safeguarding the health and well-being of the public (NMC, 2008c).

There is a mandatory requirement that all nurses re-register every 3 years and pay an annual subscription to the NMC. The standards stipulate that all registered practitioners who wish to remain active on the NMC register must have worked as a nurse or midwife for a minimum of 450 hours in the previous 3 years and undertaken a minimum of 35 hours of learning, which is relevant to the nurse's or midwife's area of practice. If the NMC requests to see evidence that the above standards have been met, then the nurse or midwife is required to provide proof that continuing professional development has been undertaken and recorded in their personal portfolio. A continuing professional development portfolio may include the following:

- **Details of your workplace:** Here this could include, for example, Band 5 staff nurse working within an adult intensive care unit
- **Your employer's details:** Details about your place of employment, for example NHS Trust, private hospital; you may wish to include the number of hours that you are contracted to work, if appropriate
- **Your role:** For example, what your role entails and to whom you are responsible. You may find it useful to look at your job description
- **Evidence of professional learning:** Study days such as moving and handling and cardiopulmonary resuscitation must be attended on an annual basis. In addition to these mandatory study days, there is a requirement for practitioners to demonstrate

evidence of continuing professional learning by attending study sessions relevant to their areas of clinical practice. For example, a district nurse may choose to attend a tissue viability study day and then write a short reflective account which enables him or her to consider how this knowledge can be applied within clinical practice. In the reflection, the date and number of hours must be recorded to ensure that the minimum of 35 hours is reached over 3 years
- **Life events:** This section may include an aspect of family life that has had some impact on an individual's working life. For instance, changing jobs or completion of a period of study that has resulted in new and challenging responsibilities
- **Critical incidents and personal reflection:** These are incidents that the nurse has observed and/or taken part which have affected him or her, for instance looking after a patient who subsequently dies. The positive aspects of learning are not always apparent at the time. However, by using a framework such as the Gibbs reflective cycle (1992), an individual can look retrospectively at the incident and analyse his or her subsequent learning (Hogston and Simpson 2002)

Duty of care

The concept of duty of care is complex. Here a brief overview is provided; however, it must be remembered that duty of care is always context dependent. *The Code* (NMC, 2008a) applies directly to registered nurse practitioners; however, the principles that it sets out of good practice and duty of care apply to all those directly involved in patient care. Duty of care, according to Lord Atkin (1932), can be seen as:

> reasonable care to avoid acts or omissions which you can reasonably foresee would be likely to injure your neighbour.

The definition of what is reasonable originated from the Bolam test in 1957, where the case of *Bolam* v *Friern Hospital Management Committee* [1957] resulted in the following legal ruling:

> The test is the standard of the ordinary skilled man exercising and professing to have that special skill. A man need not possess the highest expert skill at the risk of being found negligent. . . . It is sufficient if he exercises the skill of an ordinary competent man exercising that particular art.

The case of *Wisher* v *Essex AHA* [1988] is the current standard used to define reasonable care with respect to students and junior staff:

> The standard is that of a reasonably competent practitioner and not that of a student or junior.

Fitness to practise

Fitness to practise enables a nurse or midwife to practise as a registrant without restriction. Grounds for an individual being considered unfit to practise are identified by the NMC (2008a):

- Misconduct
- Lack of competence
- A conviction or caution (including a finding of guilt by a court martial)
- Physical or mental ill health
- A finding by any other health or social care regulator or licensing body that a nurse's or midwife's fitness to practise is impaired

Nurses and accountability

Accountability is another complex concept. This section only begins to outline some of the issues associated with accountability.

The government

In addition to their responsibilities to the regulatory body of the NMC, nurses are accountable to the 'stakeholders', that is, the general public and the government to provide effective, efficient, high-quality care.

Since the inception of the NHS in 1948, much debate has surrounded government funding and target setting. Government targets such as reductions in waiting lists and additional financial resources for certain services such as a winter bed crisis inflame political opinion and debate about the cost-effectiveness and the quality of patient's provisions. Present-day government initiatives to involve the public in the development of a health care service for the twenty-first century are discussed later in this chapter.

The general public

Nurses are accountable for the delivery of appropriate care to patients within a variety of care settings. The level of expertise at which an individual delivers this care will vary, depending upon the education that they have received. In *The Code* (NMC, 2008a), the registered practitioner's delegation of responsibility to unqualified staff, and the accountability of that registered practitioner, is stated thus:

> The delegation of nursing or midwifery care must always take place in the best interests of the person the nurse or midwife is caring for and the decision to delegate must always be based on an assessment of their individual needs.

Consequently, those involved in patient care should undertake only those tasks for which they have received appropriate education. In the case of delivering fundamental nursing care, this may be a part of formal programme of study such as the National Vocational Qualification (NVQ) in health care studies.

The employer

Finally, nurses are accountable to their employer under a contract of employment. Under terms of employment there is an understanding that the nurse will act in a responsible manner when carrying out his or her duties. NHS trusts have their own policies and procedures, which are designed to ensure that patients are protected from harm. The term 'vicarious liability' refers to situations whereby the employer accepts responsibility for the fault of its employees. However, if the employee is found not to have followed accepted procedure or protocol, for example the trust's drug administration policy, then the trust is not legally liable for the employee's error. Vicarious liability is fraught with legal technicalities and further reading in this area is encouraged.

Nursing hierarchy

Within a clinical setting it is common to find the nursing hierarchy as given in the following subsections, wherein the roles and responsibilities of nurses holding these titles are also described (see Figure 1.1). The titles used here may vary depending on the setting.

Modern matron

The modern matron is responsible for managing, leading and developing care services normally within a clinical directorate, for example community services. The modern

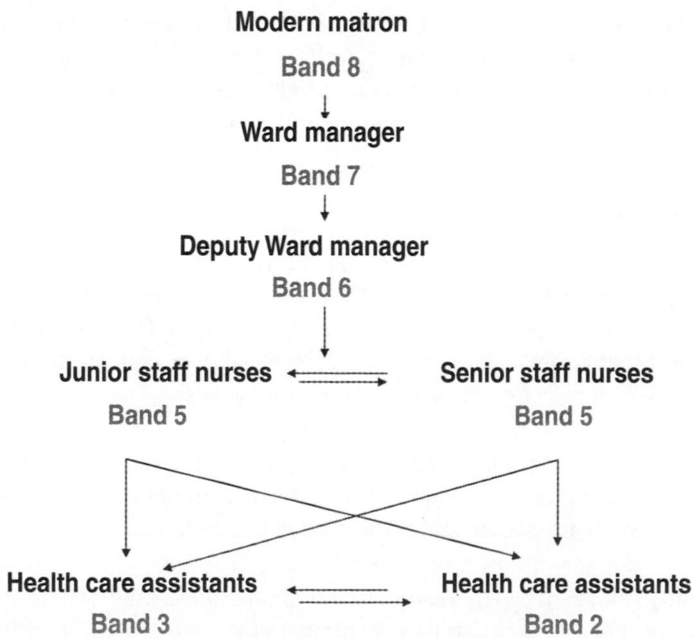

Figure 1.1 Example of nursing hierarchy.

matron will have significant experience and clinical expertise within the field that they are working, facilitating nursing developments and contributing to the Trust and Directorate Clinical Governance strategy.

Ward manager

The ward manager is responsible for the 24-hour delivery of care to patients within a designated care setting. The ward manager is sometimes referred to as sister (female) or charge nurse (male). Consequently, a ward manager will have a wide range of responsibilities: those may vary from the day-to-day management of an off-duty rota to the management of a ward's budget. The ward manager may be responsible for the recruitment and selection of new members of staff. A part of their role is to ensure that all staff members develop and retain appropriate clinical skills; thus, the ward manager must enable qualified and unqualified staff to attend clinical study days which meet their professional and academic needs. Such development objectives may be highlighted during the yearly appraisal cycle, and the ward manager is responsible for ensuring that these are met. The ward manager may also be actively involved in clinical audits and formulating policies and procedures related to their field of expertise.

Deputy ward manger

The deputy ward manager (sometimes known as the team leader) is a registered nurse with at least 2 years of experience as a Band 5 senior staff nurse, and has an appropriate secondary qualification, gained through post-graduation qualifications and experience. A deputy ward manager will be expected to undertake the management of a designated clinical environment. In addition, he or she may be involved in the implementation of government directives such as 'the fractured neck of femur pathway' (NHS Plan, 2000). A deputy ward manager will be required to supervise and develop the clinical expertise and competencies of junior members of nursing staff, for example newly qualified staff nurses, student nurses or health care assistants. It is common for a deputy ward manager to hold the mentorship and preceptorship certificate in areas where student nurses are allocated.

Senior staff nurse

A senior staff nurse is typically a registered nurse with at least 12 months of experience as a junior staff nurse. Senior staff nurses are responsible for ensuring that safe, appropriate care is delivered to patients and their families. In carrying out their duties, senior staff nurses are required to assess, plan, implement and evaluate the care that is provided to patients over a recognised time period, for instance during an early duty. In carrying out their duties, senior staff nurses are expected to take an active role in liaising with other members of the multidisciplinary team, such as doctors, physiotherapists, district nurses and general practitioners. Senior staff nurses will actively engage with student nurses, fulfilling the role of assessor/mentor, once the mentorship and preceptorship qualification has been successfully completed.

Junior staff nurse

The title of junior staff nurse relates to newly qualified staff nurses with current NMC registration and health and social care experience, albeit as a student nurse. The qualified nurse works within codes of practice and professional guidelines, planning nursing care for patients and their families and managing the work environment as required. The junior staff nurse utilises professional and clinical knowledge that he or she has acquired through registration.

Senior health care assistant

A senior health care assistant will have successfully completed the Level 3 NVQ in health care studies. The role of a senior health care assistant is to provide fundamental care to patients under the supervision and direction of a qualified practitioner, to accurately record patient information and to supervise more junior members of the team.

Junior health care assistant

The health care assistant will have successfully completed NVQ at Level 2 or will be undertaking this qualification. A junior health care assistant will deliver personal care to clients within a variety of care settings under the supervision of senior team members.

Student nurse

A student nurse will be undertaking a 3-year pre-registration nurse education programme; upon successful completion of the programme of study, the student nurse will be eligible to register with the NMC as a registered nurse. The first year of education known as the 'common foundation programme' enables all students, irrespective of their destined branch, to study together. During the second and third years of the programme of study, the student nurse will study theoretical subjects that directly relate to their chosen field of nursing. During these 3 years students will experience a variety of clinical settings and develop a sound theoretical knowledge base which enables them to apply theoretical knowledge to practice, equipping them for their role as registrants.

District nurse

A district nurse assesses patients within a community setting; it may be the client's home, general practice setting or a residential care home. A district nurse will plan and implement care, maintain associated records and coordinate the workload of the team of which he or she is a member. District nurses are registered nurses who have successfully completed a specialist practitioner programme at degree level.

Health visitor

A health visitor usually works with families with specific health and social needs, and consequently liaises as and when appropriate with other health professionals and agencies such as social services. Health visitors run child health clinics, providing advice and health education to parents of babies and young children; they also work with patients who suffer from a disability or chronic illness. Health visitors are registered nurses or midwives who have successfully completed a health visitor programme at degree level.

Practice nurses

Practice nurses work in general practitioner surgeries as part of a team, which will include doctors, and, depending upon the size of the practice, may involve working with other members of a multidisciplinary team, such as physiotherapists, pharmacists, dieticians and other nurses. Practice nurses are registered nurses who have undertaken an additional training as identified by the general practitioner who is their employer.

Nurse consultants

These nurses are experienced registered nurses who have chosen to specialise in a particular area of health care. Nurse consultants spend 50% of their time on direct patient care, ensuring that the high level of nursing expertise that they possess is utilised in the direct delivery of care. Nurse consultants are also actively engaged in the education, training and development of colleagues and are involved in research and evaluating care that is delivered.

Government directives

In this section current government directives are described; the government lays down statutes in law which relate directly to clinical practice.

Clinical governance

Each individual NHS Trust's board of governors is responsible for ensuring that safe and acceptable standards of care are delivered in all areas of clinical and non-clinical practice. They are required to do this through framework (DH, 1998). NHS organisations are accountable for continuously improving the quality of their services.

Data Protection Act 1998

This Act sets out eight principles which apply to the keeping of computerised data and certain types of manual records that includes health records; personal data is clearly defined as data 'which relates to a living individual'. Employers are responsible for ensuring that data collection systems comply with the provisions as set out within the Act.

Dimond (2008) notes that the principles are designed to ensure that any personal data must be accurate, relevant, held only for specific defined purposes for which the user has been registered, not kept for longer than necessary and not disclosed to those who are unauthorised.

Our Healthier Nation

An action plan to tackle poor health was provided in the form of the government report *Our Healthier Nation* (DH, 1999); aims were set out to improve the health of the nation as well as the health of the worst off in particular.

In this document the government had put forward the following four targets to be achieved by 2010:

1. Reduction in the death rate associated with cancer, in those under 75 years by at least a fifth
2. Reduction in the death rate associated with coronary heart disease and stroke, in those under 75 years by at least two fifths
3. Accidents and serious injury to be reduced by a tenth
4. Reduction in the death rate associated with suicide to be reduced by at least a fifth in line with overarching objectives related to the treatment of mental illness

The government explained how they intended to achieve these objectives, principally by increasing funding and encouraging the development of local health initiatives (DH, 1999); there was to be a 'new balance' in which people, communities and the government would work in partnership to improve the health of the nation.

National Institute for Health and Clinical Excellence

One of the functions of NICE, which was set up in 1999, is to disseminate good clinical practice throughout the NHS, and offer guidelines in relation to research-based practice. In England, NICE produces guidance in three areas of health through the following three centres:

- **Centre for Public Health Excellence:** Develops public health guidance on the promotion and the prevention of ill health
- **Centre for Health Technology Evaluation:** Develops technology appraisals and interventional procedure guidance. Technology appraisals are recommendations on the use of new and existing medicines and treatments within the NHS. Interventional procedure guidance evaluates the safety and efficacy of such procedures which are used for diagnosis or treatment
- **Centre for Clinical Practice:** Develops clinical guidelines. These are recommendations based on the best available evidence on the appropriate treatments and care of people with specific diseases and conditions (NICE, 2007)

National Health Service Plan (a plan for investment, a plan for reform)

This plan sets out specific targets for NHS trusts to achieve within documented time frames. For example, 'the fractured neck of femur pathway' is the integrated care pathway that aims to effectively and efficiently manage the patient's progression from accident and emergency department to discharge. Within the provision of this 'fast-track care' is the involvement of members of the multidisciplinary team, such as physiotherapists, occupational therapists, social workers, doctors, nurses, district nurses and hospital-at-home services. The ultimate aim, according to Komaromy (2001), is for those patients to have a shorter inpatient time and an improved community support network on discharge.

Health Care Commission 2004

The Health Care Commission's remit is to review the quality of care that is at present provided across the NHS and the independent sector. With the aim of ensuring that the care that is provided meets the prescribed recognised standards, for instance benchmark statements, NICE has set out standards of clinical excellence. The Health Care Commission informs patients, the general public, health service employees and health professionals about changes and improvements to local health care provision (DH, 2004a).

Standards for Better Health

The document *Standards for Better Health* (DH, 2004b) outlines the seven domains of care against which all providers of health care are measured:

1. Safety
2. Clinical and cost-effectiveness
3. Governance
4. Patient focus
5. Accessible and responsive care
6. Environment and amenities
7. Public health

In each of the above domains noted are the 'core standard', which sets a minimum level of service, and the 'developmental standard', which provides a framework for the improvement of care delivery.

The Health Care Commission and the Commission for Social Care inspection utilise these domains and standards to ensure that minimum standards of care are delivered across all providers of care, irrespective of whether the care is delivered within NHS, Foundation Trust, or private or voluntary sector (DH, 2004b).

NHS's *Job Evaluation Handbook*

This handbook (DH, 2004c) sets out the job evaluation scheme, which is to help 'ensure that all staff are rewarded fairly and that the NHS respects the principles of equal pay for work of equal value', thereby enabling employers, employees and staff representatives to determine the point of transfer from clinical grades to pay bands (DH, 2004c; Royal College of Nursing [RCN], 2005), for example from 'E grade' staff nurse to Band 5, Point 24 staff nurse. The handbook considers job evaluation factors and the skill level required to fulfil a named post.

Agenda for Change

The underpinning principles of *Agenda for Change* are the harmonisation of terms and conditions for all NHS employees (DH, 2004d). *Agenda for Change* was implemented across the UK on 1 December 2004. It aimed to address the issue of equal pay for work of equal value; central to the *Agenda for Change* is the Knowledge and Skills Framework (KSF).

Knowledge and Skills Framework

The KSF is integral to the government's *Agenda for Change* policy (DH, 2004b). It is designed to support career progression and the personal development of staff working within patient care, ensuring that developmental objectives are clear and appropriate. Doctors and dentists are not included in this framework. The KSF defines and describes the knowledge and skills that are required by staff and are appropriate to their role and level of professional responsibility. The KSF enables individuals to identify skills acquisition that will support their career progression. It is envisaged that all staff will progress through a named band on an annual incremental basis. Each pay band has a series of incremental pay points and two gateways, which are identified in job descriptions. The KSF is made up of core and specific dimensions; each dimension comprises at least four levels or indicators (DH, 2003, 2004c; RCN, 2005).

Core dimensions

These dimensions are core to the work of everyone who works in the NHS:

1. Communication
2. Personal and professional development
3. Health, safety and security
4. Service and developments
5. Quality
6. Equality, diversity and rights

Specific dimensions

These dimensions can be applied to define parts of different posts. They are grouped into four categories:

1. Health and well-being
2. Information and knowledge
3. General
4. Estates and facilities

Gateways

Foundation gateway

This gateways falls within the first 12 months of appointment to any post irrespective of the band, and aims to ensure that the individual is able to fulfil the role concerned.

Second gateway

This occurs at a fixed point, normally near the top of a pay band, for example Band 5 staff nurse (DH, 2004c; RCN, 2005). This gateway is a formal review; its purpose is to ensure that the individual is able to fulfil the roles and responsibilities consistently as set out in the job description.

National Service Frameworks

National Service Frameworks (NSFs) are 'long-term strategies for improving specific areas of care'. Currently there are ten NSFs. Within each of these frameworks, the DH has set out a national standard and identified key interventions, for example long-term conditions (DH, 2005). The DH (2000) states that the NSFs will set out standards to suggest how care can be improved, for example, with regard to neurological services across the board so that a first-class service can be delivered over the next 10 years to everyone who has a neurological condition.

High Quality Care for All: NHS Next Stage Review

This report (DH, 2008a) sets out the challenges facing the delivery of effective, efficient and appropriate health care in the twenty-first century. Key challenges are identified, which are summarised as an increase in expectations, demand that is driven by demographics, a continuing development of an 'information society', advances in treatment and care, the changing nature of disease as well as the changing expectations of the health workplace.

An NHS is needed that provides patients and the public with more information and choice, works in partnership with local health authorities and has high-quality care at its heart. The NHS must be flexible, responding to the needs of local communities.

The structure of the NHS in England

Department of Health

This Department supports the government in its plans to reform and provide an integrated and comprehensive range of services that is based on clinical need, not the ability to pay.

Modernisation Agency

Established in 2001 the agency's remit is to develop 'patient-centred service that gives power to its staff and patients at all levels' (DH, 2008c). This agency has two core functions: firstly, to ensure that the NHS meets the needs of its patients in the twenty-first century; and secondly, to modernise services in an appropriate and meaningful manner so that the services that the general public require are easily accessible and available. The Modernisation Agency is expected to achieve this objective by the integration of services and the development of best practice throughout the NHS.

Primary care trusts

Primary care trusts (PCTs), according to the DH (2008b), have a key role to play in assessing local needs and also have a responsibility to commissioning care. PCTs manage local health care services; within a primary care group are general practitioners, dentists, opticians, pharmacists and NHS Direct. The function of PCTs is to ensure that there is adequate provision of services for the general population, and this could be NHS hospital services and the inpatient and outpatient provisions, or the NHS walk-in centres and mental health services. They control 80% of the total NHS budget.

Strategic health authorities

In 2002, 28 strategic health authorities were created. Following re-organisation in 2006, this number decreased to 10. At present, their function is to manage local health care services; strategic health authorities achieve this by developing local improvement plans and ensuring that national priorities such as the development of an integrated stroke care pathway are actively supported (DH, 2008b).

Care trusts

At present, only a small number of care trusts are in existence (DH, 2008b). Their function is that of joint collaboration between the NHS and local health authorities, specifically where a closer working relationship is considered to be of benefit for the provision of local health care services.

Mental health trusts

They provide a range of psychological therapies such as bereavement counselling, general health screening within the local community and inpatient health care provision for clients, with a range of mental health diagnoses (DH, 2008b).

NHS trusts

Acute trusts

Acute trusts manage hospitals and formulate strategies for the improvement of hospital services. They are also the employers for hospital staff such as doctors, nurses, midwives, health visitors and allied health professionals, for example physiotherapists and radiographers.

Foundation trusts

Foundation trusts are NHS hospitals which have been given a degree of financial and operational independence (DH, 2008b). The trusts remain under the overarching umbrella of the NHS; however, they are run by members of the public, staff and locally based managers who are able to tailor the services that they provide to the needs of the local population.

Ambulance trusts

Thirty-three ambulance services cover England, providing access to emergency health care for the general population (DH, 2008b). The ambulance service operates on three levels, ranging from immediate life-threatening to non-emergency response. Under government strategic plans, certain criteria are set which relate to the response time.

The structure of the NHS in Scotland

In Scotland the Scottish Government Health Directorate is responsible for NHS Scotland and the provision and development of community-centred care. The responsibilities of the Scottish Government Health Directorate also include the ambulance service; the state high security hospital; NHS 24, which provides 24-hour telephone advice service within Scotland; NHS Health Scotland; NHS Education for Scotland; NHS Quality Improvement Scotland, which monitors clinical standards; and the National Waiting Times Centre Board (DH, 2008d).

The structure of the NHS in Wales

Within Wales, NHS services are delivered to the Welsh people via local health boards and NHS trusts. Primary, secondary, tertiary and community care services are provided in a format similar to that of England.

The Welsh Assembly allocates resources to the local health boards. The Health Commission Wales finances inpatient and outpatient care. Health of Wales Information Service provides an NHS Wales Directory, which includes contact details of health providers, health watchdog, public health information and an online health encyclopaedia (DH, 2008e).

The structure of the NHS in Northern Ireland

There are four health boards within Northern Ireland: Eastern, Northern, Southern and Western Health, as well as Social Services Board. The responsibility of commissioning services is to meet the ever-changing needs of the population who lives within Northern Ireland.

Acute and community NHS services are provided to the population via five health and social care trusts (DH, 2008f):

1. Belfast
2. Northern
3. Southern
4. Western
5. South Eastern

Conclusions

In this chapter a generalised overview of the nurse's roles and responsibilities in the twenty-first century has been discussed. The role of the NMC in relation to the regulation of pre- and post-registration nurse education has been explained, as has the nurse's fourfold responsibility: firstly, to the general public; secondly, to their professional organisation (NMC); thirdly, to the government; and finally, to their employer.

The importance of lifelong learning and reflective practice has been introduced and the causes and consequences of changing government directives in relation to the patient's choice have been briefly discussed.

Glossary

Acute trusts	Responsible for NHS hospitals
Agenda for Change	Terms and conditions for all NHS employees
Ambulance trusts	Provide emergency health care
Band 5 senior	Senior staff nurse, previously known as an 'E' grade
Band 5 junior	Junior staff nurse, previously known as a 'D' grade
Care trusts	NHS and local health authorities working in partnership
Clinical governance	Framework through which NHS is accountable
Code of conduct	Standards of conduct and performance
Data Protection Act	Principles of ensuring that data are held safely and used for defined purposes
Duty of care	Reasonable care to avoid acts or omissions
Elective	Planned hospital admissions
Emergency	Unplanned hospital admissions
Gateways	Points within a band designed to ensure that individuals are fulfilling their role
Health Care Commission	Review quality of care delivered within NHS and private sector
High Quality Care for All	Lord Darzi report, challenges facing health care in the twenty-first century
Higher education institution	Providers of pre-registration nurse education
Job Evaluation Handbook	Evaluation document used by employers and employees to ensure fair and equitable pay
Knowledge and Skills Framework	Defines and describes knowledge and skills appropriate to role and level of responsibility
Mental health trusts	Providers of inpatient and outpatient services for patients suffering from mental health problems
Modernisation Agency	Modernising services to meet the needs of the general public
National Health Service Plan	Specific targets to achieve within documented time frames
National Institute for Clinical Excellence	Research-based guidelines
National Service Frameworks	Long-term strategies for improving specific areas of care, e.g. long-term neurological conditions
Nursing and Midwifery Council	Professional regulatory body for registered nurses and midwives

Our Healthier Nation	Four government targets to be achieved by 2010
Personal portfolio	Evidence that continuing professional development has taken place
Primary care trusts	Managing local services, e.g. general practice and commissioning NHS hospital services
Secondary care	Acute care
Sign-off mentor	Mentor who makes final clinical assessment at the end of pre-registration programme
Standards for Better Health	Seven domains of care against which all providers of care are measured
Student nurse	Individual undertaking a 3-year programme of study leading to registration
Strategic health authorities	Manage local NHS services
Unfit to practise	Criteria under which a nurse may be referred to the NMC
Vicarious liability	Employer accepts responsibility for the fault of its employees, proving that they have followed recognised protocol

Post-chapter quiz

1. Explain the key functions of the Nursing and Midwifery Council, giving an example of each
2. What action would you take if you considered that someone was not 'fit to practice, fit to purpose'?
3. Who is accountable for the actions of a health care assistant?
4. Who is accountable for the actions of a staff nurse?
5. What do you understand by the term 'Agenda for Change'?
6. What do you understand by the term 'Data Protection Act'?
7. What does the term 'promotion gateway' mean?
8. List how you might empower an individual
9. Why is the Bolam test (1957) important?
10. What do you understand by the term 'vicarious liability'?

References

Department of Health (1998) *A First Class Service: Quality in the New NHS*. London: HMSO.
Department of Health (1999) *Saving Lives: Our Healthier Nation*. London: HMSO.
Department of Health (2000) *National Health Service Plan*. London: HMSO.
Department of Health (2003) *Job Evaluation Handbook*, 1st ed. London: HMSO.
Department of Health (2004a) *Healthcare Commission: Inspecting, Informing Improving*. London: HMSO.
Department of Health (2004b) *Standards for Better Health*. London: HMSO.
Department of Health (2004c) *Job Evaluation Handbook*, 2nd ed. London: HMSO.
Department of Health (2004d) *Agenda for Change*. London: HMSO.

Department of Health (2005) *The National Service Framework for Long-Term Conditions.* London: HMSO.
Department of Health (2008a) *High Quality Care for All: NHS Next Stage Review Final Report.* London: HMSO.
Department of Health (2008b) About the NHS in England 2008. Available at http://www.nhs.uk/aboutnhs/CorePrinciples. Accessed 24 June 2009.
Department of Health (2008c) NHS choices: your health, your choices. Available at http://www.nhs.uk/Pages/homepage.aspx. Accessed 12 December 2008.
Department of Health (2008d) About the NHS in Scotland. Available at http://www.show.scot.nhs.uk/. Accessed 10 January 2009.
Department of Health (2008e) About the NHS Wales. Available at http://new.wales.gov.uk/topics/health/nhswales/. Accessed 10 January 2009.
Department of Health (2008f) Health and social care in Northern Ireland. Available at http://www.n-i.nhs.uk/. Accessed 10 January 2009.
Dimond, B. (2008) *Legal Aspects of Nursing*, 5th ed. England: Pearson Education Limited.
Hogston, R. and Simpson, P. (eds) (2002) *Foundations of Nursing Practice: Making the Difference.* London: Palgrave McMillan.
Komaromy, C. (2001) *Dilemmas in UK Health Care.* Buckingham: Open University Press.
National Institute for Health and Clinical Excellence (2007) Available at http://www.nice.org.uk/aboutnice. Accessed 10 December 2008.
NHS Plan (2000) *The NHS Plan: A Plan for Investment, A Plan for Reform.* London: HMSO.
Nursing and Midwifery Council (2006a) *Standards for Mentors, Practice Teachers and Teachers.* London: NMC.
Nursing and Midwifery Council (2006b) *Standards to Support Learning and Teaching in Practice.* London: NMC.
Nursing and Midwifery Council (2008a) *The Code: Standards for Conduct, Performance and Ethics for Nurses and Midwives.* London: NMC.
Nursing and Midwifery Council (2008b) *Advice on Delegation for Registered Nurses and Midwives.* London: NMC.
Nursing and Midwifery Council (2008c) *The Prep Handbook.* London: NMC.
Royal College of Nursing (2005) NHS Knowledge and Skills Framework outlines for Nursing Post. *RCN Guidance for Nurses and Managers in Creating KSF Outlines in the NHS.* London: Royal College of Nursing.

Chapter 2
Safeguarding Vulnerable Adults

Victoria Darby

Learning opportunities

This chapter will help you to:

1. Define the key terms used within safeguarding vulnerable adults
2. Describe the types of abuse that can occur
3. Identify the ethical concepts of beneficence, non-maleficence, justice and autonomy
4. Begin to understand the legal statutes and policies which surround safeguarding vulnerable adults
5. Describe the nurses' duty of care in safeguarding vulnerable adults
6. Identify the fundamental principles of referral when abuse of a vulnerable adult is suspected

Pre-chapter quiz

1. List your health values
2. How would you define a vulnerable adult?
3. List all the types of abuse you think a vulnerable adult could encounter
4. Identify how often you think abuse occurs in vulnerable adults
5. Why should nurses have an understanding of ethics?
6. What procedure should you follow if you suspect a vulnerable adult is being abused?
7. Describe what you understand by the word 'confidentiality'
8. List any Acts, policies or reports that are related to safeguarding the vulnerable adult
9. How does the Nursing and Midwifery Council's Code of Conduct (NMC, 2008a) guide nurses to protect the vulnerable adult?
10. In what ways can working 'interprofessionally' enhance patient care and safeguard vulnerable adults?

Introduction

Safeguarding vulnerable adults is essential in ensuring that individuals are empowered, respected and given the opportunity to make autonomous decisions about their health care needs (Department of Health [DH], 2000). The ability as a nurse to ensure that every individual is made aware of their rights lies at the heart of protecting the public. In order to safeguard vulnerable adults, it is essential to have an understanding of ethical frameworks, legal policies and statutes, alongside professional guidance.

The government has used (DH, 2000) several terms such as protection of adults, safeguarding adults and adult protection, but the standard term being adopted currently is safeguarding vulnerable adults (Mandelstam, 2009). A variety of the terms will be used interchangeably throughout the chapter, but the key term adopted is safeguarding vulnerable adults.

Defining a vulnerable adult and abuse

Adult

The Family Reform Act (1969) identified the age of majority (becoming an adult) as 18 years or older within England, Wales and Northern Ireland and 16 years or older in Scotland.

Vulnerable adult

The definition of a vulnerable adult therefore refers to anyone of 18 years or older in England, Wales and Northern Ireland or 16 years or older in Scotland:

> who is or may be in need of community care services by reason of mental or other disability, age or illness: and who is or may be unable to take care of him or herself, or unable to protect him or herself against significant harm or exploitation. (DH, 2000)

The definition identifies that anyone over the age of 18 years (16 years in Scotland) who is being abused or is at risk of another person taking advantage or harming them in some way constitutes a vulnerable adult. This covers a huge array of individuals within British society:

- A 94-year-old lady who has just become blind and turns to a voluntary carer to spend her pension for her
- A 23-year-old man with severe learning disabilities who needs all his personal care needs met by health care professionals
- A 54-year-old lady who is admitted for surgery for a ruptured appendix and is in excruciating pain on arrival in the accident and emergency department

Each of these individuals is reliant on nurses and other health care professionals who, it is anticipated, will protect their rights and ensure they are given every opportunity to make autonomous decisions about their health care needs.

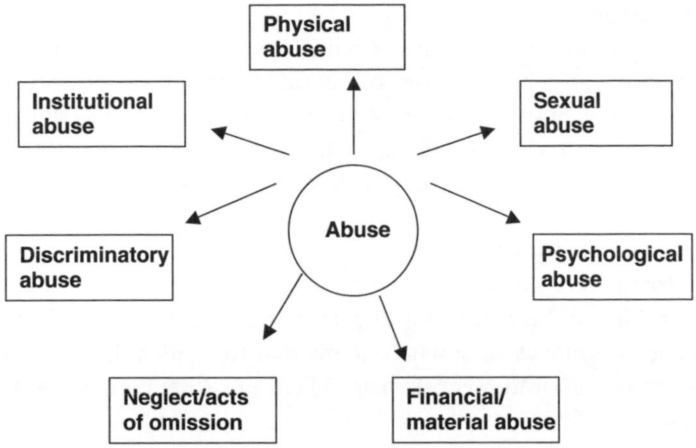

Figure 2.1 Types of abuse.

Abuse

There are several definitions of abuse available and one of those is cited by the DH (2000) as:

> a violation of an individual's human and civil rights by any other person or persons.

When receiving any health care input, individuals have human and civil rights that have to be maintained. When any of those rights are ignored or infringed, abuse has taken place. There are many types of abuse that can occur and each will now be defined with examples.

Types of abuse

There are several types of abuse that can occur; being aware of these can help you to help your patients. Figure 2.1 identifies the various types of abuse.

Physical abuse

This is where a vulnerable individual's body is harmed. Examples of physical abuse are kicking, slapping, biting, hitting, misuse of medication and excessive use of restraint. For a relative to tie a person to their bed so they cannot wander off in the night is physical abuse.

Sexual abuse

An individual who has been pressured into a sexual act, could not consent or did not consent to a sexual act, is said to have been sexually abused. This covers abuse such as rape and sexual assault. When an individual has sexual intercourse, for example, with a patient without their consent, it is deemed sexual abuse.

Psychological abuse

Psychological abuse is a non-physical attempt to emotionally undermine or damage vulnerable adults' well-being. To use words to undermine someone's self-worth by informing them they are useless or using the threat of violence are just two examples of psychological abuse. For a carer to constantly demand an individual get up at 0530 hours using threatening language is an example of psychological abuse.

Financial or material abuse

To steal or attempt to steal money or material goods from a vulnerable individual is financial abuse. This can take many forms such as stealing jewellery from a locker in the ward, using patient's money to purchase items that the patient is unaware of and was not intended for, or deliberately isolating an individual so that their financial matters are controlled and abused by another.

Neglect and acts of omission

Neglect is defined as a failure to implement care that would meet clients' needs, such as physical or medical needs (DH, 2000). This may constitute not providing basic necessities such as food, heat or medication. It may also include a limiting or denying access to appropriate health care services. Access to health care services is a basic human right, the interference in which constitutes neglect.

Discriminatory abuse

To abuse another by discrimination is to verbally or physically harm another due to specific characteristics, attributes or beliefs of an individual. There are many characteristics or attributes that abuse can be directed to, such as race, gender, age, ethnicity, disability and sexuality (DH, 2000).

Institutional abuse

Institutional abuse relates to any organisation knowingly harming any individual in its care. Hospitals and care homes have many demands to meet, but this must not be knowingly detrimental to the care they offer. If a hospital knows they have an outbreak of methicillin-resistant *Staphylococcus aureus* (MRSA) and continue to take patients into that area, then it would be an example of institutional abuse.

Identification of abuse of the vulnerable adult

Statistics for abuse of the vulnerable adult are broken down into many differing categories, which makes it difficult to identify the scale of adult abuse in the UK. Categories of adult abuse include elder abuse, domestic violence, racial abuse and sexual abuse. There is a clear understanding and statistical analysis for child abuse with the child protection and at-risk register, yet there appears to be little clarity when it comes to adult abuse (The House of Commons Health Committee, 2004). The segregation of data into different categories for vulnerable and abused adults can only serve to dilute the impact of the scale of abuse that vulnerable adults experience. Data that are collected and reported must be used with caution as it is clearly an underestimation of the problem.

Action for Elder Abuse (2008) identified that approximately 4% of the elderly population in the UK experience abuse. This equates to approximately 342 000 people over the

Table 2.1 Some health values.

Health values	Agree	Disagree
A carer should be able to access all the financial affairs of the patient if the patient lacks capacity		
Voluntary euthanasia should be legalised for the terminally ill patients		
Alcoholics should have access to liver transplants		
Gender reassignment operations should not be funded by the NHS		

age of 65 years having experienced some form of abuse (Mowlam et al., 2007). Domestic violence is another category of abuse of the vulnerable adult. Although the incidence of domestic abuse has fallen from 23% in 1995 to 16% in 2006/2007 (Office for National Statistics, 2008), it still equates to a large number of people experiencing abuse. The reality is that adult abuse occurs within the UK and therefore nurses need to ensure their clinical care attempts to protect the vulnerable adult. This begins with nurses having an awareness of their own health values and beliefs and ensuring professional health values are maintained in the clinical environment.

Health values

Values exist within everyone, as a set of attitudes that guide actions towards others and objects within society. They are socially constructed and malleable in the face of changing circumstances (Hawley, 2007). Many of the values individuals have are acted upon but not often consciously thought through. So a person may value the sanctity of life, but when confronted with a terminally ill patient asking for their life to be prematurely ended, it may cause a nurse to reflect whether he or she would change his or her values.

By reading the provocative statements given in Table 2.1, you may become aware of some personal health values. In Table 2.1, you are invited to review the health values and decide why you agree or disagree with the statements.

By exploring personal values, it can become evident that some vulnerable adults in society may be at a disadvantage because of the values you hold. When personal values are consciously thought through and discussed, it can create a review and reshaping of individual values. Therefore, it is vital to become aware of personal values and begin to understand that in the clinical setting, differences in individual values will often cause debate and dilemmas. Developing an understanding of ethics may help guide the student through the myriad of opposing values in society, especially those concerning safeguarding vulnerable adults (Holm, 2006).

Ethics and safeguarding the vulnerable adult

Ethics is a branch of philosophy that focuses on the study of morals. What is right and wrong, good and bad, the right way to live, the wrong way to behave? The complexities of delivering nursing care often call into question what is right and wrong, good and bad. In clinical practice, ethical dilemmas will present themselves and it is necessary to be aware of ethical principles in order to inform the decision-making process. The Code (NMC, 2008a) is a set of ethical and professional principles identified by the NMC that directs registered nursing and midwifery practitioners to conform to a specific standard of practice.

Clinical dilemmas in safeguarding vulnerable patients can be as simple as walking down the ward and three people calling out for help at the same time, but only one person can be seen first. The Code (NMC, 2008a) guides the nurse to 'delegate effectively', 'work effectively as part of a team' and 'manage risk'. To apply these principles to the scenario of walking down the ward and three people asking for help, the nurse has to:

- Identify which patient is at the greatest risk and need
- Prioritise patients in order of risk and then attend to the patient with the greatest risk first
- If there are patient needs that can be delegated to another member of the care team who is competent and available, then the nurse needs to delegate appropriately so that patients have their needs met as efficiently as possible
- Ensure effective communication between the nurse, patients and all the staff so there is clear understanding as to why certain patients had to wait and why staff have been asked to assist

It is essential that student nurses have an understanding of nursing ethics in order to identify ethical questions and to create a systematic approach when attempting to reach a decision to the ethical dilemma (Allmark, 2005). In order to create a structure with respect to a complex and often emotive decisions, ethical principles can support this. There are many ethical concepts and frameworks, but Beauchamp and Childress (2001) identified a set of principles as a starting point for understanding ethics. The four ethical principles identified by Beauchamp and Childress (2001) are:

- Autonomy
- Non-maleficence
- Beneficence
- Justice

Autonomy

Autonomy is the ethical principle of free choice. Every patient must be given the freedom to think and act freely and independently. An autonomous patient is one who is allowed to voice their own opinion about the health care treatment that they are receiving. To be in a health care setting can feel intimidating, and reliance on health care professionals for information can feel like the patient has no choice in their health care treatment.

Tuckett (2006) argues that it is essential for the nurse to reflect on whether the patient is being given the opportunity to voice their individual thoughts or if the patient is being led into decisions by health care professionals. Decision-making on someone else's behalf is known as professional paternalism. Ensuring that every patient hears and understands all the treatment options along with the advantages and disadvantages is the key to ensuring autonomy is upheld and paternalism is avoided.

Daniel James was a 23-year-old rugby player who was paralysed from the chest down in a training session. His friends and family helped him travel to Switzerland where assisted suicide is legal and Daniel died at the assisted suicide clinic. His parents and friends were not prosecuted back in the UK as the Director of Public Prosecutions deemed it not in the public interest (BBC, 2008). Throughout the case, there was detailed involvement with all health care professionals who reported Daniel's unfailing desire to die since the injury, with Daniel stating 'not a day has gone by without hoping it will be my last' (BBC, 2008). The family could argue that they were acting to uphold the autonomy of their son.

In the UK, assisted suicide is illegal. The Assisted Dying for the Terminally Ill Bill was rejected in May 2006 and therefore nurses cannot participate in voluntary euthanasia or they will be called to account by the legal system and the NMC. Therefore, the nurse is able to listen to the patient express their autonomous thoughts but is unable to participate in any steps supporting voluntary euthanasia. In this case, the nurse would attempt to maximise the quality of life for Daniel in his paraplegic state. By supporting and meeting the autonomous decisions of Daniel that do constitute criminal or professional misconduct for the nurse, ethical sensitivity is maintained (Weaver et al., 2008). The steps that the nurse could take are:

- Use active listening skills so the patient and family feel they are able to express their views
- Provide all the support services necessary that the patient and family want to access, such as counselling, physiotherapy, occupation health, financial services and paraplegic support groups
- Document all the factual information about the patient's desire of assisted suicide
- Provide evidence-based quality care in each nursing interaction with the patient, so the nurse is attempting to maximise the patient's free will
- Ensure the nurse seeks support from other staff and organisations with this emotive situation. All health care professionals involved need to provide all the information about the procedure, at a level the individual can comprehend
- Ensure the individual's decision has been reached voluntarily and no coercion is taking place with family, friends or other health care professionals
- Review the patient's decision with them when it is felt appropriate. Consent or refusal is not a one-off decision that the patient cannot change, so it is essential to identify with the patient if their autonomous decision remains the same

It can be argued that by not supporting the patient's desire to commit suicide, the nurse is not allowing him the right to act autonomously. However, in order to practise as a registered nurse in the UK at this moment in time, the nurse has to be guided by the Code (NMC, 2008a) and the legal requirements. To promote free will and independence for each action that is legal and permissible under the Code is the professional and correct course of action for a registered nurse.

Non-maleficence

Non-maleficence is to never knowingly cause harm to any individual (Hawley, 2007). Nurses have to abide by a duty of care to ensure that they never consciously abuse their patients (NMC, 2008a). All nursing care should be concerned with working with the patient to provide effective and appropriate care where the nurse does not consciously cause harm.

It is important to understand that in the course of routine care certain procedures may be uncomfortable, such as receiving chemotherapy. The nursing action is non-maleficent as nurses are attempting to ensure no harm is caused to the patient. When the patient receives the chemotherapy, there may be some discomfort but the nurse is providing the correct course of treatment and not knowingly causing harm.

If a health care professional filled a syringe with a massive overdose of diamorphine, which would result in death, as Harold Shipman (a general practitioner) did, then it would be knowingly harming the patient and be deemed maleficent. Harold Shipman knowingly caused harm by murdering about 250 patients (The Shipman Inquiry, 2005) through consciously administering massive doses of diamorphine to them.

Many ethical dilemmas are fraught with emotionally charged issues, especially about terminal prognosis. The ethical dilemma of relatives asking nurses not to tell the patient if the prognosis turns out to be terminal is often raised. Patients about to receive information about a terminal prognosis are vulnerable adults as they are reliant on others to impart information and meet certain care needs. It is easy to get caught up in the emotional plight of the relatives who may be struggling to come to terms with the disease process that might result in a terminal prognosis. Time has to be invested in listening and providing support mechanisms for the family and friends involved as well as the patient. However, the nurse has a duty of care to the patient and has to follow robust guidelines for disclosing confidential patient information.

The key steps to acting in a non-maleficent way in this situation are:

- The nurse cannot agree to give a relative confidential information before the patient. Nurses are bound by case law, their employment contract and their code of conduct to maintain confidentiality (Dimond, 2008). Therefore, the nurse is knowingly doing no harm by ensuring the patient has access to their confidential information and not withholding the information from them.
- The patient has the right to receive any confidential information first. Effective communication skills and support structures will need to be offered alongside the giving of any terminal prognosis.
- The patient has the right to give their consent or refusal for anyone else to have the confidential information disclosed to them. Therefore, the nurse would have to ask the patient if they consent to their relative being present when receiving confidential information.
- All the health care professionals who have direct need for access to medical and confidential information are involved so that it is clear who has access and understanding about the confidential information (in terms of friends and family) and who does not.

The Code (NMC, 2008a) guides the nurse to respect confidentiality and ensure people are cared for as individuals. By acting in a non-maleficent manner, the nurse ensures that the vulnerable patient is at the centre of all decisions. It protects them from friends or family taking control of certain situations and directing the health care of the patient according to their health values.

Beneficence

Beneficence is the moral duty to do good and maximise good. The nurse has a duty of care to follow this principle as beneficence is intertwined throughout the Code (NMC, 2008a). Individuals receiving care must be respected, treated with dignity and provided with a high standard of care, all of which are acts of beneficence. This ethical principle helps empower the vulnerable adult as the nurse seeks to provide care that is in the patients' best interest. However, not everyone seeks to be beneficent and there are many areas where health care professionals have to safeguard the vulnerable adult. Vulnerable patients can be exposed to many risks of abuse within the health care setting and it is essential they have health care professionals advocating on their behalf.

Mr Steven Hoskin was admitted to an accident and emergency department several times with injuries consistent with physical abuse. He was known to social services as having learning disabilities and was living on his own in a bedsit with all support from social services discontinued (Cornwall Adult Protection Committee, 2007). In order to be beneficent, the accident and emergency nurse should do good and maximise good. The key steps to maximising good in this situation are:

- Treat the patient as an individual and respect dignity while providing care
- Provide evidence-based care to meet the physical injuries of the patient
- Ensure effective communication is used to ascertain a factual account of the situation
- Document the clinical care given according to the record keeping guidelines (NMC, 2007)
- Reflect on the situation and ask the question 'Is there a safeguarding vulnerable adult concern?'
- Follow the local policy guidelines if a safeguarding vulnerable adult suspicion is raised. It is essential to work with other agencies in a coordinated and comprehensive manner in order to protect individuals

Mr Hoskin was eventually murdered by people who had singled him out as a vulnerable adult. He suffered physical, psychological and discriminatory abuse and eventually had his hands stamped on and fell from a viaduct to his death. In the years leading up to his murder, Mr Hoskin was known to a housing association, the police, adult social care, the NHS and the Youth Service as a vulnerable adult. He was also known to several agencies as someone who carried out abuse as he had been convicted of assault. Yet at no time since Mr Hoskin was placed in a bedsit was an adult protection concern made or acted upon, even though he had been in contact with so many health care agencies. This account highlights the need to be beneficent and to work interprofessionally.

Justice

Justice is the moral duty to offer the same standard of care to each individual regardless of their economic status, ethnic origins, political views, religion, gender or sexuality. If the nurse was in charge of serving lunches, she or he would need to ensure that each patient had been given the opportunity to select something they are able to eat. The vegetarian patient is offered a vegetarian option and the Islamic patient who has stated they only eat halal food is offered appropriate food. Therefore, it is important to remember that justice is not about treating people as carbon copies of each other. Justice is about understanding the patient as an individual but offering the same standard of care. If one patient requires a bed bath and one requires a shower, they should both receive the same standard of care by the nurse in terms of professionalism in meeting personal hygiene needs.

A nurse had started work in a care home and began to notice that a patient was not receiving adequate nutrition due to neglect by other staff (DH, 2008). Justice was not being maintained as some patients were assisted with their food to ensure they had their nutritional needs met while others were not. To ensure justice was being maintained, the nurse needed to ensure all of the patient's nutritional needs were being met. By acting as the patient's advocate, the nurse must attempt to protect the individual's rights and interests (NMC, 2008a); for justice to be upheld it is vital that the nurse adheres to the following points:

- Ensure nursing care is given in an unbiased and professional manner. Therefore, the nurse needs to ensure that patients receive the same standard of care for all their needs.
- Take into account language barriers, cultural sensitivity and physical impairments (such as hearing loss and sight loss) when meeting the care needs of the patient. The nurse needs to assess if there were any barriers to meeting the patient's nutritional needs and create strategies to overcoming these barriers. If the patient, for example, had dentures that were causing them so much pain that they could not eat, then this barrier could be overcome by mouth care and a dental review.
- Reflect on the situation and ask the question 'Is there a safeguarding vulnerable adult concern?'
- Follow the local policy guidelines if a safeguarding vulnerable adult suspicion is raised. It is essential to work with other agencies in a coordinated and comprehensive manner in order to protect individuals.

The nurse involved decided, based on the evidence seen, that there was a suspicion of abuse of a vulnerable adult and reported the suspicion in line with the care home's vulnerable adult policy. From the single report of abuse by a nurse, the care home was investigated by the Department of Work and Pensions and the local authority fraud team. Carers within the home were prosecuted for physical and financial abuse along with neglect (DH, 2008). Ensuring justice is being upheld is often a clear indicator that nurses are upholding their duty of care.

Allmark (2005) contends that students should focus on entering into debates, challenging and consolidating their health beliefs in order to gain a deeper insight and understanding of ethics rather than following strict principles. Debating ethical dilemmas and learning from each ethically challenging clinical experience will enhance the quality of care offered by the nursing profession (Weaver et al., 2008).

Policies and legislation for safeguarding the vulnerable adult

Policies and legislation can be seen to work in several ways to support and attempt to safeguard the vulnerable adult's rights and needs. The first way is to have a clearly defined process to access information to ensure the vulnerable adult's rights are maintained. The second way is to ensure that no one, except those with designated authority, has access to confidential information. Thirdly, there needs to be a clear process to vet individuals who work with vulnerable adults. Finally, the fourth way is to have a stringent process of referral when a suspicion of abuse of a vulnerable adult is suspected. Nurses need to be aware of the policies and legislation that safeguard vulnerable adults and the specific policies identified by the clinical area they work within.

No Secrets

No Secrets (DH, 2000) is the key document that outlined the principles of good practice in safeguarding vulnerable adults. It defines a vulnerable adult and states the procedures to safeguard them from abuse. It consists of recommendations to create interagency frameworks, interagency policy and procedures to respond to suspicions of vulnerable adult abuse. No Secrets (DH, 2000) has empowered the vulnerable adult by identifying frameworks that can create a system to identify, investigate and call to account those found to be abusing adults. However, it is now widely accepted that to offer guidelines did not go far enough and that legislation is required to support the vulnerable adult (DH, 2008; Mandelstam, 2009).

Review of No Secrets, October 2008

It has been identified that although No Secrets (DH, 2000) has gone a long way in providing guidance on safeguarding vulnerable adults, there is much more that could be achieved. Therefore, the Department of Health, Department of Criminal Justice and the Home Office have begun a review of the No Secrets guidance. The review is seeking to pull together information from investigations where abuse and the breakdown of safeguarding principles have occurred. It also seeks to highlight examples of excellent safeguarding initiatives and the views of those professionals involved in safeguarding vulnerable adults. The focus is to learn how to enhance empowerment of the vulnerable adult and identify the mechanisms necessary to improve the safeguarding systems already in place.

Human Rights Act (1998)

The Human Rights Act (1998) came into force in October 2000 in the UK. It consists of 16 human rights and freedoms that can be grouped into three sections:

- Absolute rights
- Limited rights
- Qualified rights

Absolute rights are rights that cannot be withheld by the government, such as the right not to be tortured or the right not to be treated as a slave. Limited rights are rights that in certain circumstances can be withheld by the government, such as the right to liberty and the right to life. Finally, there are qualified rights where rights of the individual are judged against the rights of the wider society, such as freedom of expression and the right to manifest one's religion or beliefs. The rights and freedoms afford the vulnerable individual the knowledge that they live in a society that empowers people to assert their human rights. The vulnerable adult, however, is often unable to empower themselves to utilise their rights and is reliant on advocates to support and enable them to act autonomously.

Freedom of Information Act (2000)

Local authorities and the NHS have a duty to acknowledge or deny that they hold specific information that is requested by an individual. They then have to provide the information they hold upon request and have a clear publication scheme. However, there is much information that is exempt from this Act including personal information, court records and public authority investigations. The Freedom of Information Act (2000) alongside the Data Protection Act (1998) can assist vulnerable adults or advocates acting on behalf of vulnerable adults to locate information.

Data Protection Act (1998)

All personal health records, written and computerised, come under the domain of the Data Protection Act. For any sensitive personal data to be released, it has to meet a stringent set of criteria laid down in the Act. Breaches of either the Freedom of Information Act (2000) or the Data Protection Act (1998) are investigated by the Information Commissioner. Anyone can be called to account for breaches of the Data Protection Act. In November 2008, the Information Commissioner's Office (ICO) identified that NHS Tayside and NHS Lanarkshire breached several principles of the Data Protection Act, when health records were found in an old site of a former hospital. They were found to be keeping information for longer than was deemed necessary and not storing sensitive information in the correct manner. The NHS bodies were ordered to comply with the Data Protection Act (ICO, 2008).

Confidentiality

It is vital that nurses protect confidential information at all times unless an exception has been created. Confidential information is created 'when one person discloses information to another (e.g. patient to clinician) in circumstances where it is reasonable to expect that the information will be held in confidence' (DH, 2003). A nurse is bound by an employment contract, the Code (NMC, 2008a) and the Data Protection Act (1998) to ensure confidentiality is maintained.

A guide to confidentiality was created by the DH (2003) called *Confidentiality: NHS Code of Practice*, which offers a detailed insight into how and why confidentiality should be maintained by all health care professionals and introduced the confidentiality model (DH, 2003). The model highlights the need to protect patients' information, to ensure patients have the choice about confidential disclosure of information. The model also highlights the need to inform patients how and when their confidential information is used and finally to constantly strive towards improving confidentiality processes.

Exceptions to the duty of confidentiality

There are several exceptions to the duty of confidentiality and the nurse needs to be fully cognisant of them. Dimond (2008) outlines these:

- The consent of a patient
- Any court order that states the duty of confidentiality can be breached
- A statutory duty to disclose confidential information such as the Misuse of Drugs Acts
- Disclosure made in the interests of the patient
- Public interest
- Police
- Data Protection Act 1998

Caldicott guardians

Since 1999, each local authority and health organisation has to appoint a Caldicott guardian. It is the role of the Caldicott guardian to identify ways in which the organisation can improve the way it stores, organises and shares confidential information. If nurses have any concerns whether to release confidential information then they can approach the Caldicott guardian.

Mental Capacity Act (2005)

The Mental Capacity Act came into effect in 2007 and seeks to both empower and protect people (Mandelstam, 2009). Some of the underpinning principles of the Mental Capacity Act (2005) are listed below, but it is not an extensive review of the Act:

- Individuals are empowered through the principle that capacity is assumed unless it has been proven a person lacks capacity. Therefore, health care professionals have to offer evidence of lack of capacity so that the lack of capacity cannot just be assigned to an individual without any evidence.
- Health care professionals must take all practicable steps to help the individual make a decision. It is not enough for a health care professional to ask a question and then determine that an individual cannot decide. They need to use every available communication skill from pictures to appropriate level and tone of voice.
- Lack of capacity is defined when a person 'is unable to make a decision for himself because of an impairment of or a disturbance to the functioning of the brain' (Mental Capacity Act, 2005).
- If an individual makes an unwise decision, it does not automatically indicate that he or she lacks capacity. Some individuals will have capacity and still make decisions that shorten their life expectancy or appear unwise to others.
- Lasting power of attorney created where an individual (donor) with capacity can authorise the attorney (someone they know) to take financial and health-related decisions on their behalf if they later lack capacity.
- Advanced decisions (living wills) are defined as decisions made by individuals with capacity regarding refusal of certain medical treatment. If the individuals lack capacity at a later stage in their life, their autonomous decision would be respected.

- The independent mental capacity advocacy (IMCA) service was created to ensure local authorities and NHS bodies have to appoint an advocate before certain complex decisions are made.
- Acts carried out to those who lack capacity must be done in the 'best interests' of the individual and the least restrictive for the individual.

Already criticisms are being made towards the Mental Capacity Act (2005). Some argue, for example, that it has created a set of specific criteria that the vulnerable adult has to be measured against in order to benefit from protection (Dunn et al., 2008). With any legislation, it will be case law that identifies if amendments or whole-scale changes will be necessary in the future to protect the vulnerable adult.

Protection of Vulnerable Adults (2004)

The Care Standards Act (2000) stated that there was to be a Protection of Vulnerable Adults (POVA) list of people, who were barred from working with vulnerable adults. This could be because they had previously harmed a vulnerable adult or had placed a vulnerable adult at risk of harm. When anyone completes a Criminal Records Bureau (CRB) form, his or her name is checked against the POVA list. The POVA list does not apply to NHS staff.

Safeguarding Vulnerable Groups Act (2006)

The Safeguarding Vulnerable Groups Act (2006) introduced the universal vetting and barring scheme for all those unsuitable for working with adults or children. The Bichard Inquiry (2004) recommended the setting up of such a scheme after the Soham murders. This vetting and barring scheme replaces and enhances the POVA list by including NHS staff. The Independent Safeguarding Authority (ISA) will operate the scheme for both adults and children from October 2009.

Safeguarding vulnerable adults from unprofessional nurses

The NMC has identified that 99.8% of registered nurses and midwives abide by the Code (NMC, 2008a) as their professional duty of care throughout their careers (NMC, 2008b) and with legal requirements. It is essential for the NMC to have processes in place to ensure nurses who abuse vulnerable adults are called to account. The Fitness to Practise (FtP) Directorate is the section of the NMC that monitors and processes allegations that a nurse or midwife is not fit for practice. Allegations related to misconduct or lack of competence can often involve abuse of a vulnerable adult by a qualified practitioner.

Fitness to practise panels

There are two panels that investigate fitness to practise. They are the Conduct and Competence Committee (CCC) and the Professional Conduct Committee (PCC). A panel uses the average expectation of a nurse's practice to review a case, not the lowest or highest expectations of nursing practice. Depending on the final sanction identified by the panel, the following decisions could be made in relation to the nurse's ability to continue practising. The nurse could (NMC, 2008c):

1. Have their name removed from the register with effect that they cannot practise as a registered nurse
2. Be suspended for a year or less
3. Have conditions of practice imposed on them for 3 years or less
4. Have a caution imposed from 1 to 5 years
5. State that the nurse was investigated and no further action was taken
6. Take no action

Interprofessional collaboration

The key to the success of any investigation into safeguarding the vulnerable adult is to have an interprofessional organisational framework (DH, 2000). Recommendations from No Secrets (DH, 2000) identified that each professional must be aware of their role in adult protection as well as how to share information and work with other professionals and agencies. Sharing information and liaising with all the health care professionals involved ensures investigations into adult abuse being carried out in a methodical, professional and effective manner.

Many investigations into the failure to safeguard vulnerable adults identify a breakdown in interprofessional collaboration (DH, 2008). The setting up of adult protection committees, such as the multi-agency management committee , were recommended by the DH (2000), but there is no statutory obligation. This means the local authorities can choose whether or not to set up such agencies and therefore there may be a lack of consistency and uniformity in the organisations across the country (DH, 2008). Penhale et al. (2007) identified that there was a demand for a statutory requirement for safeguarding vulnerable adults to ensure consistency of roles and responsibilities and to give adult protection the same status as child protection.

Reporting suspicions of abuse as a nurse

Reporting abuse is essential, and safeguarding vulnerable adult policies must be followed. If any nurse has a suspicion that harm or abuse is occurring to a vulnerable adult they have to report those suspicions. The nurse has a duty of care to follow procedures identified for reporting suspected abuse and if they do not then the nurse will be held accountable by the NMC for an omission of care to a vulnerable adult (NMC, 2008a). The steps to follow if a nurse has a suspicion of adult abuse are:

- Act on any suspicions of abuse and report those suspicions
- Follow the clinical area guidelines for reporting abuse. Check each year for any changes to the policies so the correct and up-to-date policy is utilised. The guidelines should include:
  - The nurses' role in reporting suspected adult abuse
  - The nurses' responsibilities in reporting suspected adult abuse

- Steps on how to act in emergency abuse situations, who, when and how to contact adult protection and support services
- What to do if necessary action is not taken
- Nurses will not be involved in running the investigation unless they have a designated adult protection role; however, a nurse may well be asked to report and record any information that may be used within the investigation. Therefore, the recording of information must adhere to the NMC's record keeping guidelines (NMC, 2007). Principles of record keeping involve recording factual information in a clear and accurate manner, which is legible, timed, dated and signed. It is essential that the account is objective, with no speculation or abbreviations or jargon

Students and registered nurses can advocate for an individual by ensuring that the vulnerable adults' rights and interests are protected (NMC, 2009). Students must adhere to the Code (NMC, 2008a) and promote patients' rights and interests alongside the registered nurse.

Key guidelines for safeguarding vulnerable adult abuse cases are to have a recognised coordinator and lead to ensure that the interprofessional framework is followed to a specific time frame. It is also essential that the decision-making process is shared in an interprofessional arena such as a case conference (DH, 2000). The investigation will focus on establishing all the relevant facts surrounding the suspicion and assessing the needs of the vulnerable adult now and in the future (DH, 2000). The investigation will also seek to identify what action should be taken against the abuser of the vulnerable adult.

Assessing the seriousness of abuse

When the adult protection team investigates a suspicion of adult abuse, they need to investigate the seriousness of the abuse. The criteria they use to assess the severity of adult abuse are those published by the DH (2000):

- Vulnerability
- Nature and extent of abuse
- Impact of the abuse
- Length of time the abuse has occurred
- The risk of repeated or increasing seriousness of the abuse

Reporting suspicions of abuse as a student nurse

Student nurses have to abide by the Code (NMC, 2008a) throughout their education alongside the policies identified by the university or college they are attending (NMC, 2005). Therefore, a student nurse has a duty to report any abuse they see to a qualified member of staff and then observe the steps that are taken following up the suspicion of abuse. It is essential to seek support during this time from people such as mentors, link lecturers, personal tutors and the university or college counselling department. This will ensure that students can gain a full understanding of the process that was followed and have time to express their feelings about the challenging situation they have been faced with.

It is important to remember that if the vulnerable adult has capacity and they state that they do not want any help then it will limit or stop the support that can be offered. However, if the investigation feels that other individuals are at risk of abuse then action can be taken to prevent the potential abuse of others.

Conclusions

Safeguarding vulnerable adults is essential in a society that is recording a rising level of abuse towards adults. There are many types of abuse that can occur and it is important for nurses to be aware of types and signs of abuse that the vulnerable adult may display. There are local policies and government guidelines on how to protect the vulnerable adult. However, there is a call for a review on the lack of statutory guidance for adult protection that is available for child protection. Only with the introduction of statutory legislation will a consistent interprofessional approach to safeguarding the vulnerable adult come into being.

Glossary

Abuse	A violation of an individual's human and civil rights by any other person or persons.
Advocate	To advocate for an individual is to protect the individual's rights and interests.
Autonomy	Autonomy is the ethical principle of free choice. Every patient must be given the freedom to think and act freely and independently.
Beneficence	Beneficence is the moral duty to do good and maximise good.
Confidentiality	When one person discloses information to another (e.g. patient to clinician) in circumstances where it is reasonable to expect that the information will be held in confidence (DH, 2003).
Justice	Justice is the moral duty to offer the same standard of care to each individual regardless of their economic status, ethnic origins, political views, religious affiliations or gender.
Non-maleficence	Non-maleficence is to never knowingly cause harm to any individual.
Service user, client, patient	An individual receiving care in a health care setting. Usually, learning disabilities use the term 'service user', mental health settings use the term 'client' and adult settings use the term 'patient'.
Vulnerable adult	Someone 'who is or may be in need of community care services by reason of mental or other disability, age or illness: and who is or may be unable to take care of him or herself, or unable to protect him or herself against significant harm or exploitation' (DH, 2000).

Post-chapter quiz

1. List four exceptions to the duty of confidentiality
2. Review the principles associated with the role of Caldicott guardians
3. To whom is the nurse accountable?
4. Define the term 'advocate' and list four situations in which the nurse may act as an advocate
5. List members of the multidisciplinary team who may be involved in the care of a vulnerable adult
6. To whom does the Human Rights Act apply?
7. What do you understand by the term 'capacity'?
8. Can a health care professional consent on a patient's behalf?
9. List four ethical principles
10. What is evidence-based care?

References

Action on Elder Abuse (2008) Protecting older people and other adults at risk of abuse. Available at http://www.elderabuse.org.uk/No%20Secrets%20AP%20consult/GF%20Questions%20and%20Answers.doc. Accessed 18 November 2008.

Allmark, P. (2005) Can the study of ethics enhance nursing practice? *Journal of Advanced Nursing* 51(6): 618–624.

BBC (British Broadcasting Corporation) (2008) No charges over assisted suicide. Available at http://news.bbc.co.uk/1/hi/england/hereford/worcs/7773540.stm. Accessed 18 November 2008.

Beauchamp, T.L. and Childress, J.G. (2001) *Principles of Biomedical Ethics*, 6th ed. New York: Oxford University Press.

Cornwall Adult Protection Committee (2007) *The Murder of Steven Hoskin: Serious Case Review*. Cornwall: Cornwall Adult Protection Committee.

Department of Health (2000) *No Secrets: Guidance on Developing and Implementing Multi-Agency Policies and Procedures to Protect Vulnerable Adults from Abuse*. London: DH.

Department of Health (2003) *Confidentiality: NHS Code of Practice*. London: DH.

Department of Health (2008) *Safeguarding Adults: A Consultation on the Review of the 'No Secrets' Guidance*. London: DH.

Dimond, B. (2008) *Legal Aspects of Nursing*, 5th ed. London: Pearson Education.

Dunn, M.C., Clare, I.C.H. and Holland, A.J. (2008) To empower or to protect? Constructing the 'vulnerable adult' in English law and public policy. *Legal Studies* 28(2): 234–253.

Hawley, G. (ed.) (2007) *Ethics in Clinical Practice: An Interprofessional Approach*. Harlow: Pearson Education Limited.

Holm, S. (2006) What should other health care professions learn from nursing ethics. *Nursing Philosophy* 7: 165–174.

ICO (Information Commissioner's Office) (2008) Enforcement 26th November 2008. Available at http://www.ico.gov.uk/what_we_cover/data_protection/enforcement.aspx. Accessed 28 December 2008.

Mandelstam, M. (2009) *Safeguarding Vulnerable Adults and the Law*. London: Jessica Kingsley Publications.

Mowlam, A., Tennant, R., Dixon, J. and McCreadie, C. (2007) *Comic Relief UK Study of Abuse and Neglect of Elder People*. London: Comic Relief and Department of Health.

Nursing and Midwifery Council (2005) *An NMC Guide for Students of Nursing and Midwifery* . London: NMC.

Nursing and Midwifery Council (2007) *Record Keeping*. London: NMC.

Nursing and Midwifery Council (2008a) *The Code of Conduct*. London: NMC.

Nursing and Midwifery Council (2008b) Fitness to practice. Available at http://www.nmc-uk.org/aSection.aspx?SectionID=7. Accessed 27 December 2008.

Nursing and Midwifery Council (2008c) Professional conduct committee panels. Available at http://www.nmc-uk.org/aArticle.aspx?ArticleID=3033. Accessed 27 December 2008.

Nursing and Midwifery Council (2009) *Guidance for the Care of Older People*. London: NMC.

Office for National Statistics (2008) *Social Trends 38*. London: Palgrave Macmillan.

Penhale, B., Perkins, N., Pinkney, L., Reid, D., Hussein, S. and Manthorpe, J. (2007) Partnership and regulation in adult protection. The effectiveness of multi-agency working and the regulatory framework in adult protection. Available at http://www.prap.group.shef.ac.uk/PRAP_report_final_Dec07.pdf. Accessed 5 November 2008.

The Bichard Inquiry (2004) *The Bichard Inquiry Report*. London: The Stationery Office.

The Care Standards Act (2000) *Statutory Instruments 2000 2544 (C.72)*. London: The Stationery Office.

The Data Protection Act (1998) *Statutory Instruments 1592 (C.71)*. London: The Stationery Office.

The Family Law Reform Act (1969) *Statutory Instruments 1971 1857 (C.50)*. London: HMSO.

The Freedom of Information Act (2000) *Statutory Instruments 2002 2812 (C.86)*. London: The Stationery Office.

The House of Commons Health Committee (2004) Health: second report. Available at http://www.publications.parliament.uk/pa/cm200304/cmselect/cmhealth/111/11105.htm. Accessed 27 December 2008.

The Human Rights Act (1998) *Statutory Instruments 1998 2882 (C.71)*. London: The Stationery Office.

The Mental Capacity Act (2005) *Statutory Instruments 1897 (C.72) 2007*. London: The Stationery Office.

The Safeguarding Vulnerable Groups Act (2006) *Statutory Instruments 3204 (C.145) 2008*. London: The Stationery Office.

The Shipman Inquiry (2005) The Shipman Inquiry: sixth report: the final report. Available at http://www.the-shipman-inquiry.org.uk/home.asp. Accessed 16 December 2008.

Tuckett, A.G. (2006) On paternalism, autonomy and best interests: telling the (competent) aged-care resident what they want to know. *International Journal of Nursing Practice* 12: 166–173.

Weaver, K., Morse, J. and Mitcham, C. (2008) Ethical sensitivity in professional practice: concept analysis. *Journal of Advanced Nursing* 62(5): 607–618.

Chapter 3
Assessing Needs and the Nursing Process

Lynda Sibson

Learning opportunities

This chapter will help you to:

1. Understand how care is organised
2. Define the terms assessment, planning, implementation and evaluation
3. Appreciate the importance of measurement, observation and communication in any care setting
4. Outline issues associated with patient education and health promotion
5. Describe what is meant by models of care
6. Devise plans of care in relation to an individual's needs

Pre-chapter quiz

1. Can you list Roper et al.'s activities of living?
2. Name three other nursing models
3. What are the four components of the nursing process?
4. What is task-orientated nursing?
5. How many activities did Henderson envisage?
   a. 16
   b. 18
   c. 19
   d. 14
6. What is theory?
7. Describe a conceptual framework
8. What is model?
9. What is meant by holistic?
10. What were Nightingale's elements in nursing?

Introduction

The chapter aims to focus on the generic assessment of need from a broad perspective, particularly on some of the key concepts that support and inform practice in today's health care. This chapter does not intend to include detailed discussion relating to some of the conceptual models of care, but rather to focus on some of the key components that underpin health care practice. It will provide a background to the organisation of nursing care, based on the Activities of Living approach by Roper et al. (2000), with specific reference to Florence Nightingale, considered by many to be the founder of nursing. The chapter will also refer to the medical model of assessment.

Models of nursing

The original Roper et al. (1980) model of nursing was based upon activities of living and is seen as forming the basis of nursing care in the UK, particularly in the secondary care sector. The model is based loosely upon the activities of daily living, evolving from the research of Virginia Henderson (1966). Whereas Henderson identified 14 activities that 'people engage in', Roper et al. only use 12. The current model seeks to define what living means and it breaks it down into the categories outlined in Figure 3.1.

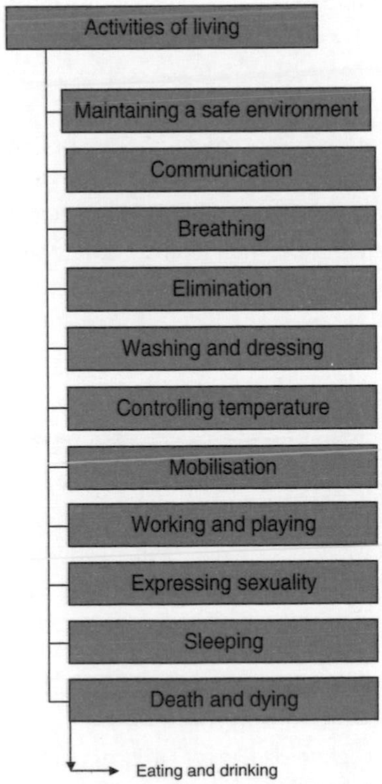

Figure 3.1 Activities of living.

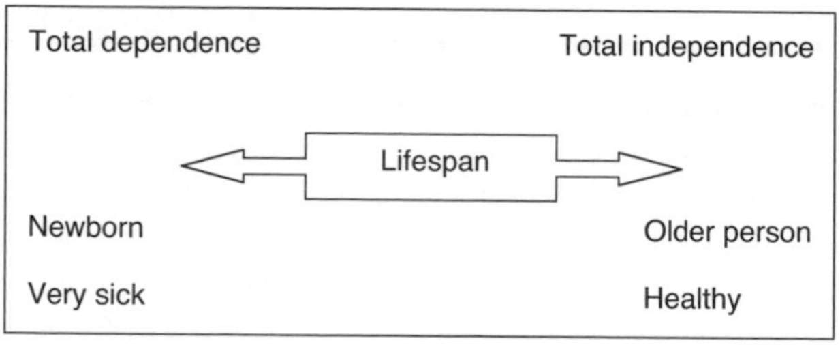

Figure 3.2 Dependence-independence continuum.

These 12 activities should also be considered within what Roper et al. defined as the 'dependence-independence continuum'. This continuum is closely related to the lifespan (see Figure 3.2). At each end of the lifespan, i.e. newborn and older patient, dependence is usually greater than in the middle of the lifespan. Dependence will vary, depending on illness and disease, and it is the assessment of the level of dependence and independence that is the cornerstone of nursing care, referred to conception through to birth and death.

Activities of living

The activities of living are often used in the initial assessment of a patient upon admission or initial assessment and are reviewed as the patient's care plan evolves. To provide effective care, all of the patient's needs, those that are set out by investigating the patient's specific requirements relative to each activity, must be met as practicably as possible.

This chapter aims to dispel some of the myths and confusion surrounding the nursing process, providing readers with a clear overview of this fundamental concept in nursing. Throughout this chapter, the term 'individual' will be used instead of patient. This reflects the fact that not everyone who is nursed is necessarily ill (e.g. individuals in the community and primary care setting), but they do need some form of nursing intervention, perhaps as a health promotion measure.

Organisation of nursing care

Crucial to the delivery of quality individualised nursing care is a method of organising care, such as the nursing process (Kemp and Richardson, 1994). The nursing process was introduced into the UK in 1980. It was initially regarded with some scepticism, partly due to it being adopted from America, where it had been implemented some years earlier. However, it has now been fully accepted into UK nursing practice and is present, in one form or another, in the majority of clinical areas.

Although the concept of the nursing process has been the cornerstone of professional nursing practice for a number of years, it has been open to misinterpretation, causing confusion amongst students and novices of nursing practice. However, it is generally recognised as describing a systematic approach to nursing that comprises a series of steps or stages which refer to the assessing, planning, implementing and evaluation of nursing care (Roper et al., 2000). In this sense, the nursing process is essentially what nurses do when providing individual nursing care. In other words, the nursing process is a *thinking* and *doing* approach that nurses use in their work (Wilkinson, 1996).

Nursing in itself is a unique blend of art and science applied to our professional practice as nurses. Nursing was initially task-orientated - often a list of tasks to be carried out. This approach was favoured practice for many years, as nurses were considered the 'doctor's handmaiden'. As nurses have emerged as professionals in their own right, the 'science of nursing' has taken precedence, with nursing theory and knowledge seen as essential to achieving a scientific knowledge base in nursing practice (Chinn and Kramer, 1995).

Nursing practice

Nursing practice in the UK has developed rapidly in the last 30 years. The changes to nurse education, from a hospital to a university setting, nurses undertaking diplomas, degrees and doctorates are examples of professional nursing development. Nursing is currently organised into four specialisms or branches: adult, mental health, learning disabilities and children's nursing. During the first part of a course, nursing students are introduced to the generic, core knowledge and theory that underpin all branches of nursing, such as communication, anatomy and physiology, applied pathophysiology and pharmacology. The second and third years focus on the knowledge, theory and practice required for the branch of choice. Midwifery and health visiting are regarded as separate professions, although still within the nursing family.

Further nursing roles have developed, particularly the speciality role, e.g. public health nursing, infection control nursing, and disease-focused roles, such as respiratory and cardiac nurse specialists, to name just a few. The latter roles have evolved from the generic nurse practitioner and nurse consultant roles. Some nurses work in an independent capacity, developing social enterprise initiatives. Social enterprises are businesses set up to tackle social and environmental needs, some of which are related to health.

Nursing history

Whilst superficially this may be viewed as dynamic and innovative, in fact Florence Nightingale, considered by many retrospectively as the founder of nursing theory, based her theories on her own experiences during the Crimean War. During Nightingale's era of the late nineteenth century, unsanitary conditions posed an enormous health hazard and she correctly concluded that external influences and conditions can prevent, suppress or contribute to death and disease. This was revolutionary at the time, since nurses then were not employed to think, just to do - back to the task-orientated approach. Although now highly regarded and respected, during her career her important observations, which she published widely, were largely ignored by the government of the time (McDonald, 2002).

Florence commenced her nursing training at age 31; much to her parents' disquiet, since at the time a career in nursing was associated with working-class women and Florence was from a wealthy and privileged background. After qualifying, she was appointed resident lady superintendent of a hospital for invalid women in Harley Street, London.

With the commencement of the Crimean War in 1853, British soldiers sent into battle were contracting cholera and malaria. Within weeks an estimated 8000 men were suffering from these diseases and Florence, amongst others, offered their services to assist with the epidemic. Her offer was initially rejected, but when a national newspaper (alerted by Florence) publicised the huge cholera death rate amongst the British soldiers there was a public outcry, and the government was forced to change its mind. Florence again volunteered her services, and with 38 colleagues, she was appalled at the conditions that she faced. Injured soldiers were housed in rooms without clean blankets or decent food and water. Unwashed, they were still wearing their dirt-encrusted army uniforms. In such appalling conditions, it was perhaps not surprising that in army hospitals, the subsequent overwhelming infections contracted by their war wounds actually accounted for one death in six, rather than the initial injury itself. Infectious diseases such as typhus, cholera and dysentery contributed to the death rate, easily overwhelming soldiers already weakened through infection and blood loss.

At the same time Mary Seacole, a Black British woman, born in Jamaica, provided health care services to soldiers of the Crimean War. Seacole worked at the front and at the docks helping to care for and tend to men who were injured in the war.

Against strong military objection for Florence to radically reform these field hospitals, she was again forced to use the British media to highlight the terrible conditions of these wounded soldiers, and after a great deal of publicity, Florence was given the task of organising the nursing care and by improving the quality of the sanitation she was able to dramatically reduce the death rate of the soldiers.

After the war, Florence returned to the UK as a national heroine. She had been deeply moved by the lack of basic hygiene and elementary care that the men received in the British Army and she decided to begin a campaign to improve the quality of nursing in military hospitals.

She published widely on her findings and with the support of friends raised money to improve the quality of nursing, founding the Nightingale School and Home for Nurses at St. Thomas's Hospital. She also became involved in the training of nurses for employment in the workhouses that had been established as a result of the 1834 Poor Law Amendment Act. Before her death in 1910, at the age of 90, Florence championed women's rights and campaigned ardently for women to have careers, then unheard of and frowned upon in the paternalistic society of the day (Nightingale, 1969).

The reason that Florence's work was so important was that she developed her own form of nursing process to improve the quality of care for the soldiers. Her basic theory was that there was a link between health and the environment, which at the time had not been considered.

Elements in nursing

Florence suggested that there were five essential elements important in restoring health. These were simply:

- Pure air
- Pure water
- Light
- Cleanliness
- Efficient drainage

She concluded that the *environment* in which her patients were nursed had an impact on health and she suggested that it was the physical, psychological and social environment that impacted on health need. Today, we still refer to these three elements, in addition to some others. Figure 3.3 outlines the current categories, whilst the *italic* text demonstrates those elements that Florence alluded to in her early publications. As you can see, they are not so different from modern-day thinking.

Theories, concepts and models

Theory

A theory provides a way of looking at a discipline, such as nursing. It is clear and explicit, in terms that can be communicated to others. Therefore nursing theories help to explain the unique place of nursing within the health care profession - e.g. how nursing differs from the role of a doctor or physiotherapist. Theory is the best effort taken to describe and explain a phenomenon or experience (Hungler et al., 2000).

Models

The word 'model' refers to a system that is not necessarily written in 'tablets of stone', but is flexible, varies over time and should reflect current practice and research. A model should:

- Be systematic, e.g. have clear basic systems in place
- Be based on evidence, e.g. should include the latest research findings, current thinking and possess a theoretical base
- Be related to concepts
- Be related to theories and values, e.g. include the relevant theory and accepted professional values (this includes acting professionally, respecting the individual and ensuring confidentiality)

Concepts

A 'concept' is used to refer to a formal view or image of something such as conceptual models.

Conceptual models

Conceptual models for nursing are therefore formal presentations of some nurses' private views or images of nursing. Conceptual models should:

- Identify essential components of the discipline (in this case, nursing)
- Show relationships between concepts or other views
- Introduce current established theories from other disciplines (such as psychology and sociology)

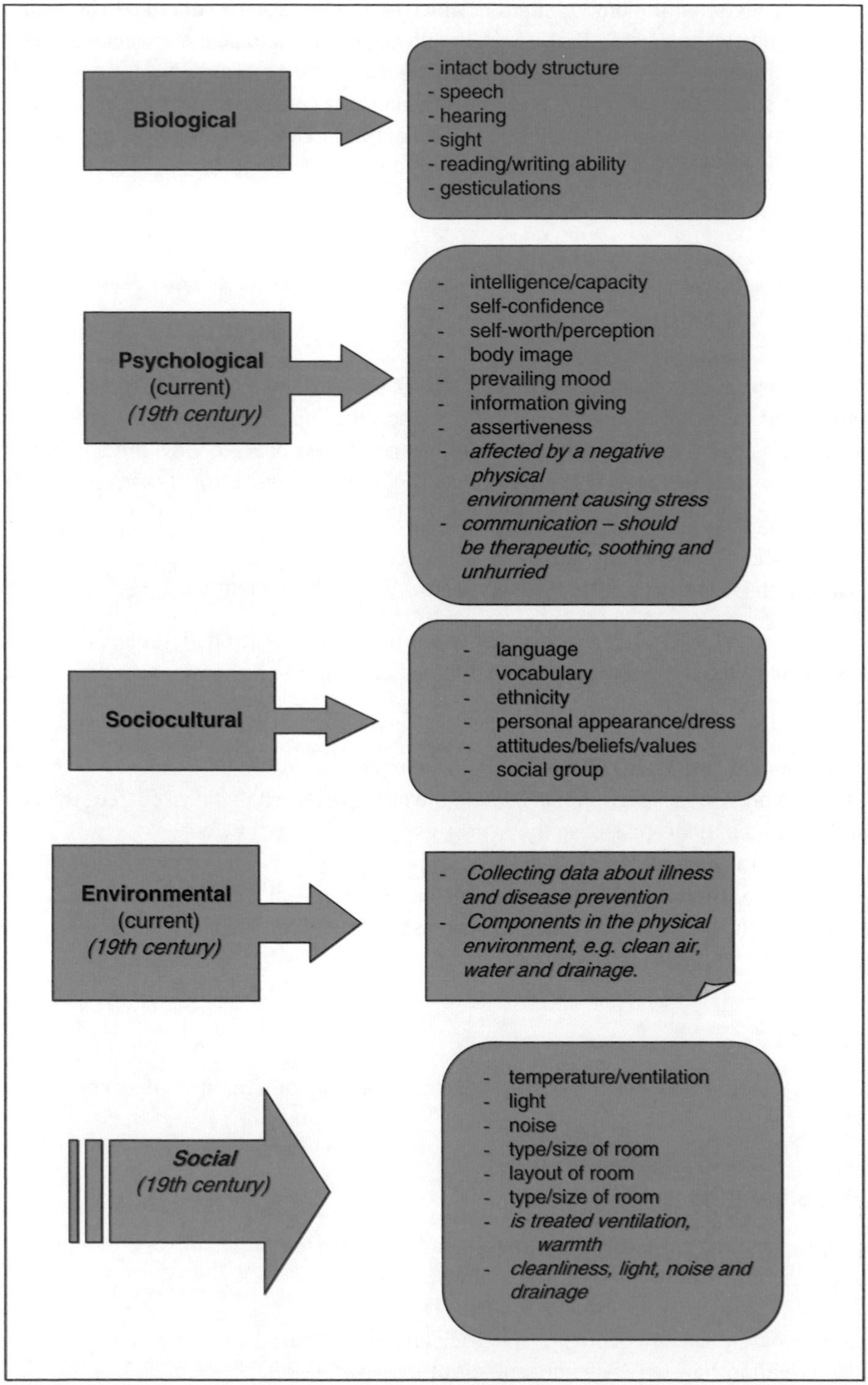

Figure 3.3 Factors influencing assessment of need.

There are a number of conceptual models that demonstrate the nursing process, but examples include the following:

Roper's Activities of Living Model (ALs) (Roper et al., 2000)

- Development model - emphasising growth and development
- Person orientated
- Focus on change
- Views a range of activities of living changing with maturation
- Supporting and enabling
- Heavily based on Henderson's work

Roy's Adaptation Model (Roy, 1984)

- Systems model - individual is made up of systems
- Systems interact with the environment
- Nursing is supporting adaptation to environment
- Holistic, purposeful and unifying
- Health is a process of responding positively to environmental change

Peplau's Interpersonal Model (Peplau, 1988)

- Inter-actional model
- Concerned with interpersonal relationships
- Nursing is organised through building relationships to support communication
- Nurse must be able to sue self-therapeutically

Orem's Model of Self Care (Orem, 1980)

- Nursing is part of a social care paradigm
- Aims at supporting individual to self-care
- Caring is an art of moral consciousness
- Care is considered to be the core and essence of nursing
- Based on a collective responsibility to support and enable

Neuman's Health Care System Model (Neuman and Young, 1972)

- Individual is a unique, holistic system
- Individuals are a dynamic composite of psychological, sociocultural and spiritual variables
- Individuals' reaction to, and relationship with, stress
- Nursing acts to impede the status of disorganisation caused by illness/disease

Figure 3.4 summarises the theories, models and concepts outlined above.

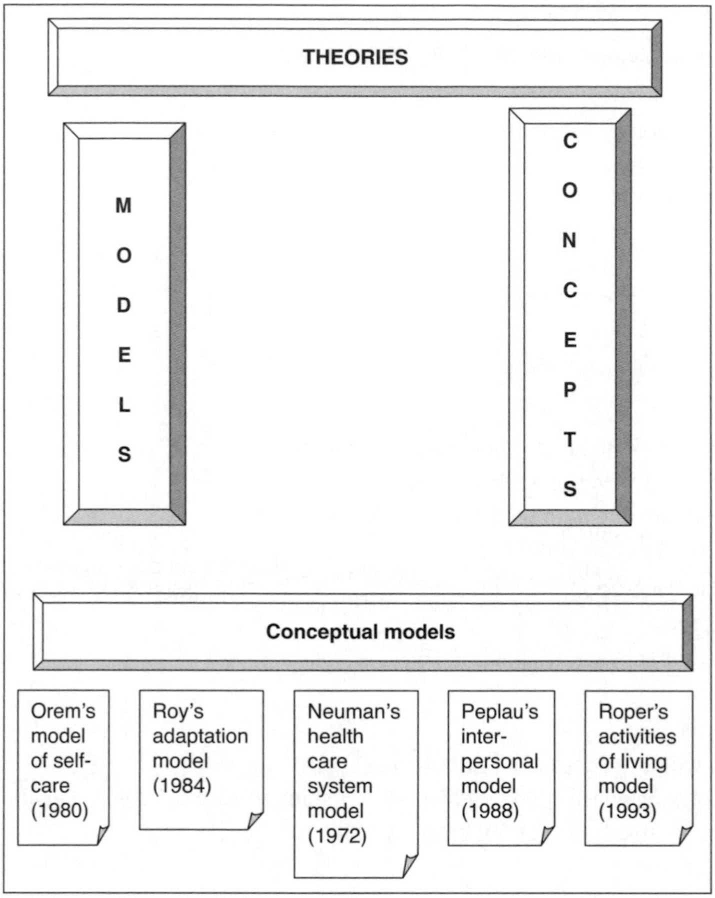

Figure 3.4 Theories, models and concepts.

Putting the two components together, we have the 'nursing process'. As outlined earlier, this chapter will focus on the key components that make up the nursing process rather than look at individual conceptual models.

Nursing process

When dealing with a new concept, definitions are always a useful starting point. So the term 'nursing process' is worth separating into its two components – 'nursing' and 'process'. The organisation and background to nursing consists of a Chief Nursing Officer (CNO) employed by the Department of Health (DH) to provide guidance to the government on matters relating to nursing practice nationally. Nursing's professional bodies are the Royal College of Nursing (RCN), a nursing union which represents the interests of nurses and nursing. The RCN also provides an educational role, lobbies government on policy and raises the profile of nursing in the UK.

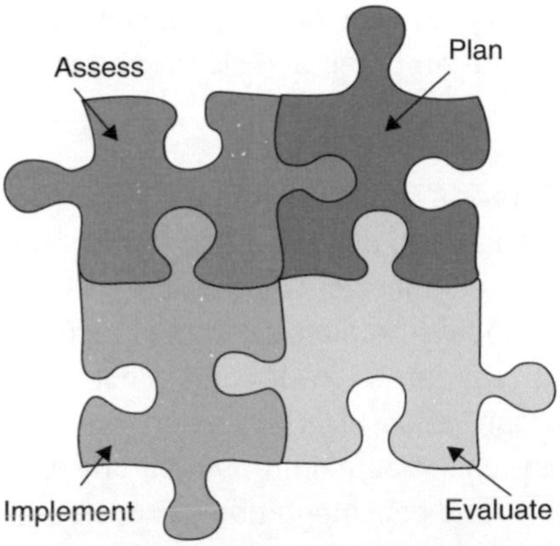

Figure 3.5 Key steps in the nursing process.

The Nursing and Midwifery Council (NMC) is an organisation set up by Parliament to protect the public by ensuring that nurses, midwives and health visitors provide high standards of care to people. The NMC maintains a register of qualified nurses, midwives and health visitors. It sets standards for education, practice and conduct, provides advice for nurses, midwives and health visitors and considers allegations of misconduct or unfitness to practise due to ill health. The NMC also produces a number of practice guidelines.

A 'process' can be defined as a procedure, method or course of action. It is often used to describe a series of interrelated events that result in an outcome of one kind or another. A process can be applied to practically any aspect of life. The process by which we use a cashpoint machine, e.g. to withdraw money from our bank accounts, is one example. We have a plastic card, with personalised information stored on it, which we insert into a machine. By entering a four-digit assigned number (sometimes called a PIN number) and then selecting a number of options, we can withdraw cash, check our bank balance or perhaps order a bank statement. A sequence of events (possession of a card, a PIN number and a computerised machine) has occurred which results in an outcome – in this case – money. The nursing process works in similar ways.

Assessment, planning, implementation and evaluation of care

It is worth remembering that all the stages in the nursing process are continuous and interlink with each other as identified in Figure 3.5.

For example, although assessment is the first stage, the individual should be assessed continuously throughout the episode of care – whether that is in a hospital or a community setting. There are essentially four steps to the nursing process (whichever conceptual model is adopted) and these will be looked at in detail. These steps are assessment, planning, implementation and evaluation. The four key steps are:

- Assess
- Plan
- Implement
- Evaluate

Each step should lead to the next and this should be an ongoing process, constantly being evaluated. To assess the individual's need is the first step and clearly forms the basis of the process.

Assessment (what is the problem and what needs to be done?)

The first stage in assessing need is to collect, organise and document the information about an individual. Information can be collected in a number of ways, using a variety of methods. The aim is to clearly identify the individual's problem(s) so that care can be planned. This information is usually recorded in a care plan of some kind, which often takes different formats and varies from organisation to organisation, but they are usually paper or electronic forms that contain fundamental information. The NMC produces guidelines on standards for record keeping and documentation (NMC, 2008).

Assessing need can take the form of an interview. Although informal, it is a very essential part of the process and should therefore be undertaken in an area or room which respects individual confidentiality – not within direct earshot of other people that is quiet and calm. This can often be difficult to achieve in a busy hospital ward, clinic or accident and emergency department, but by ensuring privacy such as at least pulling the curtains around the bed and keeping your voice to a reasonable level, you, the nurse, should be able to offer the required privacy. After introducing yourself to the individual, you should then ensure that the individual provides their consent to talk to you. This can be verbal consent and any refusal should be documented and respected.

The assessment usually starts with the essential information about the individual themselves and includes name, address, date of birth, National Health and hospital number (if known), telephone number, next of kin (or who to contact in an emergency) and their contact details, contact details of their general practitioner and any other health care professionals involved with the individual, e.g. district nurses, health visitors and physiotherapists.

The form will also require nurses to record information of the individual's occupation, ethnic background, language, religious beliefs and any specific cultural/ethnic requirements. It is important to document these details accurately, to ensure that all the patients' ethnic needs are respected.

Next, the assessment should focus on clinical aspects of the individual – providing a background of their health history to date. The required clinical information usually addresses the key issues, and is commonly known as the medical model. At this point, it is worth a brief description of the medical model, which adopts a more systematic approach to individual assessment (Simon et al., 2005). It may not necessarily be that the nurse undertakes such an approach (although more advanced nurses such as nurse practitioners are also educated in this approach). It is always worth having awareness and observing how other health care professionals assess individuals. As mentioned earlier, the layout of the form may vary, but the information documented will remain the same whether as a nursing or medical record.

- Past medical history
  - Chronological list of major illnesses, injuries and operations
  - Any current diagnosed health problems, e.g. diabetes mellitus, asthma and heart disease

  - Reason for admission (or referral) – it is important to establish that the individual is aware of the rationale for their admission or referral
  - Any other health issues
- Medications/drug history
  - Prescribed and over-the-counter drugs (including contraception)
  - Any illegal/non-prescribed drugs
  - Alternative and complementary therapies being taken
  - Known allergies – type of reaction, action taken and outcome
- Family and social history
  - Marital status
  - Children
  - Housing
  - Occupation
- General
  - Alcohol and tobacco consumption
  - Dietary preferences
  - Known food allergies
  - Bowel habits
  - Mobility – any aids used, e.g. walking stick, zimmer frame or crutches
- Specific
  - Sight – do they wear glasses or contact lenses
  - Hearing – any aids used
  - Taste – any dentures or bridges
  - Skin – noting any problems with skin integrity or skin problems
  - Sensory – any deficits in the touch sensation
- Gender related
  - Males – noting any prostate or testicular problems
  - Women – note date of last menstrual period , any concerns regarding menstruation or breast lumps/discharge and record obstetric history

Usually the next step is recording and documenting baseline observations. These are essential to provide all health care professionals with a starting point of the individual's basic biophysical measurements, which are useful comparisons for the future. These measurements are recorded in the care plan or notes and on the relevant observation charts and should include:

- Blood pressure
- Pulse
- Respirations
- Temperature
- Weight
- Body mass index
- Height
- Urinalysis
- Other specific observations, e.g. blood sugar and peak flow measurements for individuals with specific known health problems such as diabetes mellitus and respiratory problems, asthma and chronic obstructive pulmonary disease .

This information is comprehensive and initially when nurses start undertaking assessment - such as the above - it can seem to take forever. However, this is a very useful teaching tool and, with practice, nurses become much more accomplished and efficient with documenting information (Benner, 1984). During assessment, the information may come from the individual themselves and/or a carer or family member. Information may also be available in the form of patient-held records - such as individuals with specific health problems, e.g. diabetes mellitus, asthma, epilepsy, and those taking certain medications.

There may also be a referral letter from a doctor or other health care professional outlining the individual's medical history. The individual may already have a set of medical and/or nursing notes available, but it is always worth checking the details to ensure that the information is factual, accurate and up-to-date.

During the assessment, the nurse has an excellent opportunity to observe the individual both verbally and non-verbally. From a non-verbal perspective, much can be gained from just observing the individual. Noting the manner in which they walk, their eye contact with you, tone and colour of their skin, facial expression, body language and general demeanour can provide a wealth of information - before they have uttered a word. These cues can be subtle - you might note that the skin and lips appear dry, suggesting dehydration. More stoical individuals may not like to admit they have pain - but appear pale, in obvious discomfort perhaps holding or rubbing the affected area. In some senses the nurse becomes a detective - searching for clues and looking for evidence to solve what may be a mystery as to the individual's health problem.

Obviously a lot of information can be obtained from the verbal responses. However, if the individual continually asks you to repeat the questions, then you may conclude that they have a hearing problem, or if their speech is slurred, it might suggest that they have suffered a stroke or have had some other neurological event.

There are some special circumstances that nurses encounter during assessment and it is outside the remit of this particular chapter to go through them in detail, but they include:

- Individuals who are unconscious
- Individuals who do not speak English
- Individuals who are mentally disturbed
- Individuals with a learning disability/special needs
- Babies and children
- Aggressive individuals

In addition to documenting this information in the relevant care plan, any unusual or untoward findings should be reported to the nurse-in-charge and/or medical team promptly. Once all this information has been recorded, the next stage is planning the care to be delivered.

Planning (how may these needs be met?)

During this stage, it is important to establish how the needs of the individual may be met, that these needs are prioritised, that the best way of achieving the goals is established and what the alternatives might be.

The care plan should allow for individualisation at this point, since although there may be generic needs, individuals do respond differently to both disease processes and nursing interventions. The nurse also needs to determine what care will be undertaken to prevent or manage problems. This includes:

- Solving existing, presenting problems
- Preventing identified potential problems from becoming actual problems
- Alleviating those problems which cannot be solved and assisting the individual to cope positively with these problems
- Preventing recurrence of a treated problem
- Assisting in ensuring that an individual is pain free and as comfortable as possible when death is inevitable

The sample care plan (see Table 3.1) provides a simple overview of the information that is required to assess, plan, implement and evaluate care (Roper et al.'s ALs have

Table 3.1 Sample care plan.

Assess[a]	Plan	Implement	Evaluate
When assessing an individual's needs, the following factors should be taken into consideration: • List individual problems in order of priority • Number each problem • Date each problem • Assess each problem in association with Roper et al.'s Activities of Living	When writing goals, some factors to remember are: • They must be written in terms of individual achievement, e.g. 'Mr X will state that he feels less anxious' • Write at least one short-term goal • Make each goal measurable e.g. 'Mr X will show lessened pain with the use of a pain chart' • Each goal should state a target date and time for evaluation	This part of the care plan needs to show all the nursing interventions. Points to remember are: • List specific actions in relation to working towards the set goals • In most cases several actions are required to achieve just one goal • It is often a good idea to cite a rationale for actions	This aspect of a care plan is ongoing until a problem has been resolved. Some important facts to remember are: • State clearly the time and date of evaluation • Use any measures that were mentioned in the plan, e.g. 'Mr X states that his pain is now reduced from 7 to 2 on the pain scale'[b] • For long-term goals, explain how much nearer to achieving that goal an individual is • Consider any changes or additions to nursing actions that might have come about

[a] May need to be repeated on an hourly basis in critical care settings.
[b] http://www.britishpainsociety.org/pain_scales_eng.pdf.

been used here) and each stage will now be described in more detail. A practical example will also be used to demonstrate the stages involved in the nursing process. Remember these are generic and can apply to any conceptual model that is adopted in the particular area of health care you find yourself working.

To demonstrate this more clearly, a practical example (see Box 3.1) will be used to demonstrate the nursing process and subsequent care plan.

Box 3.1 Practical example.

Mr Smith is a 76-year-old widowed gentleman who has been admitted to the ward with a sudden onset of shortness of breath. He had a heart attack 2 years ago and has been taking medication for heart failure for the last 3 months.

Once he is in bed, he is obviously having trouble breathing and cannot complete a sentence without gasping for breath. As the nurse admitting Mr Smith, you notice that his ankles are very swollen and his breathing sounds 'bubbly'.

Mr Smith also suffers from diabetes and has not been taking his prescribed tablets for the last 2 days, because of feeling unwell.

The referral letter from his general practitioner, who requested that Mr Smith be admitted to hospital, expressed concern that his house was untidy with little food available.

Immediate problems need to be identified and dealt with urgently. For example Mr Smith will need to have his respiratory problems dealt with immediately. His symptoms (breathlessness, swollen ankles and 'bubbly' breathing) suggest that he is suffering from heart failure and will need prescribed oxygen therapy and medication to help him excrete the excess fluid from his circulatory system thereby relieving his symptoms (DH, 2000).

Less urgent problems can wait – in this example Mr Smith's diabetes may become a cause for concern since he has not been taking his medication regulating his blood sugar. This needs to be dealt with in the next hour or two, but once his acute breathing problem has been managed effectively (DH, 2007a, 2007b).

Other problems, in this case, Mr Smith's potential social problem related to his housing, will require referral to other health care professionals. Social services or the intermediate care team should be made aware of Mr Smith's problems so that a better home environment can be established prior to his discharge from hospital.

At this stage the expected outcomes or results need to be established. Some thought needs to be given to how the individual will benefit from nursing care. What will the individual be able to achieve and in what time frame?

Mr Smith therefore has initially three identified problems:

Problem 1 – inability to breathe due to heart failure
Problem 2 – potentially uncontrolled diabetes
Problem 3 – poor and inadequate housing

Problem 1 must be dealt with immediately and the administration of prescribed oxygen and a diuretic medication (which speeds up fluid elimination from the body) will rapidly improve his condition.

Problem 2 needs to be addressed within the next hour or two and will involve some initial measurement and observation of his blood sugar levels with some further health promotion and education on how to manage his diabetes.

Problem 3 is a long-term problem that will require the input of other health care professionals. Whilst this problem is not immediate, it will potentially have an impact on his long-term health. For example Mr Smith may find climbing the stairs in his house increasingly difficult if he is out of breath. His shortness of breath may also account for why the house was untidy and little food was evident. He would find it very difficult to walk around his house or go shopping with such shortness of breath.

So each problem here is important and has an effect on his health - but there is clearly a priority or order in which they need to be dealt with.

Implementation

Implementation focuses on what care has actually been delivered. The care plan now requires implementation - there is no point in writing a comprehensive care plan if no one actually implements it. Nurses also need to keep in mind *what* they are doing and *why* they are doing it. It is very easy to get carried away with writing and thinking about an individual's problems without relating it back to what is achievable in a given time frame. Implementation, therefore, focuses on the actual steps taken to deliver care.

During this stage, nurses should continuously assess the individual's current health status before acting - as some problems do resolve without any intervention or may change dramatically and quickly. Nurses then undertake the care or intervention - perhaps applying a dressing to a wound, and then assess the response. All interventions should be accurately recorded and documented, with any adverse or unexpected outcomes to be reported immediately. Nurses need to decide what is going to be documented and where. The care plan allows for some free-text writing so that any additional notes can be added as necessary.

Crucial to this stage (and indeed every stage of the nursing process) are some key assessment skills in order to consider how the individual is responding to treatment (see Box 3.2). It may sound very obvious but simply observing the patient may provide you with the answer you need. If we use our example of Mr Smith, the nurse would be *observing* and *measuring* that his respiratory rate has reduced from 50 breaths per minute to

Box 3.2 Key assessment skills.

- Observing
- Measuring
- Listening
- Talking

25 breaths per minute and *listening* to hear that he is able to complete a sentence without getting breathless. These are two simple observations that allow the nurse to assess his first problem and determine whether the treatment has been successful. The nurse would also be *talking* to Mr Smith to ask how he is feeling generally.

Evaluation

Evaluation focuses on whether the aims of the intervention have been met and is the part of the cycle when the nurse judges the effectiveness or otherwise of a nursing intervention in terms of the expected outcome (Kemp and Richardson, 1994). Evaluation should also assess the intervention from a broader perspective, to understand if it has measured up against a standard, perhaps the related National Service Framework (NSF) or similar clinical guidelines (Downie et al., 1990). Evaluation is part of good clinical practice and nurses should always evaluate their interventions or actions. Several questions need answering at this stage:

1. How does the individual's health and ability compare with the expected outcome?
2. If he or she achieved their stated outcomes, is the person now ready to manage on their own and become independent?
3. Is the outcome measurable against a set standard?

One of the key features of the nursing process is to encourage individuals to move from total dependence towards total independence - the dependence-independence continuum referred to earlier in the chapter (see Figure 3.2). This is not always achievable with every individual, but on the scale between these two points, the nursing process can assist the individual to achieve a degree of independence, no matter how small that may be.

Essential in evaluating our interventions is to review whether the goals have been achieved and decide on alternative action if required. This may mean revisiting the beginning of the nursing process, starting with assessment, and start again. Nurses need to observe, question, test and measure the activities undertaken so far. These activities are essential to allow the nurse to reflect on the care given and to ask some questions:

- Have the goals been met?
- Was the action appropriate?
- Are new goals required?

Since individuals respond differently to illnesses, disease processes and their treatment, it is not always possible to predict that everyone will have similar outcomes. For example Mr Smith may not have responded well to the diuretic medication and required a further dose before his respiratory rate was reduced. Some diuretic medications have side effects and other drugs have to be given to counteract these effects. Therefore the nurses' assessment of his treatment is vital in providing the doctors with the relevant information to treat his heart failure.

Similarly, for Mr Smith's second problem of potentially uncontrolled diabetes, the plan may have been to provide Mr Smith with more information regarding his diabetes as part of health promotion. In this way we would be encouraging him to develop greater independence in self-managing his diabetes, but we may discover that Mr Smith has a good understanding of his diabetes, but had simply forgotten to take his tablets. This information is therefore useful on which to evaluate his care and plan for a different goal.

It is essential that the information regarding the individual's needs is factual, relevant and comprehensive. Documentation of nursing care is very important and the next section addresses some of the important issues related to documentation and record keeping in general.

Documentation

Documenting what care has taken place is essential for a number of reasons:

1. Communicates with others what has been observed or done
2. Identify roles of individual health care professionals
3. Provides a record of clinical actions taken
4. Organisation and dissemination (or sharing) of information with other health care professionals
5. Demonstrates the order of events relating to individual care

Individuals now not only have a legal right to see their records, but increasingly are participating in writing them. With regard to documentation, there are legal frameworks that apply to all health care professionals, including nurses. The Data Protection Act (OPSI, 1984) gave patients/clients access to their computer-held records in certain circumstances and is underpinned by eight Data Protection Principles (1984). The Data Protection Act requires anyone who handles personal information to comply with a number of important principles. It also gives individuals rights over their personal information. In addition, the Freedom of Information (FoI) Act (OPSI, 2000) gives individuals the right to ask any public sector body, including the NHS, for all the information they hold on any subject of their choice, as well as any personal information they hold on the individual, unless there is a good reason, and the organisation must provide the information within a month.

In addition, the Access to Health Records Act (OPSI, 1990) gives patients and clients the right of access to manual (paper) records about themselves that were made after 1 November 1991. There are both legal and professional issues to be aware of when compiling care plans (NMC, 2008).

Nursing care plans

These documents should represent all the nursing activity carried out for individuals wherever they are being nursed. In some clinical areas these may be referred to as Kardex's, patient assessment forms, patient profiles, nursing notes or history. Whatever the name or format given, what is essential is that the documentation adheres to the NMC's Code (NMC, 2008) and as per Trust policy and provides a comprehensive, accurate and holistic overview of the individual in question.

Table 3.2 Sample care plan for Mr Smith.

Date: 20 December 2008	**Time: 14.30**	**Nurse: Suzy Smith**	**Ward: 7B medical admission unit**
Assess	**Plan**	**Implement**	**Evaluate**
Problem 1: Breathing – shortness of breath due to probable heart failure	• Mr Smith's respiratory rate to decrease from 50 to 25 breaths per minute within 2 hours • Mr Smith to be able to complete sentences without getting out of breath within 2 hours	• Administer prescribed oxygen and diuretic therapy • Sit Mr Smith upright • Monitor fluid balance • Observe cannula • Document basic observations every 30 minutes for 4 hours	• Respiratory rate now 25 • Continue to monitor basic observations • Ensure Mr Smith receives prescribed medication • Perform electro-cardiograph (ECG)
Problem 2: Eating and Drinking – potential uncontrolled diabetes mellitus	• Mr Smith's blood sugar to be maintained within recommended guidelines (NICE, 2008)	• Measure and document Mr Smith's blood sugar hourly and urinalysis twice daily	• Blood sugar remains elevated • Commence new insulin regime • Ensure low-sugar diet adhered to • Check if Mr Smith can monitor his own blood sugar
Problem 3: Maintaining a safe environment – poor home environment and potential social issues related to Mr Smith's coping mechanisms at home	• Ensure safe home environment on discharge	• Call general practitioner • Refer to social services • Contact district • Nurse/ intermediate care team	• Social worker to visit Mr Smith on ward in 3 days • Liaise with hospital social worker and discharge team

Some areas will have paper records, some will be electronic and some will have a combination of both. Whatever format, the records should be stored safely and securely. At all times the nurse should ensure that confidential clinical information remains just that – confidential. It should not be shared with any other patients/clients or member of the individuals' family unless they specifically request it. It should, as far as possible, be written with the individual (NMC, 2008).

To demonstrate a care plan, we refer back to the case of Mr Smith and document his care in the sample care plan (see Table 3.2). In this instance, Roper et al.'s (1993) ALs have been adopted, but any of the conceptual models will have a similar format.

Conclusions

This chapter has focused on the broader perspective of the nursing process and considered the four key stages of assessment, planning, implementation and evaluation of care with reference to measurement, observation and communications that are essential for the nursing process to work effectively. Issues related to documentation, both professionally and legally, and a sample care plan has hopefully provided the reader with a clear summary of the nursing process.

There are several advantages of the nursing process - one of these is that its focus is not only on medical problems but also on the human response of individuals. Each individual will react differently to medical problems - some will be stoical and others will adopt a 'sick role' taking to their bed at the first hint of a cold or minor illness such as flu. Individuals will also respond differently to interventions and their care plans need to reflect this.

Nurses need to adopt a holistic approach to care. Holism is a term widely used in health care and it refers to the fact that nurses should treat each individual as a whole - taking into account all the ALs but should not ignore the component parts that contribute towards the individual, nor the impact that society and the environment has on the individual.

Florence Nightingale and her theory of nursing was discussed at the beginning of the chapter; she theorised that a systematic approach to care, which took into account the basic elements of a clean environment, in terms of air, water, light, cleanliness and sanitation, was essential in achieving health and independence. Now some 150 years later, we continue to use these basic concepts of assessment, planning, implementing and evaluating care that she used to nurse the soldiers in her care, a wise woman indeed. Florence provided advice for nursing students in 1873 by stating:

> Nursing is most truly said to be a high calling, an honourable calling. But what does the honour lie in? In working hard during your training to learn and to do all things perfectly. The honour does not lie in putting on Nursing like your uniform. Honour lies in loving perfection, consistency, and in working hard for it: in being ready to work individually: ready to say not 'How clever I am!' but 'I am not yet worthy'; and I will live to deserve to be called a Trained Nurse.

Glossary

Activities of Living	Based on Roper, Logan and Tierney's model of Activities of Living and is based on everyday things we all do as part of everyday life, e.g. washing, dressing, eating and drinking.
Concepts	Major components of theory, conveying the abstract ideas within a theory.
Guidelines	Written statements outlining best decisions about treatment or care for a particular condition or situation, typically written in statement form by a reputable organisation.

Health promotion	The process of enabling people to exert control over the determinants of health and thereby improve their health. It is an essential guide in addressing the major health challenges faced by developing and developed nations, including communicable and non-communicable diseases, and issues related to human development and health.
Heart failure	A condition related to the structure or function of the heart and its impaired ability to supply sufficient blood flow to meet the body's needs. Common causes of heart failure include myocardial infarction and other forms of ischaemic heart disease, hypertension, valvular heart disease and cardiomyopathy.
Models	General term referring to a symbolic representation of a phenomenon in words, letters of numbers. Models provide an understanding of how theoretical relationships work.
Nursing process	Process by which nurses deliver care to patients, supported by nursing models or philosophies. The nursing process was originally an adapted form of problem-solving and is classified as a deductive theory.
Paradigm	A generally accepted structure or a worldview within a discipline that organises the theory aspect.

Post-chapter quiz

1. How does a model of care help nurses help patients?
2. Why is an individual approach to care advocated?
3. What is a nursing history?
4. What is a medical history?
5. List three types of measurement associated with patient care
6. How can the nurse ensure privacy during history taking?
7. Who was Virginia Henderson?
8. List the key features associated with documentation as per the NHS Code of Practice
9. What are the four key assessment skills?
10. Describe six principles underpinning protection

References

Benner, P. (1984) *From Novice to Expert: Excellence and Power in Clinical Nursing Practice.* California: Addison-Wesley Publishing Co.

Chinn, P.L. and Kramer, M.K. (1995) *Theory and Nursing – A Systematic Approach*, 4th ed. St Louis, Baltimore: Mosby.

Department of Health (1997) *Review of Patient – Identifiable Information* (Caldicott Report). London: HMSO. Available at http://www.dh.gov.uk/en/Publicationsandstatistics/Publications/PublicationsPolicyAndGuidance/DH_4068403. Accessed 19 January 2009.

Department of Health (2000) *Coronary Heart Disease: National Service Framework for Coronary Heart Disease – Modern Standards and Service Models.* London: HMSO. Available at http://www.dh.gov.uk/en/Publicationsandstatistics/Publications/PublicationsPolicy And Guidance/DH_4094275. Accessed 5 January 2009.

Department of Health (2003) *Confidentiality: NHS Code of Practice*. London: HMSO. Available at http://www.dh.gov.uk/en/Managingyourorganisation/Informationpolicy/Patient confidentialityandcaldicottguardians/DH_4100550. Accessed 5 January 2009.

Department of Health (2007a) *NSF Diabetes Delivery Strategy*. London: HMSO. Available at http://www.dh.gov.uk/en/Publicationsandstatistics/Publications/PublicationsPolicyAnd Guidance/Browsable/DH_4097539. Accessed 5 January 2009.

Department of Health (2007b) *National Service Framework for Diabetes*. London: HMSO. Available at http://www.dh.gov.uk/en/Healthcare/NationalServiceFrameworks/Diabetes/ index.htm. Accessed 5 January 2009.

Downie, R.S., Fyfe, C. and Tannahill, A. (1990) *Health Promotion – Models and Values*. Oxford: Oxford University Press.

Henderson, V.A. (1966) *The Nature of Nursing*. New York: Macmillan Publishing.

Hungler, D.F., Beck, B.P. and Polit, C.T. (2000) *Essentials of Nursing Research: Methods, Appraisal, and Utilization*. Philadelphia: Lippincott Williams and Wilkins Publishers.

Kemp, N. and Richardson, E. (1994) *The Nursing Process and Quality Care*. London: Edward Arnold.

McDonald, L. (ed) (2002) *The Collected Works of Florence – An Introduction to Her Life and Family*. Ontario: Wilfrid Laurier University Press.

National Institute for Health & Clinical Excellence (2008) *The Management of Type 2 Diabetes*. London: NICE. Available at http://www.nice.org.uk/nicemedia/pdf/CG66Full Guideline0509.pdf. Accessed 19 January 2009.

Neuman, B. and Young, R.J. (1972). A model for teaching total person approach to patient problems. *Nursing Research* 21: 264–269.

Nightingale, F. (1969) *Notes on Nursing: What It Is and What It Is Not*. New York: Dover Publications Inc.

Nursing and Midwifery Council (2008) *The Code Standards of Conduct, Performance and Ethics for Nurses and Midwives*. London: NMC. Available at http://www.nmc-uk.org/aFrameDisplay.aspx?DocumentID=3954. Accessed 5 January 2009.

Office of Public Sector Information (1990) Access to Health Records Act. Available at http://www.opsi.gov.uk/acts/acts1990/ukpga_19900023_en_1. Accessed 5 January 2009.

Office of Public Sector Information (2000) Freedom of Information Act. Available at http://www.opsi.gov.uk/acts/acts2000/ukpga_20000036_en_1. Accessed 5 January 2009.

OPSI (Office of Public Sector Information) (1984) Data Protection Act. Available at http://www.opsi.gov.uk/Acts/Acts1998/ukpga_19980029_en_1. Accessed 5 January 2009.

Orem, D. (1980) *Nursing: Concepts of Practice*, 2nd ed. New York: McGraw-Hill.

Peplau, H. (1988) *Interpersonal Relations in Nursing: A Conceptual Framework of Reference for Psychodynamic Nursing*. Basingstoke: Mcmillan Education.

Roper, N., Logan, W. and Tierney, A.J. (1980) *Elements of Nursing*. Edinburgh: Churchill Livingstone.

Roper, N., Logan, W. and Tierney, A.J. (2000) *The Roper-Logan-Tierney Model of Nursing: Based on Activities of Living*. Edinburgh: Churchill Livingstone.

Roy, C. (1984) *Introduction to Nursing: An Adaptation Model*. New Jersey: Prentice Hall.

Simon, C., Everitt, H. and Kendrick, T. (2005) *Oxford Handbook of General Practice*. Oxford: Oxford University Press.

Wilkinson, J. (1996) *Nursing Process – A Critical Thinking Approach*. California: Addison-Welsey Publishing Co.

Chapter 4
Promoting Safety

Janet G. Migliozzi

Learning opportunities

This chapter will help you to:

1. Understand the importance of maintaining patient safety
2. Define some common risks in health care
3. Understand your role in relation to medicine administration
4. Understand the factors that increase the risk of patient falls
5. Outline the measures needed to minimise transmission of infection risk
6. Discuss the correct technique for hand washing

Pre-chapter quiz

1. What is an adverse event?
2. Outline two pieces of legislation that govern safety in health care
3. What do you understand by the word 'hazard'?
4. Outline four potential risks in health care
5. What is the nurse's role in patient safety?
6. List five common factors that affect patient safety
7. What is the Morse Scale used for?
8. Describe five steps that promote the safe dispensing of medicines
9. What are standard infection control precautions?
10. When should hand hygiene be carried out?

Introduction

'The hospital should do the sick no harm' (Nightingale, 1859) and yet patients are harmed when in hospital, with 850 000 'adverse events' happening each year – this equates to one in ten patients who are admitted to hospital and whilst most patients who receive health care are 'safe', adverse events cost the NHS around £3 billion a year in additional hospital stays, health care-associated infections (HCAI) and the settlement of negligence claims (Parish, 2003).

Maintaining a safe environment in hospitals depends on not only the infrastructure, but also the equipment and materials used on the premises, and all health care personnel, irrespective of the setting, are responsible for maintaining a safe environment. However, 'health care relies on a range of complex interaction between people, skill, technologies and drugs. Sometimes things can - and do - go wrong' (Department of Health [DH], 2006a). Consequently, health professionals need to be aware of factors that affect the safety of patients and staff, what constitutes a safe environment for a particular person or for a group of people in a health care setting, and act to minimise risk appropriately.

This chapter considers the minimisation of risk to both patients and staff in the health care setting. The importance of risk assessment and risk minimisation will be discussed in order to promote safe and effective care. Common risks to health care staff and patients will then be outlined. The second part of the chapter focuses on three areas of practice: drug administration, prevention of falls and infection prevention and control and will explore methods to minimise risk relating to these themes in the health care setting.

Risk assessment

As all health care involves risk and although risk cannot be totally eradicated, health professionals have a duty to ensure that the necessary action is taken to reduce the risk to patients and much can be done to ensure that it is kept to a minimum (Curran, 2001). The Health and Safety Executive (HSE, 1998) defines a hazard as 'anything that can cause harm' where harms includes injury, ill-health, damage to plant, equipment, property and the environment and interruption to service delivery (HSE, 1997). A risk is the probability that harm will arise, i.e. 'the chance, high or low, that someone will be harmed by the hazard' (HSE, 1998), and is therefore, as argued by Mayatt (2002), 'something that can be changed'.

Risk assessment helps to identify and manage workplace hazards which may pose a threat to the health, safety and welfare of people, or to the delivery of care (McCulloch, 1999). The HSE (1997) describes risk assessment as a structured process involving five steps.

Step 1: Hazard identification

The first step addresses hazard identification and those hazards that could result in significant harm under the conditions of the workplace - these would include:

- Slipping/tripping hazards from poorly maintained floors or stairs
- Fire from flammable materials
- Chemicals that are harmful to health, e.g. disinfectants and laboratory solutions
- Electricity, e.g. poor wiring
- Dust

- Fumes
- Manual handling
- Noise
- Poor lighting
- Low or high temperature
- Machinery and equipment used in day-to-day practices

Step 2: Identification of who might be harmed and how

This step recognises those who may be harmed and the ways in which they might be harmed:

- People sharing the workplace
- Operators
- Cleaners
- Office staff
- Members of the public, e.g. visitors
- Staff and patients with disabilities
- Inexperienced staff
- Lone workers

Step 3: Risk evaluation

This step includes a consideration of how likely it is that each hazard could cause harm and deciding for each significant hazard whether the risk is high, medium or low and whether or not the risk has been reduced as far as is reasonably practicable.

Step 4: Documentation of risk assessment

Written documentation of the precautions to be taken, e.g. guidelines and procedures that should be made are considered in Step 4. If the risk is not adequately controlled, then an indication of what needs to be done, e.g. an 'action list', should be documented.

Step 5: Risk assessment review and revision

The final step outlines issues associated with review and this involves checking that each hazard is still adequately controlled. If not, then an indication of the action to be taken must be made.

Key legislation for managing a safe environment is the Health and Safety at Work Act 1974, which specifies the general duties of employers towards employees and others, which includes members of the public and patients in health care, and also the duties of employees to themselves and each other.

However, as argued by Mayatt (2002), the Health and Safety at Work Act 1974 also forms the basis for all other occupational health and safety legislation and these are outlined in Box 4.1.

Box 4.1 Health, safety and environmental legislation relating to the health care sector.

Health and Safety at Work Act (1974)
Management of Health and Safety at Work Regulations (1999)
Control of Substances Hazardous to Health Regulations (COSHH) (2002)
Manual Handling Operations Regulations (1992)
Display Screen Equipment Regulations (1992)
Personal Protective Equipment Regulations (1992)
Ionising Radiation Regulations (1999)
Electricity at Work Regulations (1989)
Noise at Work Regulations (1989)
Genetically Modified Organisms (Contained Use) Regulations (1992) and 1996 Amendment
First Aid at Work Regulations (1981)
Consultation with Employees Regulations (1996)
Safety Representative Regulations (1977)
Reporting of Injuries, Diseases and Dangerous Occurrences Regulations (RIDDOR) (1995)
Working Time Regulations (1998)
Provision and Use of Work Equipment Regulations (1998)
Lifting Operations and Lifting Equipment Regulations (1998)
Workplace (Health, Safety and Welfare) Regulations (1992)
Construction (Design and Management) Regulations (1994)
Construction (Health Safety and Welfare) Regulations (1996)
Control of Asbestos at Work Regulations (1987)
Control of Lead at Work Regulations (1998)
Environmental Protection Act (1990)

Source: Adapted from Mayatt (2002).

Common risks in health care

Individuals employed in health care settings can be exposed to a broad range of risk that may result in harm. Mayatt (2002) identifies commonly encountered risks and these include:

- Manual handling
- Hazardous chemicals and biological agents
- Aggression and violence
- Stress
- Ionising and non-ionising radiation

Patients in health care settings are at risk of:

- Pressure ulcers
- Infection

- Falling
- Malnutrition
- Constipation

Common factors affecting patient safety

Similarly, due to illness or disability, certain groups of patients are unable to protect themselves and are inherently more at risk to injury (Table 4.1).

Minimising the risk of medication error

> The administration of medicines is an important aspect of the professional practice of persons whose names are on the Council's register ... it requires thought and the exercise of professional judgement. (NMC, 2008a)

A prescribed medicine is the most frequent treatment provided for patients in the NHS (DH, 2004). However, medication error has been identified as one of the common threats to patient safety in contemporary health care (Neale et al., 2001), and in a hospital of 400 beds, at least one patient experiences a potentially serious drug error everyday (Taxis and Barber, 2003) and the cost to the NHS is estimated to be £2–400 million per year (DH, 2004); furthermore, 4–10% of prescriptions are illegible or ambiguous (DH, 2000a).

Errors can arise in drug selection, prescribing, dispensing, administration and therapeutic monitoring (Fijin, 2002), and in 2004, the DH set out key steps to minimise the risk

Table 4.1 Factors affecting patient safety.

Age and development	The risk of injury will vary with age and level of development, e.g. the young and the elderly are particularly vulnerable
Sensory perception	Individuals with impaired hearing, sight, touch, smell and touch perception are highly susceptible to injury particularly in a strange environment
Cognitive awareness	Impaired/altered awareness due to confusion, disease, medication, impaired level of consciousness increase the risk of injury
Ability to communicate	A diminished ability to receive and convey information is a risk for injury as the individual is unable to interpret or read information
Mobility and health status	Individuals with poor mobility or impaired coordination are more at risk of injury
Safety awareness	Information is crucial to safety, particularly for an individual in an unfamiliar environment
Emotional state	Stress can alter an individual's ability to concentrate and decrease awareness of environmental hazards

Source: Adapted from Kozier et al. (2000).

of error at all stages of the medication process to build on the government's previous aim of a 40% reduction in serious errors in the use of prescribed drugs (DH, 2001a).

In seeking to minimise the risk of medication error and ensure patients' safety, the following steps should be adhered to (adapted from Hogston and Simpson, 2002).

The right medication

The label of the container should be checked against the prescription chart to ensure it is the correct prescribed medication, and medication should only be dispensed from the original container. Any instructions pertaining to the medication and the expiry date should also be noted. The person dispensing the drug should be familiar with basic information about the drug, its action, any contraindications and side effects.

The right patient

Prior to dispensing the medication, it is important to check that the right patient is receiving it. Checking the patient's identification bracelet and asking them to state their name are two ways of doing this.

The right time

In order to maintain a constant blood plasma level of the drug at an effective range, it is important to give the drug as close to the prescribed time as possible. Similarly, certain drugs need to be given before, with or after a meal in order to maximise the drug's effect; therefore, it is important that this is adhered to and that an explanation is given to the patient in order to ensure compliance with the drug regimen.

The right dose

When drugs are prescribed at different strengths to that required, it is important that the right amount of drug is calculated and this will require a basic knowledge of arithmetic. Similarly a calibrated medicine pot or syringe may be required for liquid medications/ injectable preparations. Where the dose to be given is in doubt or a complicated calculation is required, this should be double checked with another health professional.

The right route

Drugs may be administered in a number of ways including by mouth, rectally, via injection either intramuscularly or intravenously, topically or via inhalation, but not all drugs can be administered by all the possible routes. Indeed some medications can prove fatal if given via the wrong route. Therefore, it is important to check the route of administration prior to administration.

Vincent (2006) suggests that there are practices that help to reduce the risk of medication errors for patients and health care professionals and these include:

- Patient self-administration
- Uninterrupted medicine administration to individual patients
- Standardisation and colour coding of packaging
- Pre-filled syringes and pre-filled individualised tablet containers
- Using barcodes, scanners and Wi-Fi

Minimising the risk of falls

The National Service Framework (NSF) for Older People identifies fall prevention as a priority as stated in key standard six (DH, 2001b). Death, injury, increased dependency and impaired self-care are possible physical consequences of a fall; the psychological effects, e.g. a fear of falling and loss of confidence in being able to move about safely, can also be harmful (National Institute for Health and Clinical Excellence (NICE), 2004). There is an increasing risk of falling with increasing age and falls are the leading cause of death from injury among the over 75-year age group (Scuffham and Chaplin, 2002) with over 14 000 deaths each year as a result of an osteoporotic hip fracture (DH, 2001b). Factors contributing to increased risk of falling, as identified in the literature (Perell et al., 2001), can be divided into two groups: intrinsic, i.e. a particular characteristic of the individual and extrinsic, i.e. an external characteristic (Box 4.2).

Box 4.2 Factors associated with increased risk of falling.

Risk factor

- Internal characteristics
  - Those people aged over 80 years
  - History of previous falls
  - Gender
  - Cognitive impairment
  - Visual impairment
  - Reduced capability to carry out the activities of living
  - Those with arthritis
  - Muscle weakness
  - Those who use assistive devices
  - Gait/balance deficit
  - Depression
  - Those suffering widespread pain
  - Those who consume high levels of alcohol
  - Low body mass index
  - Parkinson's disease
  - Diabetes mellitus
  - Cerebrovascular accident
- External characteristics
  - Drugs
  - Certain groups of prescription drugs have been associated with increased risk of falling, e.g. sedatives, analgesics, laxatives and diuretics, hypnotics, tranquillizers and antidepressants (Effective Healthcare Bulletin, 1996)
  - Environmental hazards
  - Between a third and a half of falls among the elderly occur due to environmental hazards and include
  - Poor lighting, ill-fitting shoes, poorly maintained flooring, e.g. loose carpets/rug (Effective Healthcare Bulletin, 1996)

Source: Adapted from Perell et al. (2001).

The purpose of assessment is to identify those individuals who are at risk of falling with a view to implementing an effective preventative intervention(s) (NICE, 2004). Therefore, an assessment of the risk of falling is an essential part of safe practice and there are many falls assessment tools that have been developed. Cannard (1996) developed the Falls Risk Assessment Scale for the Elderly (FRASE) and this provides an easy and quick tool for assessment (Table 4.2) which can then be used in conjunction with the individual care plan.

Table 4.2 Falls Risk Assessment Scale for the Elderly (FRASE).

Risk factor	Score	Action Total score
Male	1	
Female	2	
Age (years)		3-8 = Low risk
60-70	1	9-12 = Medium risk
71-80	2	13+ = High risk
81+	1	
Gait		
Steady	0	
Hesitant	1	
Poor transfer	3	
Unsteady	3	If score > 1 for mobility/gait, sensor deficit or medication refer to physiotherapy/OT/medical staff as appropriate
Sensory deficit		
Sight	2	
Hearing	1	
Balance	2	
Falls history		
None	0	
At home	2	
In ward	1	
Both	3	
Medication		
Hypnotics	1	
Tranquillisers	1	
Hypotensives	1	
Mobility		
Full	1	
Uses aid	2	
Restricted	3	
Bed bound	1	
Medical history		
Diabetes	1	
Dementia/confusion	1	
Seizures	1	

Source: Reproduced from Cannard (1996), with permission from *Nursing Times*.

A list of practical interventions that may reduce the risk of falls for elderly patients in a health care setting is provided in Box 4.3.

Box 4.3 Practical steps to reduce the risk of falls.

Close supervision of high-risk patients
A means of calling for assistance, e.g. patient call bell
Address the patient's individual elimination needs and ensure that a urinal or commode (if needed) is available at the bedside at night
Adequate lighting
Correct use of mobility aids
Appropriate and well-fitting footwear and clothing
Keep the patient's essential items (drink, spectacles, tissues) within easy reach
Keep the bed height at the lowest level and check the brakes
Use a chair of an appropriate design and height for the patient
Exercise to improve muscle strength and balance
Adequate nutritional intake

Source: Adapted from Anthony (2007).

Minimising the risk of health care-associated infection

In health care, infection presents a hazard and is a risk for both patients and staff. In order to minimise these risks, principles of infection prevention and control must be implemented and adhered to by all concerned. Therefore, in seeking to reduce the risk of health care-associated infection (HCAI), both environmental and clinical factors need to be considered (Figure 4.1).

The hospital environment can become contaminated with microorganisms responsible for HCAI (Barker et al., 2004); therefore, the importance of the environment to the well-being of the patient should not be ignored. Since the launch of the NHS Plan (DH, 2000b) national investment to improve the cleanliness, tidiness and appearance of hospitals has been implemented. Similarly, national cleaning standards for hospitals have also been developed (DH, 2001c).

Environmental cleaning

Any health care environment presents an infection risk to patients and staff such as dust, soil and organic matter which are potentially infectious, quickly accumulate in the environment if it is not properly and regularly cleaned. Cleaning procedures should concentrate on areas with greater environmental risk, such as toilets, patients' beds and lockers and kitchens, and maintaining high standards of environmental cleaning is key in preventing the spread of infection such as *Clostridium difficile* and methicillin-resistant *Staphylococcus aureus* (MRSA) (DH, 2007).

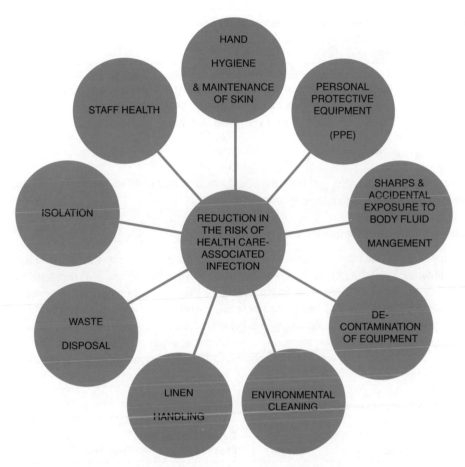

Figure 4.1 Key principles of infection prevention and control to reduce the risk of health care-associated infection.

Cleaning the environment has two purposes (Parker, 1999):

- Improve/restore the appearance, maintain function and prevent deterioration
- Reduce the number of microbes present and remove substances that will support their growth or interfere with subsequent disinfection or sterilisation processes

Cleaning involves the use of detergent and water to remove visible organic material from equipment but also a significant number of the microorganisms that may be present (Wilson, 2006). Chlorine-releasing granules or hypochlorite solutions should be used to remove spills of body fluids as they will destroy the microorganisms present and thus reduce the risk of infection to the person clearing up the spillage (Gould and Brooker, 2008). However, hypochlorite solutions should only be used in well-ventilated areas for clearing large urine spills, as an irritant chlorine vapour may be released (Gould and Brooker, 2008). The use of a disinfectant following cleaning is also recommended where there is a high level of environmental contamination, e.g. during an outbreak of infection (Barker et al., 2004), although care should be taken with the use of chlorine compounds near fabrics or carpet as they will damage these materials (Wilson, 2006). Equipment

Table 4.3 Aims of different levels of decontamination.

Method	Aim
Sterilization	Removes or destroys all microorganisms including spores
Disinfection	Reduces the number of microorganisms to a level at which they are not harmful. Spores are not usually destroyed
Cleaning	Physical removal of contamination and many microorganisms

Source: Adapted from Wilson (2006).

used for cleaning, e.g. mops and buckets, should be decontaminated and stored dry to prevent multiplication of microorganisms.

Decontamination of equipment

Confusion often surrounds the decontamination of equipment used in health care and the decision to clean, disinfect or sterilise depends on the risk of the equipment transmitting infection or acting as a source of infection (Wilson, 2006). Decontamination is a general term meaning the process of removing microbial material and an outline of the aims of the different levels of decontamination is given in Table 4.3. Risk assessment can be used to select the appropriate method of decontamination and Table 4.4 provides an indication of the level of decontamination required depending on the risk of the item used.

Table 4.4 Categories of risk and level of decontamination required.

Category	Indication	Examples	Decontamination process	Methods
High risk	Items that penetrate the skin or mucous membranes, or that enter sterile body areas	Surgical instruments, needles	Sterilization	Autoclave or sterile single-use disposable
Medium risk	Items that have contact with mucous membranes or are contaminated by microbes that are easily transmitted	Endoscopes, bedpans, vaginal speculum	Disinfection or sterilization	Chemically disinfect, pasteurise, autoclave
Low risk	Items used on intact skin	Mattresses, washbowls, floors	Cleaning	Wash with detergent and hot water and dry

Source: Adapted from Wilson (2006).

Table 4.5 Classification of waste.

Hazardous waste	Non-hazardous waste
Infectious waste (sharps, anatomical waste)	Offensive/hygiene waste (incontinence pads and other human hygiene, sanitary waste, nappies)
Cytotoxic and cytostatic medicines	Non-cytotoxic and cytostatic medicines
Health care chemicals and hazardous properties	Domestic waste
Batteries	Packaging waste
X-ray photochemicals	Recyclable materials
Radioactive waste	Food waste

Waste disposal

The recently published Hazardous Waste Regulations (Statutory Instrument, 2005) place a duty on waste producers to segregate hazardous and non-hazardous waste at source and proposes a unified approach to ensure compliance with all regulatory requirements. As health care-generated waste can harbour microorganisms and is therefore potentially harmful to staff, patients, the public and the environment (Wilson, 2006) in order to minimise risk it is important that all waste is properly segregated according to type. There are two types of health care waste (Table 4.5) and a new national colour-coded system is now recommended for the segregation of health care waste into streams that are linked to an appropriate disposal path (Table 4.6).

Table 4.6 The national colour-coding system for the segregation of health care waste (DH, 2006b).

Colour	Description/disposal method
Yellow stream	Infectious waste which requires disposal by incineration
Orange stream	Infectious waste which may be treated to render it safe prior to disposal, or alternatively can be incinerated
Purple stream	Cytotoxic and cytostatic waste which must be incinerated in a permitted or licensed facility
Yellow/black stream	Offensive/hygiene waste which may be land filled in a permitted or licensed site
Black stream	Domestic waste which does not contain infectious materials, sharps or medicinal products and may be land filled in a permitted or licensed site. Recyclable components should be removed through segregation. Clear or opaque receptacles can also be used for domestic waste

Linen handling

Used linen is a potential infection risk especially if it is contaminated with body fluids or has been used in the care of a patient with an infectious disease. Health service used linen must be washed at the highest possible temperature, quickly tumble dried and/or ironed to ensure that microorganisms are destroyed. Guidelines for the management of used or infected linen (NHS Executive, 1995) state that laundries that process hospital linen must comply with DH guidance on disinfection, staff protection and effluent control in order to minimise the risks of personal contamination when handling used linen. Consequently, laundering at a ward level is not advised, as most health care settings are not able to comply with DH guidance because there is no safe means of monitoring control measures.

In minimising risk from used linen, guidelines for the safe handling of linen are summarised in Box 4.4. Similarly, Table 4.7 outlines the national colour coding system for the segregation of used linen into linen skips/containers.

Box 4.4 Guidelines for safe handling of linen.

- Wear a plastic apron for bed making
- When handling contaminated linen, gloves and plastic apron should be worn and hands washed after contact
- Linen which is contaminated with body fluid should be placed firstly, into a dissolvable liner, secured tightly and then placed into an appropriate linen bag
- Linen should be bagged at the bedside
- Use the national colour-coding system
- Securely fasten the linen bag when full

Source: Adapted from Barrie (1994).

Sharps and accidental exposure to body fluid management

A 'sharp' includes needles, scalpels, broken glass or other items that may cause a laceration or puncture and may be contaminated with body fluid. Sharp instruments frequently cause injury to health care workers (Wilson, 2006), and the main hazards of a sharps injury are hepatitis B, hepatitis C and HIV. There were 914 incidents of blood-borne virus exposure in health care workers between 2006 and 2007 and four health care workers

Table 4.7 National colour-coding system for hospital linen (NHS Executive, 1995).

Category	Bag colour	Description
Used	White linen or plastic	Used, soiled and foul linen
Infected	Water-soluble bag, with red outer linen or plastic bag	Linen used by patients who have an infectious disease
Heat labile	Orange stripe	Fabrics that are likely to be damaged by a hot wash

were reported as having acquired hepatitis C infection as a result of their injury (Health Protection Agency, 2008).

Accidental exposure to body fluids can occur by:

- Percutaneous injury, e.g. needlestick injury
- Exposure of broken skin
- Exposure of mucous membranes

The reporting of injuries and dangerous diseases (RIDDOR) imposes a duty of care on the employer to report certain types of incident to the HSE (1995), and this includes sharps injuries and accidental exposure to blood-borne viruses.

However, the risk of a sharps injury can be minimised by adhering to safe practice when using or disposing of sharps and complying with Control of Substances Hazardous to Health Regulations (COSHH) regulations (see Box 4.5) (HSE, 2002).

Box 4.5 Measures to minimise the risk of sharps injury.

- Wear appropriate personal protective equipment (PPE)
- Assemble devices with care
- Do not re-sheath needles unless unavoidable in which case, a commercial re-sheathing device should be used
- Do not carry used sharps by hand or pass to another person
- Do not disassemble sharps prior to disposal – discard as one unit
- Discard used sharps in a sharps box that complies with UN3291 and BS7320 standards
- Take sharps boxes to the point of use to enable immediate disposal
- Ensure sharps boxes are available at all locations where sharps are used
- Sharps boxes should be placed on a level surface or wall mounted below shoulder height
- Close sharps box aperture between use
- Never overfill sharps boxes – adhere to the 'fill to' line
- Lock sharps box when full
- Do not place sharps boxes into clinical waste bags

Below Figure 4.2 are the steps that the nurse should take following accidental exposure to body fluids.

Personal protective equipment

The correct use of personal protective equipment (PPE) is an essential component of safe practice and the minimisation of hazard exposure. Within the context of infection prevention and control, PPE include:

- Disposable gloves
- Disposable aprons

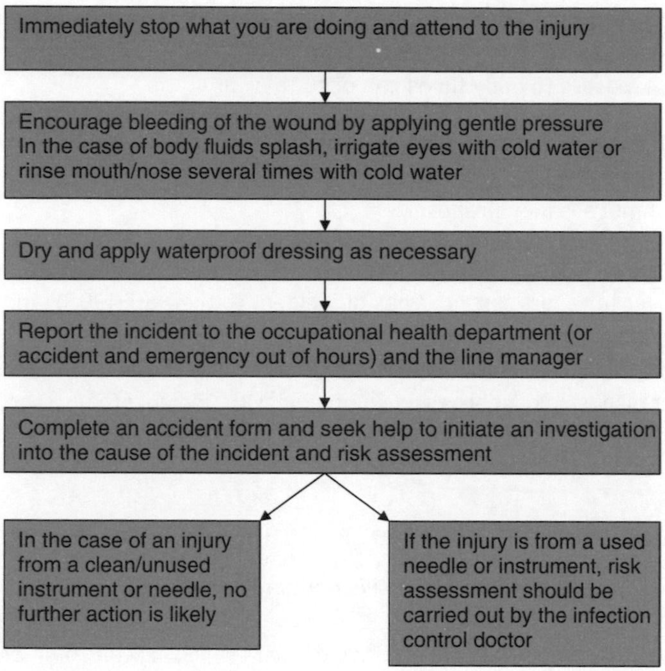

Figure 4.2 Actions to take following accidental exposure to body fluid. (Adapted from RCN, 2004.)

- Eye protection
- Mouth protection
- Food protection
- Fluid-repellent gowns

Staff need to ensure that a risk assessment approach is used to ensure that the correct amount/type of PPE is worn (Figure 4.3), and this should be based on the possible risk of contamination, rather than the infection encountered. Similarly, the principle of standard infection control precautions (Box 4.6) requires that staff take precautions to protect themselves from contact with any potentially infectious substances encountered during

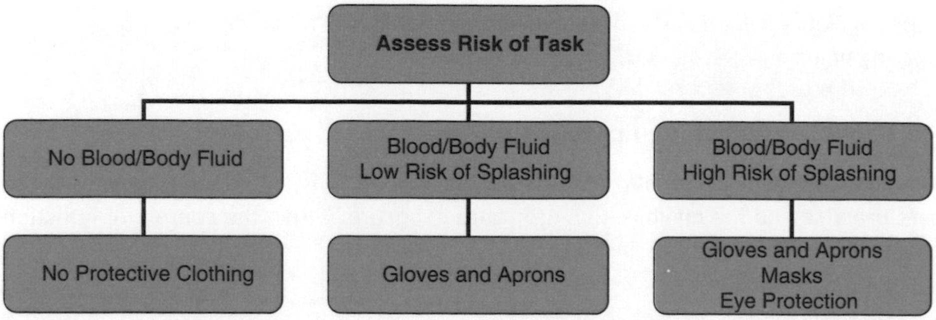

Figure 4.3 Risk assessment tool for the use of personal protective equipment (PPE).

their course of work and there is an onus on employers to ensure that a supply of the types of protective clothing are readily available.

Box 4.6 Standard infection control precautions.

Hand washing
- Before and after contact with patients
- After gloves are removed
- After contact with body fluids

Maintain skin integrity
- Cover cuts with waterproof dressing
- Dry skin properly and use hand cream

Protective clothing
- Use to protect against direct contact with body fluid
- Assess risk of procedure and select appropriate protection

Sharps safety
- Use equipment with safety devices
- Use safe handling and disposal procedures
- Provide hepatitis B vaccination for staff at risk
- Report exposure to blood or body fluid

Safe handling of clinical waste
- Use safe handling and disposal procedure
- Discard excreta directly into drainage system
- Incinerate contaminated disposable material

Decontamination of equipment
- Clean and decontaminate equipment after use
- Disinfect used linen by laundering
- Use protective clothing whilst handling and cleaning

Decontamination of environment
- Keep environment clean and free from dust
- Disinfect spills of body fluid

Source: Adapted from Wilson (2006).

Isolation

The aim of isolation is to minimise the risk of microorganisms from the affected person being transferred to others (known as source isolation formerly barrier nursing) or to prevent the spread of infection to a patient who has reduced resistance to infection (protective isolation formerly known as reverse barrier nursing). Isolation procedures are the outcome of a risk assessment, which includes the source of infection, route of transmission (Box 4.7) and the susceptibility of others (Wilson, 2006); therefore, the principle of isolation is to isolate the microorganism not the patient.

Box 4.7 Routes for possible transmission of microorganisms.

Contact: The most common route of transmission of infection is via direct (skin/body fluid) or indirect (instruments or equipment) contact
Respiratory: The infection is spread via respiratory secretions generated by coughing and sneezing
Airborne: Microorganisms are transferred by droplet nuclei (minute particles) or by dust particles. Air currents will carry these particles and disperse them in the environment
Food or waterborne: Some infections can be transmitted via the ingestion of contaminated food or water resulting in gastrointestinal symptoms
Vector borne: Diseases can be transmitted by vectors such as lice, mosquitoes and ticks

Physical segregation from other patients is particularly recommended where an infection is transmitted by airborne particles or respiratory droplets, or there is likely to be gross contamination of the environment, e.g. if a patient has profuse diarrhoea.

Staff health

Health care workers have always been at risk of both acquiring and transmitting infection (May, 2000). Access to an occupational health service should be available to all staff working in health care, and in order to minimise the risk of occupational exposure, guidelines for safe practice include (May, 2000):

- Covering lesions on hands with waterproof dressings
- Appropriate management of skin conditions, e.g. psoriasis, eczema
- Immunisation, e.g. hepatitis B, rubella
- Pre-employment health screening
- Reporting of accidents and adverse events
- Restriction of non-immune/pregnant staff in certain situations
- Counselling and support

Hand washing

The hands of health care personnel are the most common vehicle by which microorganisms are transmitted between patients and hands are frequently implicated as the route of transmission in outbreaks of infection (Wilson, 2006). Hand hygiene is an easy and proven means of protecting patients from infections. Furthermore, as each health care professional has a duty to promote and safeguard the interest of their patients, identify the risks and take the appropriate action to minimise them (NMC, 2008b), hand hygiene is paramount.

Indications for hand hygiene

Hands should be decontaminated before every direct patient contact and after any contact that has resulted in hands potentially becoming contaminated with blood, body fluids or microorganisms or when gloves have been worn.

The World Health Organization (2006) identifies 'five moments for hand hygiene' and these include:

1. Before patient contact
2. Before aseptic task
3. After body fluid exposure risk (and after glove removal)
4. After patient contact
5. After contact with patient surroundings

The term 'hand hygiene' includes:

- Hand washing with liquid soap and water
- Hand washing with a surgical scrub and water
- Use of an alcohol-based hand rub or gel

The choice of hand-cleansing solution used is dependent on what the episode of care has entailed.

Liquid soap and water will remove transient microorganisms and is sufficient for most care activities (Pratt et al., 2007) and must be used for hands that are visibly soiled or heavily contaminated with organic matter and on removal of gloves.

Alcohol-based hand rub or gel can be used for hand hygiene when the hands are not visibly soiled/contaminated or when hand-washing facilities (a sink, running water) are not readily available. However, alcohol products are ineffective against spores; therefore, if caring for a patient with *C. difficile*, hands should be washed with liquid soap and water.

The use of surgical scrubs should be restricted to situations where the removal of resident microorganisms on the hands is necessary, e.g. in operating theatres and before undertaking invasive procedures (Pratt et al., 2007). Table 4.8 provides a guide as to the indication for use of each of the hand-cleansing solutions.

Hand-washing techniques

Hands should be washed using a technique that ensures that all parts of the hand and wrists are decontaminated.

Alcohol-based hand hygiene products

The same technique used for hand washing should also be used for applying hand hygiene products. Repeated use of some alcohol-based hand hygiene products can lead to a possible build-up of residue on the skin; therefore, some manufacturers recommend that hands should be washed with soap and water after four to five uses of an alcohol-based product (Pratt et al., 2007). Figure 4.4 outlines the correct methods for hand washing using soap and water and a hand rub.

Table 4.8 Indication for use of hand-cleansing solutions.

	Liquid soap	Alcohol-based hand rub or gel	Antiseptic solution/ surgical scrub
Hands are visibly soiled or grossly contaminated	√		
On removal of gloves	√		
Removal of transient microorganisms	√	√	
Visibly clean hands		√	
Hand preparation prior to undertaking an invasive procedure			√
Preoperative hand preparation			√
Removal of resident microorganisms			√

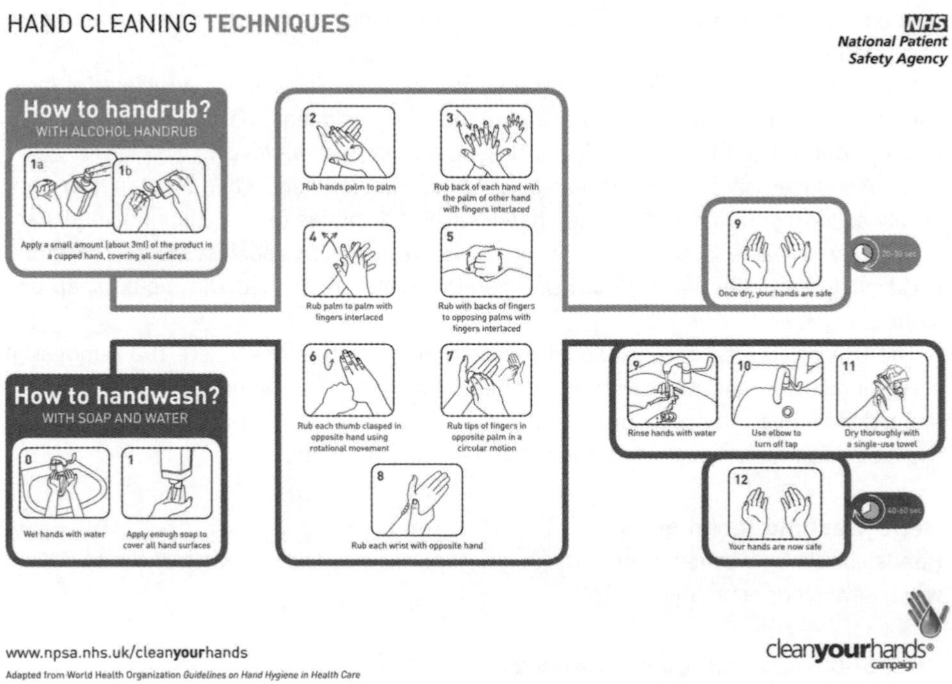

HAND CLEANING TECHNIQUES
NHS
National Patient Safety Agency
How to handrub?
WITH ALCOHOL HANDRUB
1a
1b
Apply a small amount (about 3ml) of the product in a cupped hand, covering all surfaces
How to handwash?
WITH SOAP AND WATER
0
Wet hands with water
1
Apply enough soap to cover all hand surfaces
2
Rub hands palm to palm
3
Rub back of each hand with the palm of other hand with fingers interlaced
4
Rub palm to palm with fingers interlaced
5
Rub with backs of fingers to opposing palms with fingers interlaced
6
Rub each thumb clasped in opposite hand using rotational movement
7
Rub tips of fingers in opposite palm in a circular motion
8
Rub each wrist with opposite hand
9
Once dry, your hands are safe
9
Rinse hands with water
10
Use elbow to turn off tap
11
Dry thoroughly with a single-use towel
12
Your hands are now safe
www.npsa.nhs.uk/cleanyourhands
Adapted from World Health Organization Guidelines on Hand Hygiene in Health Care
cleanyourhands campaign

Figure 4.4 Hand-washing techniques. © National Patient Safety Agency material is reproduced with the permission of the National Patient Safety Agency.

Hand drying

Thorough drying is important to ensure that any remaining moisture is removed and that the skin does not become dry and cracked, which increases the risk of harbouring microorganisms on the hands. Hands should be dried using disposable paper towels and a foot-operated waste bin should be used to dispose of used paper towels as this will reduce the risk of contaminating the hands.

Nail care

Nails should be kept short, free of nail polish and well groomed. Long or artificial nails should not be worn during health care practice as these interfere with glove usage and make adequate hand washing difficult (Jeanes and Green, 2001).

Jewellery

Rings, bracelets and wristwatches worn by health care workers can become grossly contaminated with microorganisms during health care practice and should, ideally, not be worn during working hours. However, flat wedding bands are permissible as long as they can be moved/removed during hand hygiene practice to ensure that all areas of the hands can be thoroughly decontaminated.

Skin care

The skin is the first and primary defence against infection; therefore, it is important healthcare workers take care of their hands as frequent hand washing and use of hand hygiene products can cause skin dryness and irritation. The regular use of a good quality skin moisturiser should be encouraged and any skin problems reported to the occupational health department.

Conclusions

This chapter has explored the importance of risk assessment to the promotion of patient and staff safety and measures to minimise risk relating to three areas of practice have been explored and outlined. Maintaining a safe environment will impinge upon all aspects of patient care.

The nurse must consider both the safety of the patient as well as his/her own safety. Promoting patient safety and minimising risk should be paramount in all care settings - community and institutional.

Risk assessment can help to identify and prevent risk or harm occurring. The nurse owes a duty of care to the patient and that duty of care will encapsulate safe nursing practice. Each registered nurse must remember that he or she is accountable for his or her actions or omissions.

Glossary

Cleaning	A process to remove microorganisms in order to maintain the appearance and function
Decontamination	A term that encompasses cleaning, disinfection and sterilisation
Disinfection	A process that destroys microorganisms but not their spores

Extrinsic	Originating due to causes or factors from outside of a body or organ
Gait	A manner of walking
Intrinsic	Originating due to causes or factors within a body or organ
Ionising radiation	A term used to describe electromagnetic rays (X-rays and gamma rays) or particles (alpha and beta) that occur naturally from the radioactive decay of natural radioactive substances, e.g. radon gas, or those produced artificially, e.g. X-ray set
Isolation	The physical separation of a person with an infectious disease from non-infected people
Non-ionising radiation	A term used to describe the part of the electromagnetic spectrum that includes optical radiation (ultraviolet, visible and infrared) and electromagnetic fields (microwaves, power and radio frequencies)
Microorganism	Any organism too small to be visible to the naked eye. Includes bacteria, viruses, some fungi, mycoplasmas, protozoa and rickettsiae
Protective isolation	The physical separation of an immunocompromised person
Sharps	Any item that is able to cut or puncture the skin or mucous membranes
Sterilisation	A process that destroys all microorganisms including their spores

Post-chapter quiz

1. What is the purpose of a risk assessment?
2. Describe the five steps to safer medicine administration
3. Outline four legislative Acts that govern safety in health care
4. What is RIDDOR?
5. Outline four factors that would increase a patient's risk of falling
6. What is the most frequent treatment given to patients in the NHS?
7. Outline the measures required (standard infection precautions) to minimise infection risks to both patients and staff
8. Define the term 'hand hygiene'
9. What is the body's primary defence against infection?
10. What do 'adverse events' cost the NHS each year?

References

Anthony, L. (2007) Falls prevention and assessment. *British Journal of Healthcare Assistants* 1(1): 10–14.

Barker, J., Vipond, I.B. and Bloomfield, S.F. (2004) Effects of cleaning and disinfection in reducing the spread of Norovirus contamination via environmental surfaces. *Journal of Hospital Infection* 58: 42–49.

Barrie, D. (1994) How hospital linen and laundry services are provided. *Journal of Hospital Infection* 27: 219–235.

Cannard, G. (1996) Falling trend. *Nursing Times* 92(2): 36–37.

Curran, E. (2001) Reducing the risk of healthcare-acquired infection. *Nursing Standard* 16(1): 45–52.

Department of Health (2000a) *An Organisation with a Memory - Report of an Expert Group on Learning from Adverse Events in the NHS*. London: HMSO.
Department of Health (2000b) *The NHS Plan*. London: HMSO.
Department of Health (2001a) *Building a Safer NHS for Patients - Improving Medication Safety*. London: HMSO.
Department of Health (2001b) *National Service Framework for Older People*. London: HMSO.
Department of Health (2001c) *National Cleaning Standards for Hospitals*. London: HMSO.
Department of Health (2004) *Building a Safer NHS for Patients: Improving Medication Safety*. London: The Stationery Office.
Department of Health (2006a) *Safety First: A Report for Patients, Clinicians and Healthcare Managers*. London: The Stationery Office.
Department of Health (2006b) *Health Technical Memorandum 07-01: Safe Management of Health Care Waste*. London: The Stationery Office.
Department of Health (2007) *Clean, Safe Care: Reducing Infections and Saving Lives*. London: The Stationery Office.
Effective Healthcare Bulletin (1996) *Preventing Falls and Subsequent Injury in Older People*. Edinburgh: Churchill Livingstone.
Fijin, R. (2002) Hospital prescribing errors: epidemiological assessment of the predictors. *British Journal of Clinical Pharmacology* 53(3): 326-332.
Gould, D. and Brooker, C. (2008) *Infection Prevention and Control: Applied Microbiology for Healthcare*, 2nd ed. Hampshire: Palgrave Macmillan.
Health and Safety Executive (1995) *A Guide to the Reporting of Injuries, Diseases and Dangerous Occurrences Regulations*. London: Health and Safety Executive.
Health and Safety Executive (1997) *Successful Health and Safety Management*. London: Health and Safety Executive.
Health and Safety Executive (1998) *Five Steps to Risk Assessment*. London: Health and Safety Executive.
Health and Safety Executive (2002) *Control of Substances Hazardous to Health Regulations*. Approved Code of Practice and Guidance, 4th ed. London: HSE Books.
Health Protection Agency (2008) *Eye of the Needle: United Kingdom Surveillance of Significant Occupational Exposures to Bloodborne Viruses in Healthcare Workers*. UK: Health Protection Agency.
Hogston, R. and Simpson, P.M. (2002) *Foundations of Nursing Practice*, 2nd ed. Hampshire: Palgrave Macmillan.
Jeanes, A. and Green, J. (2001) Nail art: a review of current infection control issues. *Journal of Hospital Infection* 49: 139-142.
Kozier, B., Erb, G., Berman, A.J. and Burke, K. (2000) *Fundamentals of Nursing: Concepts, Process, and Practice*. New Jersey: Prentice Hall Health.
May, D. (2000) Infection control. *Nursing Standard* 14(28): 51-57.
Mayatt, V.L. (2002) *Managing Risk in Healthcare - Law and Practice*. United Kingdom: Butterworths Tolley.
McCulloch, J. (1999) Risk management in infection control. *Nursing Standard* 13(34): 44-46.
National Institute for Clinical Excellence (2004) *Clinical Practice Guideline for the Assessment and Prevention of Falls in Older People*. London: RCN.
Neale, G., Woloshynowych, M. and Vincent, C. (2001) Exploring the cause of adverse events in NHS hospital practice. *Journal of the Royal Society of Medicine* 94: 322-330.
NHS Executive (1995) *Hospital Laundry Arrangements for Used and Infected Linen*. HSG(95)18. London: HMSO.
Nightingale, F. (1859) *Notes on Nursing*. Revised, with additions. London: Balliere Tindall.
NMC (2008a) *Standards for Medicines Management*. London: NMC.

NMC (2008b) *The Code - Standards of Conduct, Performance and Ethics for Nurses and Midwives*. London: NMC.

Parish, C. (2003) Make no mistake. *Nursing Standard* 17(29): 12–13.

Parker, L.J. (1999) Current recommendations for isolation practices in nursing. *British Journal of Nursing* 8(13): 881–887.

Perell, K.L., Nelson, A., Goldman, R.L., Luther, S.K., Prieto-Lewis, N. and Rubenstein, L.Z. (2001) Fall risk assessment measure in analytic review. *Journals of Gerontology Series A, Biological Sciences and Medical Sciences* 56(12): M761–M766.

Pratt, R.J., Pellowe, C.M., Wilson, J.A., Loveday, H.P., Harper, P.J., Jones, S.R.L.J., McDougall, C. and Wilcox, M.H. (2007) Epic2: national evidence-based guidelines for preventing healthcare-associated infections in NHS Hospitals in England. *Journal of Hospital Infection* 65S: S1–S64.

RCN (Royal College of Nursing) (2004) *Working Well Initiative - Good Practice in Infection Control*. London: Royal College of Nursing.

Scuffham, P. and Chaplin, S. (2002) *The Incidence and Costs of Accidental Falls in the United Kingdom*. Final Report. York: York Health Economic Form Consortium. The University of York.

Statutory Instrument (2005) *The Hazardous Waste (England and Wales) Regulations*. London: The Stationery Office.

Taxis, K. and Barber, N. (2003) Ethnographic study of incidence and severity of intravenous drug errors. *British Medical Journal* 326: 684–686.

Vincent, C. (2006) *Patient Safety*. Edinburgh: Elsevier Churchill Livingstone.

Wilson, J. (2006) *Infection Control in Clinical Practice*, 3rd ed. London: Balliere-Tindall.

World Health Organization (2006) *Hand Hygiene - When and How*. Geneva: WHO.

Chapter 5
Communicating Effectively

David Briggs

Learning opportunities

This chapter will help you to:

1. Understand some of the important factors when talking to patients, carers and colleagues effectively as well as identifying some of the factors that enable patients and their carers to communicate effectively
2. Realise the importance of listening effectively especially when time is pressured
3. Be able to identify some situations where communication difficulties exist and possible methods of helping to alleviate the problems
4. Consider the importance of receiving messages by body language and to understand about different methods of communication such as the electronic dissemination of information
5. Think about some situations when it is important to know how to pass on information and who to pass that information on to and to be informed about some of the key concepts related to communication and record keeping
6. Consider how reflection can be used as a process to develop skills when communicating with others

Pre-chapter quiz

1. What aspects of verbal communication affect how the message you send is received by the other person?
2. How do you encourage someone to talk to you?
3. Why do you think listening is such an important part of communication?
4. Think of a situation where you have found it difficult to communicate with someone. What were the possible reasons?
5. Think about a friend of yours. Consider the last time you spoke to your friend on the telephone. Also visualise the last time you saw them and discussed an issue. Assuming that the general purpose of both was to 'keep in touch'; which did you find the better encounter?
6. Why is it important in the health care environment to be able to communicate with people from other cultures?

7. How did you react the last time that someone said something to you which you found 'not very nice'?
8. How would you define non-verbal communication?
9. If you use a form of electronic communication via the internet, why do you do so?
10. How do you decide if someone needs to know a fact?

Introduction

Communication is fundamental to every interaction between a health professional and a nurse. Without the ability to communicate, the consultation would probably never occur in the first place and the process would never reach an effective conclusion. Communication has many attributes at its core, for example imparting information (Pennell and Bryon, 2008). The communication needs to be effective and Hobson (2008) argues it must be 'person-centred'. In order to examine the subject effectively, the person or student must be aware that the concept is far from a simple one and therefore any definition must include factors such as these.

In this chapter, attempts are made to build on some fundamental concepts associated with communication, an example is listening which is of course important to all situations where verbal communication takes place. However the process by which it is adapted by the user within the interpersonal interaction is a much more complex arrangement. Important issues associated with the subject of communication are revisited and a story in relation to how the reader may improve their communication skills is developed.

It is appropriate to use the Department of Health's (DH's) framework on communication and its inclusion in pre-registration health and social care courses as a structure for producing this chapter (DH, 2003). Within that document, the DH cites aspects of good communication skills and it is these that would guide any attempt to define the term 'communication' (these aspects are referred to as categories). The relevant categories are included in Box 5.1. It is these that guide the development of the chapter, in so doing the reader is asked to acknowledge that in each category, examples have been used to add a direction to the general discussion (an example used is jargon and how this relates to a person's understanding of the subject matter during a process of verbal communication). The intention is to encourage discussion; each part of the work will raise other issues within the reader's mind around the particular concept.

Box 5.1 The Department of Health's (2003) statement of guiding principles for including communication within a pre-registration curriculum: examples of good communication skills.

Talk to patients, carers and colleagues effectively and clearly conveying and receiving the intended message

Enable patients and their carers to communicate effectively

Listen effectively especially when time is pressurised, i.e. skills in engaging and disengaging
Identify potential communication difficulties and work through situations
Understanding the differing methods of communication used by individuals
Understand that there are differences in communication signals between cultures.
Cope within specific situations
Understand how to use and receive non-verbal messages given by body language
Utilise spoken, written and electronic methods of communication
Know when the information received needs to be passed on to another person/professional for action
Know and interpret the information needed to be recorded in patient's records, writing discharge letters, copying letters to patients and gaining informed consent
Recognise the need for further development to acquire specialist skills

Talking to patients, carers and colleagues effectively and clearly conveying and receiving the intended message

This section of the chapter examines talking to patients, carers and colleagues effectively and clearly conveying and receiving the intended message. The ability of the student nurse to learn how to talk to all participants in a nursing environment is a fundamental prerequisite to being able to undertake their role effectively.

Talking involves using words, and Jepson (2008) suggests that health care workers have 'a language of care'. He considers three aspects of language that are particularly important in communicating with others in the caring environment. The need to avoid jargon is advisable (patients generally do not know what an MSU is when the nurse uses the term to signify a midstream specimen of urine). The use of active verbs in the conversation is advisable (e.g. using the term 'thriving' rather than the patient is just 'doing well' has more of a vibrant ring to it). Finally, the importance of stating clearly what you mean about aspects of care is helpful (the patient is not in pain rather than the patient is just comfortable is an example of this phenomenon). The words you use and the way they are used in conveying a message are essential.

Talking has several purposes (e.g. asking a patient to carry out an action in the pursuit of nursing care), but Egan (2006) highlights the important one of solving problems. Through speaking we can exert influence over people. Whilst we are conversing we may begin to form a strategy in our mind and therefore the basis of an action plan. We may also form an awareness of what others are trying to say to us and becoming self-aware is an important part of the problem-solving process. Finally we may agree to a solution with the carer or colleague to sort out their concerns. Other skills, therefore, come into play such as negotiating or empowering people, but these skills are fundamentally borne out of being able to verbally communicate with others.

In his article, Communication - getting it right, Bamforth (2007) gives us a warning. We usually communicate messages verbally to patients and carers with the aim of giving that person choices about how they may reconcile issues with their or their clients' or relative's health. For example, in talking to a chronically ill patient and the family about maintaining the patient's independence, there may be several ways of tackling the same problem. For example, when the patient is being cared for at home, the patient may see the bed being bought downstairs as a way forward to be with the family or may want their room upstairs rearranged so that the family has a place to sit and talk with them. Either way they may want their carer's view. By talking about the alternatives in care, the patient is encouraged to take ownership of any decision and is therefore more likely to act upon it.

Facilitating patients and their carers to communicate effectively

The ability to talk to patients is therefore an important nursing attribute, but the ability to create an environment in which conversation can take place is equally as important.

Bamforth (2007) relates to this concept when he suggests that the importance of communication in district nursing is very often the fact that it takes place in the patient's own home. Here, it is almost impossible to talk to the patient without the carer's either knowing or being involved, this has the potential to facilitate cooperation between patient and carer in planning the patient's care on a day-to-day basis; however, there are often issues that the patient may want to discuss with the nurse alone (e.g. they may be worried about how their carer is coping). The skill is often demonstrating to the patient or carer that only with both their input can good quality care be achieved (by giving them examples). Equally, the nurse may need to show the carer that giving the patient time alone with the professional assists both the carer as well as the patient. Putting in place procedures that allow for both these processes to happen at the patient's place of residence requires tact, empathy, understanding and assertiveness on the part of the health professional.

In order to encourage such an environment, it is clear that the nurse needs to be aware of the pitfalls. Moss (2008) reminds the nurse that he or she is not a friend (a friend has a much deeper, more personal relationship with the patient and carer) and it may be unwise for the professional to become personally involved for fear of having their decision-making compromised. The nurse cannot offer what Moss (2008) describes as general 'chat' sessions; there should always be a reason for the communication. The nurse must discuss the boundaries around the care that he or she can offer early on in the relationship as a health professional has other patients to care for and ill-defined boundaries can lead to allegations of a poor standard of care later on in the relationship. The quality of the environment in which talking to carers and patients takes place depends largely on the perceptions of the patient, carer and nurse. This means there must be agreement between them as to what those perceptions are.

In order to arrive at this agreement, the nurse needs to be careful that he or she is consistent in his or her verbal approach to the patient. A difficulty that many nurses have is that they may be asked to give health promotion advice on a behaviour detrimental to health that they themselves actually practise. Percival (2001) asks how some nurses may reconcile health education on smoking with their own smoking status within a health-promoting environment. Her advice suggests that the professional must be non-judgemental, giving clear concise information. The skill is (through verbal communication) to encourage the patient to value you as a professional and to value what you stand for as a nurse.

The importance of listening effectively

One of the important attributes that a nurse uses to assist in getting the patient to value them is to demonstrate that they are listening. This in turn shows that they are interested in what the patient or the carer has to say.

Listening is a skill in itself. Stickley and Freshwater (2006) state that 'good listening may be associated with humility rather than talkativeness'; indeed, they suggest that the best nurse listener is the one with the less ego needs. Moss (2008) cites Trevithick (2005), who details some basic attributes of a good listener. The person will maintain good eye contact. He or she will pay attention to the non-verbal cues given out by the patient (e.g. a tear in the eye suggesting that the issue is emotionally painful even though they may state they are coping with it). The good listener will have an open and attentive form of posture. These are just a few of the qualities listed, but some people may realise that some of these attributes may take years to develop (such as the ability to pick up various non-verbal cues in line with the person's speech) and so listening skills may not be developed quickly.

It is all too easy to treat listening as simplistic, especially when many nurses may see it as a 'basic nursing skill' (Gadsby, 2007). Listening can be empathic and therefore therapeutic. Newson (2006) reminds us that a common problem in elderly people is loneliness. This may have been exacerbated by bereavement; whatever the reasons, loneliness can lead to deteriorating health and the ability of the nurse to communicate with the elderly patient can help stem the problem. In a primary health care setting, a visit by a district nurse is something that the patient values and may look forward to, as he or she may be the only person the patient sees that day. Empathic listening can assist in making the most of the visit by both the participants involved.

Stott (2007) reminds the reader that whilst listening is a valuable skill, it is something that is not always done well. Whilst the nurse is listening, he or she may well be trying to place what is being said in the context of his or her own values. In order to ensure that the understanding of what is being said is complete, Stott (2007) recommends that the reader repeats what the person has said in order to attempt that clear understanding between the parties has in fact occurred.

Potential communication difficulties

The art of listening is therefore important in conversing with another individual. Unfortunately for some people, deafness makes the process of conversation a difficult task to engage in. Murphy et al. (2005) remind us that communication difficulties such as deafness amongst residents in a residential home mean that these individuals may find it difficult to form relationships with other residents. It is important that we consider some issues around communication difficulties and some ideas that may assist the participant with the difficulty to engage and participate in the discussion.

Miller (2008) considered the difficulties that some patients with dementia face in conversing with others. These include the ability to understand what other people are saying. Patients may also have difficulty in their perception of the meaning attached to the ideas expressed. Any change in the person's routine may also affect their ability to communicate. Other factors include having a vision or hearing impairment and excessive noise in the room whilst the person is trying to speak to the patient. The patient may find it difficult to talk to people who are unfamiliar with him or her and other factors such as the side effects of medication may also impair his or her ability to talk.

Allan (2006) takes the issue of dementia patients and deafness a step further. In her study involving dementia patients, their relatives and carers, the participants raised some important issues which they believed would help the situation. The value of hearing aids was raised in countering some aspects of social isolation. The concept of clear explanation by the person talking to the patient (rather than loud explanation) was thought to be important. Mealtimes around a communal table are generally to be encouraged in most environments as a way of facilitating patients to interact. In the case of patients with dementia, the study suggests these sort of activities need to be handled carefully as they may not suit every person with dementia, due to the patients becoming frustrated because of their inability to communicate with others. The lesson from studies like these may be that for patients who have specific illnesses and disabilities, there may be some very individual problems of communication, which require very specific solutions in order to solve the difficulties.

The differing methods of communication used by individuals

Examination of the issue of communication and the difficulties attached to the process has meant that people have developed their abilities to communicate by using many different methods. The use of verbal means of communication (as discussed earlier), applying non-verbal actions and undertaking written methods of sending messages are three such methods.

Oxtoby (2005) suggests that people can use several different aspects of communication at once when they interact with each other. She suggests that in terms of non-verbal communication people build rapport, show compassion, use body language to help demonstrate their concerns and also observe other people so that they can react appropriately all at the same time (see Figure 5.1). Importantly, these non-verbal aspects are vital if we are to relate to the patient as an individual. Duffy (2006) demonstrates how important it is that the health care team are aware of their body language when breaking bad news to terminally ill patients.

A further method of communication is through the written form. Just as people make judgements about us through our non-verbal gestures, so they do so through the way we relate to concepts in our writing. Evans (2002) offers us some good advice. Firstly, we need to decide on our key message and audience, and then we need to use words that are more easily understood in the text. The layout and design of what we have written on the paper is important (i.e. the structure of any communication in terms of the paragraphs must be clear and the ideas follow logically from one to another). Finally, the addition of drawings or diagrams can help increase the understanding in the reader's

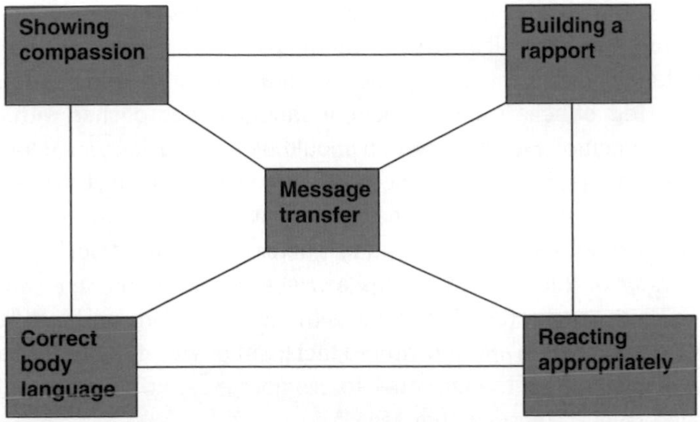

Figure 5.1 Good attributes which assist the transfer of a message.

mind and also the accuracy of any nursing notes, that accuracy being congruent with the guidance offered by the Nursing and Midwifery Council (NMC) (2007).

The use of these different methods allows various attributes of each method to be put to the best use when the sender is sending the message. To take an example, a telephone call (the use of speech and language) can be used to set up a meeting between the various participants. When people get around the table, they may watch how people react to various suggestions and get a feel of their acceptance to proposals. After the meeting, written minutes will be sent to reinforce any agreements and detailed actions to be taken (and by whom). In this scenario, each method of communication has specific purposes but taken together all methods play a part in securing an end result to the meeting.

Communicating with people from different cultures

It has been demonstrated that the methods by which people can communicate may present specific challenges. It is also the case that as Britain grows more ethnically diverse, nurses are presented with new challenges over how to communicate effectively with patients from different cultures.

Meddlings and Haith-Cooper (2008) report in their research that due to language and cultural barriers, midwives in Bradford have had difficulty in providing ethnically appropriate care to Pakistani women who may have a different ethnic and cultural background to themselves. Phillips (2003) reports that people from different cultures may have different religious and political beliefs to that of the nurse. As an example it is common for certain cultures to be stereotyped in relation to aspects of communication. People from some specific cultures in Europe are often thought to get excited very easily, while individuals from other countries may give the impression through their language of being abrupt to the native Britain. Ultimately an awareness of issues related to ethnicity and the patient's cultural needs can help the nurse in achieving a good outcome from a conversation with a patient from a different culture (Houghton, 2008).

Pullen (2007) offers advice on how to enhance strategies for this conversation. The nurse should work towards gaining trust from the patient. This can be done by minimising misunderstandings as much as possible. Communication strategies should consider the patient's system of beliefs and the patient should be approached with caution and compassion. The point of the conversation should be made quickly in as professional a way as possible. Importantly, the nurse needs to demonstrate respect to the patient from another culture and in order to do that he or she may need to involve an interpreter.

Fontes (2008) cautions us that interpreting is actually quite hard work. The interpreter is a skilled person who listens, translates and speaks all at the same time. Equally, Meddlings and Haith-Cooper (2008) remind us that untrained interpreters have omitted added, condensed, simplified and substituted facts. Either way if the nurse cannot speak the language of the patient, then in order to promote a caring environment, he or she must find an interpreter to bridge that gap.

Coping in a very specific and difficult situation

The ability to communicate with patients from different cultures can therefore present the nurse with many challenges, but there are situations involving interpersonal relationships which can be guaranteed to be difficult for the health professional involved. One such situation involves verbal abuse.

Hoban (2004) describes a typical case in which a patient in accident and emergency department shouts at a nurse 'You don't care about my foot'. Oxtoby (2004) reported on a survey in which nine out of ten nurses had suffered some form of verbal abuse during their career. Importantly, verbal abuse can take many forms including name calling, unnecessary shouting, swearing or hurtful accusations.

Rowe and Sherlock (2005) report quite worryingly that the most frequent source of verbal abuse to health professionals come from other health workers. She suggests that an underlying reason is the fact that stress occurs in the workplace. Johnson et al. (2007) gives the individual nurse some advice on how to tackle an instance of verbal abuse. These include making an appropriate response (this may be the delaying of giving an answer), following up on the abuse (this includes documenting the event and reporting it to a supervisor) and the final step is insisting on a response (even if this means taking the matter through the grievance procedure of the employer).

Crouch (2004) equally reminds us that the employer can also be proactive in taking measures to reduce the problem. The manager must be proactive in speaking to patients where staff have complained of its occurrence. Conflict resolution training can also be provided, assertiveness training offered and reporting procedures tightened up. The prevention of verbal abuse requires a 'zero-tolerance' response which is seen to be effective.

Using body language effectively

Body language can be used to emphasise or to lessen the effects of important messages. The use of effective body language is a skill which needs to be developed by the practitioner.

Hovell (2008) reminds us that body language is often seen in the context of the part of the body that is being used to aid the communication. This is important as, when communicating, the practitioner will often emphasise the use of the particular organ being employed. An example is the nurse who turns his or her ear towards the patient when listening. Such actions ultimately reinforce the view to the other conversant that the nurse is a full participant within the conversation.

McLean (2008) reminds us that these sorts of actions can 'speak louder than words'. A patient may only volunteer oral information when they are comfortable with the health professional and can view him or her with a sense of integrity and trust. What may appear on the surface to be superficial actions by the nurse can be very important to the patient. Waiting to be invited into a patient's house may seem on the surface very straightforward, but unless this occurs the patient may feel that the professional is lacking in respect for their private space and their privacy. First impressions are vitally important in making or breaking a relationship and unless the health professional is careful about that initial consultation, an effective professional-patient relationship or rapport may never develop.

Difficulties in forming a nurse-patient relationship can develop through the inability to use non-verbal communication or where non-verbal issues adversely affect its development. Richards (2007) reminds us of the importance of using non-verbal communication in addressing sensitive issues for the patients. The recall of a specific event to one person can be very amusing but to another human being who has been personally and badly affected by it, the event can be far from funny. Non-verbal cues can usually lead the communicator to deduce which one is the case. Equally, Piper (2008) relates to the issue of body image and its non-verbal effects in interactions. Most nurses would relate to some horrific scars they have seen on the faces of various patients. The patient may be very conscious of this and on the other hand the nurse is left with a decision as to whether to be open about it or to ignore its existence. It is with experience and a knowledge about the implications for non-verbal gestures that leads the nurse to decide the best way forward.

Using the electronic means of distributing information

At various times in this chapter, a number of issues concerned with speaking (e.g. listening to people) and also written communication (e.g. communication via pen and paper) have been considered. The important issue of using the electronic means as a channel of distributing messages will now be examined.

The use of the term 'information technology' which involves the use of computers may suggest to the reader a number of concepts including electronic mail, the use of the internet, various intranet systems and telemedicine (to list but a few).

The computer has become part of the caring environment seemingly on the premise that large amounts of information can not only be stored in a small place, but also be sent around the nursing and caring fraternity quickly. Some health professionals may argue that there has been no choice but to embrace their use, as patients themselves may well access them (indeed patients are now booking online appointments at a number of local general practitioners surgeries). Others will argue that the computer in many cases has replaced the very valuable and necessary 'personal touch' that nursing needs to deliver its objectives. West (2003) suggests that data can be obtained more easily whilst some tasks seem to take much longer as a result of computer use. Technology is here to stay and the way we communicate with some patients and health professionals has now changed.

Indeed Clark (2007) discusses how information technology has the potential to radically transform care. Examples are texting patients to remind them about appointments or taking medications. The situation has moved on so fast that medical consultants are now asking is the face-to-face consultation necessary (Sullivan and Wyatt, 2005). Many patients are proficient in using the internet and can ascertain the information they require. If this latter view is simplistic, then many health professionals would argue that it might also be dangerous. The value of speaking to a nurse or doctor is that the patient can ask them questions, that the information can be related to the individual's circumstances and that the health professional can try and reduce the patient's anxiety as much as possible. The computer can process large amounts of information in a systemic and logical fashion, but it cannot see those non-verbal cues in the patient that so often lead to advice that enhances the effects of treatment.

The dangers of communicating via computers are not only inherent for patients but a range of new occupational diseases are now emerging for nurses and doctors. If computers have reduced stress in one respect through the health professional obtaining sufficient and ready information, they may have increased stress through another in terms of information overload. Patten (2003) discusses the Health and Safety Executive's guidance on the issues that affect the use of computers (an example being guidance on using visual display equipment HSE, 2006). The dangers are clear but so is the principle. Any form of communication has inherent difficulties and dangers and the health practitioner ignores them at his or her peril.

The use of telemedicine can also present the user with this sort of dilemma. Kohler (2008) suggests that telemedicine can reflect the use of domestic equipment which people may use in their own homes. This item is connected to a monitoring centre which tracks the pattern of incoming information. Patients can be empowered to manage and play more of a role in their own care. The person who is suffering from a sleep disorder can be videoed at night and make health choices with the health care professional as a result of seeing the video. Dimond (2003) states that the patient must be warned of the risks of using telemedicine. The use of videoing a patient's behaviour may provoke anxiety in that person. Telemedicine can bring benefits to the patient but as in all forms of communication, the technique has to be examined for any potential pitfalls and risks for the individual person involved.

The ability to know when someone needs to know a piece of information

Whether using verbal or electronic communication, the sender needs to know when a person or institution should be given a piece of information. Voulsden (2000) highlights this when he states 'no man is a rock'. We need to share information in order to pass on ideas, disseminate good practice, give someone the basis on which to act and to ensure that the team is cohesive in its approach to patient care.

The nursing handover is often seen as the highlight of sharing patient information on a day-to-day basis in the nursing context. This allows a report to be made on the patient's condition and care and to discuss what needs to be done for the patient in future. Without such a procedure, the consistency of care could not be facilitated, but many nurses would relate to the possibility of interruptions, the tendency for nurses to forget such large amounts of received information and the large amount of time that such handovers take. The nursing handover has been subjected to a study by Pothier et al. (2005). While they state the procedure played a crucial role in providing good-quality health care in a modern health care environment, they also suggest improvement was possible. They suggest a formal handover sheet should be designed so that the sender is directed to send the pertinent information and the receiver is given the information which he or she requires to act in the best interests of the patient.

A further context in which it is necessary to provide the correct information is in giving the patient discharge advice. This requires that the nurse has significant knowledge in the particular field of care for which the advice is being given. The knowledge can then be targeted towards the patient's needs. The patient can also clarify the issues. Authors such as Smith and Liles (2007) have demonstrated in their studies how important the issue of giving information prior to hospital discharge is for the patient.

Such information needs to be kept confidential and passed only to the person that needs to have access to it. Hendrick (2000) reminds the reader of the importance of confidentiality and the fact that certain issues need to be considered when the police ask the health professional for information. The NMC in the code of conduct (NMC, 2008) makes requirements for the nurse to act appropriately in ensuring a level of trust between the patient and the nurse. This trust can only occur if the issue of confidentiality is managed appropriately.

Another area of information giving that has come under scrutiny is the issue of referrals to community nurses when a patient leaves hospital. Fellows et al. (2003) cite many studies which deal with this issue and some hospital nurses are often uncertain when they should refer people to the district nursing service. Primary care systems allow a patient to be referred to the district nurses through a number of ways (e.g. other nurses, general practitioners, social workers and by patients' self-referring). This means that a district nurse will often hear of a patient's discharge prior to receiving the hospital referral. Equally, a patient who is discharged at 1600 hours on a Friday evening with the expectation that the district nurse will visit the next day means that the referral procedures have to be carefully structured to allow for this to happen. The health professional needs to know not only what information is to be given to a colleague, but also about the processes which allow for that information to be received by them.

Information and record keeping

Part of the process that allows the correct information to be given and received is that of record keeping. Watson (2003) argues that poor record keeping may indicate a lack of care given, records allow for nurses to continue the same care given by another nurse. Omissions in the data may mean that an important aspect of care is overlooked.

The importance of record keeping has been acknowledged by the NMC (2007) and guidance has been provided in that document on how the nursing and midwifery professional should proceed. Hutchinson and Sharples (2006) summarise the recommendations. These are far-reaching and include aspects such as keeping records of events related to patient care, research-based records, maintaining confidentiality and auditing any records. Importantly, some might argue that there is an element of necessary vagueness in them such as using professional judgement as to what is included in the records (this might vary to some degree from practitioner to practitioner). Either way, the NMC reminds the practitioner that records should be written with a view to realising that they will be scrutinised sometime in the future (NMC, 2007).

McGeehan (2007) discusses best practice in record keeping. This author also appears to acknowledge that poor record keeping does exist. Good records kept by a practitioner can help in the investigation of complaints and instances where legal issues are involved. The records should be factual, consistent and accurate (NMC, 2007). Equally, where new processes of record keeping are introduced in a health care environment, it is important that health care professionals are educated in their use. Good record keeping involves a collaborative effort between the organisation and the individual nurse.

Abraham (2003) also relates to the problem of how inaccurate notes can hinder the process of investigating complaints. She reminds us that communication with patients is itself a nursing intervention and therefore this requires recording as any other nursing action. The old cliché is often an appropriate one: if you haven't written it down, you have not done it and if it has not been described, it has not been seen.

An icon which represents the question of consent and record keeping is the consent form. This document exists as a record to ensure that patients have been fully informed of what is about to occur and also have been informed of the risks associated with a procedure. On the one hand, it must be assumed that the person has the mental capacity to make those decisions, on the other, protection must be open to those who lack the capacity (given by the Mental Capacity Act, 2005) (Nazarko, 2007). Without proper advice, a patient cannot be expected to make an informed decision and the records need to show that advice has been given.

Communication and reflective practice

The ability to assist the patient to make an informed decision through having sufficient information demonstrates the importance of ethical theory to the whole subject of communication. Competent practice demands that the nurse consider the implications of good and bad communication, of becoming an autonomous practitioner (which necessitates the ability to communicate effectively) and to be able to communicate not only with many different patients but also within groups of particular patients (e.g. self-care groups or support groups). Jasper (2003) suggests that one of the best methods of considering ethical theory in relation to communication issues is through the use of reflecting with other people.

The ability to learn about communication from reflection can be extremely effective for it is possible to look at communication quite explicitly through a reflective framework. It is also safe to assume that when reflecting with others, communication must be implicit within the process to enable reflection to work. Therefore the practitioner can learn not only from the conclusions of what has been discovered about the specific issue used in the reflection but also from what has happened in the reflection itself. In terms of a practitioner's learning, this then becomes a very synergistic but also a very powerful event.

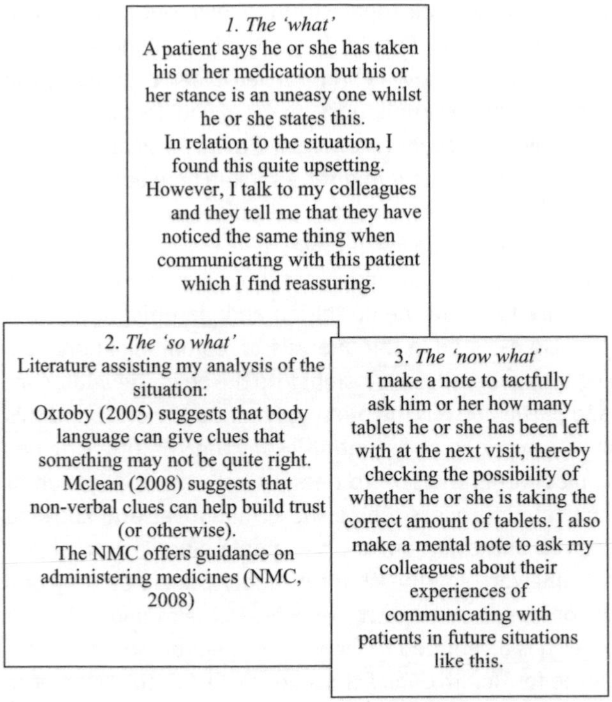

1. The 'what'
A patient says he or she has taken his or her medication but his or her stance is an uneasy one whilst he or she states this.
In relation to the situation, I found this quite upsetting.
However, I talk to my colleagues and they tell me that they have noticed the same thing when communicating with this patient which I find reassuring.
2. The 'so what'
Literature assisting my analysis of the situation:
Oxtoby (2005) suggests that body language can give clues that something may not be quite right.
Mclean (2008) suggests that non-verbal clues can help build trust (or otherwise).
The NMC offers guidance on administering medicines (NMC, 2008)
3. The 'now what'
I make a note to tactfully ask him or her how many tablets he or she has been left with at the next visit, thereby checking the possibility of whether he or she is taking the correct amount of tablets. I also make a mental note to ask my colleagues about their experiences of communicating with patients in future situations like this.

Figure 5.2 The Rolfe's reflective framework, applied through a critical incident involving communication. (Adapted from Jasper, 2003, p. 101.)

The use of a reflective framework adds both structure and depth to the process. Seed (2006) reminds us that any reflection must consider the positive and the negative aspects of any critical incident. Jasper (2003) uses Rolfe's model to demonstrate how this occurs through the application of a model. A dimension of communication to each section of the framework to demonstrate the effectiveness of the process has been added (see Figure 5.2).

This example (Figure 5.2) has been simplified to illustrate the processes of reflection involved. It has been designed to encourage the practitioner to engage in the process and to demonstrate that important conclusions can result from that engagement. McLean's (2008) phrase 'actions can speak louder than words' can be cited here.

Conclusions

This chapter has used as its basis four important themes:

1. Communication is an important topic in its own right
2. The DH's criteria for the teaching of communication in pre-registration nursing courses (2003) offers the reader a good structure for examining the topic
3. The theory underpinning communication strategies should be considered in a 'micro' and 'macro' context
4. Incorporating communication theory into a reflective process can enhance the participants' ability to communicate effectively

The first is that communication is an important topic within its own right as it transgresses all aspects of nursing care. Whether we consider the patient receiving a general anaesthetic in a theatre environment or the lady having her leg ulcer dressed in the primary health care setting; without communication, nursing care would simply not be effective, and the communication may be verbal or non-verbal as discussed earlier. It may be written, for example, in nursing records or it might be spoken between people of different cultures. Unless all these aspects of the communication are addressed in the delivery of care, the communication itself may be ineffective.

Secondly, in recognising that communication is an important topic in nursing, it seemed pertinent to use the DH's (2003) work to aid in the definition and identification of the particular component topics. This also assisted in the analysis of 'communication' as a concept in its own right. In so doing the reader is given insight into the policy development both in the health care domain and particularly in the nursing field. On the one hand this has enabled this chapter to cover a number of essential issues; on the other, it has enabled the use of specific examples within the text to demonstrate the application of important aspects of the communication process. The issue of handover and knowing which information has to be received and by whom is an example. Such a format has allowed the reader to take the framework for the chapter, apply principles for good communication and use these to conjure up some own examples in their mind.

The third issue is that the chapter has attempted to view the subject on both a 'micro' and a 'macro' level (National Institute for Health Clinical Excellence, 2006) to illicit macro and micro concepts. Information has been provided which may assist the student to deal with aspects of any verbal abuse they may experience and comment has been made asserting that the organisation has a responsibility in helping to deal with the problem of abuse. The reader might find this approach useful in future when examining any official document on communication, as it is always worth considering the role for the practitioner but also for the organisation.

Finally, after reading this chapter and assimilating its contents, the reader may be able to enhance their own communication abilities and is encouraged to do this ongoing. Aspects of the chapter have considered the advantages involved in effective non-verbal communication and the benefits of good listening and how these can be used in the health care environment. Non-verbal communication and listening, entwined within a reflective process, is advocated, demonstrating how reflection can assist when incorporating new ideas and learning about communication in everyday life.

Glossary

Body language	The use of the body in assisting in or sending a message
Communication	Transmitting or receiving messages from another person or thing
Culture	Living one's life in a certain way
Electronic mail	Messages sent via a computer
Ethnic	Refers to classify a person into a particular social group
Jargon	A stereotyped name for a concept or item
Listening	Hearing what someone else is saying
'Macro'	This sociological term is often used when referring to organisations

'Micro'	This sociological term is often used when referring to the individual person
Non-judgemental	Not reaching any judgements or conclusions about what is happening or what someone else is saying
Non-verbal communication	Communication which does not involve the use of words or verbs
Nursing handover	This term usually refers to when nurses pass information to other nurses to enable them to care for patients. The process can be formal or informal and is often defined by a specific procedure employed in a nursing environment
Patient independence	This term refers to the patient being able to care for themselves
Personal relationship	An emotional bond between people which is not based on business transactions
Rapport	Developing a relationship (business or personal) with someone else
Record keeping	Documents which are kept, usually detailing events that have occurred. In nursing, these documents generally record patient care
Referral	This term suggests that a communication is made to another professional or service, advising them that a patient will require their care
Reflection	Thought that results in learning
Self-awareness	Being aware of one's own thoughts, feelings and actions
Verbal abuse	Spoken messages which are sent with the view of insulting the other person
Verbal communication	Messages sent which involve the use of speech and verbs
Zero tolerance	A term which is used to send the message that no event of a certain type will be allowed or tolerated

Post-chapter quiz

1. Why is it important to give people as much choice as possible when talking to them about their care?
2. Why is it important that we are consistent in the verbal messages we send to someone else?
3. How can you demonstrate that you are listening to someone?
4. How can you encourage communication in a difficult situation such as caring for someone with dementia?
5. Give examples of how using several methods to communicate at once assist in enhancing the overall communication
6. What is an advantage and disadvantage of using an interpreter?
7. How should you immediately react when someone appears to say something to you which you find unacceptable?
8. Why is the phrase 'actions speak louder than words' so important when thinking about communication?
9. What are the dangers involved in using electronic mail?
10. How can you encourage someone to receive the message in the way it was intended to be received?

References

Abraham, A. (2003) Inadequate nursing care and the failure to keep nursing records. *Professional Nurse* 18(6): 347–349.

Allan, K.I. (2006) Deafness and dementia: consulting on the issues. *The Journal of Dementia Care* 14(3), 35–38.

Aronson Fontes, L. (2008) *Interviewing Clients Across Cultures: A Practitioner's Guide*. New York and London: The Guilford Press.

Bamforth, T. (2007) Communication – getting it right. *Community Living* 21(2): 18–19.

Clark, J. (2007) A digital nursing future. *Practice Nursing* 18(1): 6.

Clark, J. (2008) A digital nursing future. *Practice Nursing* 18(1): 6.

Crouch, D. (2004) Are employers tackling verbal abuse. *Nursing Times* 100(41): 24–25.

Department of Health (2003) *Statement of Guiding Principles Relating to the Commissioning and Provision of Communication Skills Training in Pre-Registration and Undergraduate Education for Healthcare Professionals*. London: Department of Health.

Dimond, B. (2003) Telemedicine and the law. *Nursing Times* 99(21): 50.

Duffy, A. (2006) Non-verbal communication in cancer and palliative care. *Nursing Times* 102(46): 30–31.

Egan, J. (2006) Listen and lead. *Nursing Standard* 20(36): 72.

Evans, S. (2002) How we can all make our written information accessible. *Living Well* 2(3): 23–24.

Fellows, D., Goodman, M., Wilkinson, S., Low, J. and Harvey, F. (2003) District nurses' referrals to home-based palliative nursing services. *Nursing Times* 99(14): 34–37.

Gadsby, A. (2007) How easy it is to forget our basic nursing skills. *Nursing Times* 103(37): 10.

Hendrick, J. (2000) *Law and Ethics in Nursing and Health Care*. Cheltenham: Nelson Thornes Ltd.

HSE (Health and Safety Executive) (2006) *Working with VDUs*. London: Health and Safety Executive.

Hoban, V. (2004) In the frontline of abuse. *Nursing Times* 100(49): 26–27.

Hobson, P. (2008) Understanding dementia: developing person-centred communication. *British Journal of Healthcare Assistants* 2(4): 162–164.

Houghton, G. (2008) Women seeking asylum: are communication needs being met? *British Journal of Midwifery* 16(3): 142.

Hovell, G. (2008) Body language. *Nursing Times* 104(26): 20.

Hutchinson, C. and Sharples, C. (2006) Information governance: practical implications for record-keeping. *Nursing Standard* 20(36): 59–64.

Jasper, M. (2003) *Beginning Reflective Practice*. Cheltenham: Nelson Thornes.

Jepson, R. (2008) The Language of care. *RN* 71(1): 52.

Johnson, C., Martin, D. and Markle-Elder, S. (2007) Stopping verbal abuse in the workplace. *AJN* 107(4): 32–34.

Kohler, M. (2008) Telemedicine seeks to empower patients to manage their care. *British Journal of Community Nursing* 13(3): 135–137.

McGeehan, R. (2007) Best practice in record-keeping. *Nursing Standard* 21(17): 51–55.

McLean, C. (2008) Building rapport with patients: actions speak louder than words. *British Journal of Primary Care Nursing* 5(3): 140–142.

Meddlings, F. and Haith-Cooper, M. (2008) Culture and communication in ethically appropriate care. *Nursing Ethics* 15(1): 52–61.

Miller, C. (2008) Communication difficulties in hospitalized older adults with dementia. *The American Journal of Nursing* 108(3): 58–64.

Moss, B. (2008) *Communication Skills for Health and Social Care*. London: Sage Publications.

Murphy, J., Tester, S., Hubbard, G., Downs, M. and MacDonald, C. (2005) Enabling frail older people with a communication difficulty to express their views: the use of Talking Mats as an interview tool. *Health and Social Care in the Community* 13(2): 95-107.

National Institute for Health and Clinical Excellence (2006) *Four Commonly Used Methods to Increase Physical Activity*. London: National Institute for Health and Clinical Excellence.

Nazarko, L. (2007) The mental capacity act and care documentation. *Residential Care* 9(5): 227-229.

Newson, P. (2006) Loneliness and the value of empathic listening. *Nursing and Residential Care* 8(12): 555-558.

Nursing and Midwifery Council (2007) *Record Keeping*. London: Nursing and Midwifery Council.

Nursing and Midwifery Council (2008) Standards from Medicine Management, Nursing and Midwifery Council, London. Available at http://www.nmc-uk.org. Accessed 5 December 2008.

Oxtoby, K. (2004) How to tackle verbal abuse. *Nursing Times* 100(43): 20-22.

Oxtoby, K. (2005) Reaching a clear understanding. *Nursing Times* 101(20): 20-22.

Patten, N. (2003) Looking for guidance. *Occupational Health* 55(4): 12.

Pennell, M. and Bryon, L. (2008) When giving information. *End of Life* 2(2): 27.

Percival, J. (2001) Burning issue. *Nursing Standard* 15(25): 24.

Phillips, D. (2003) 'Race' and the difficulties of language. *Advances in Nursing Science* 26(1): 17-29.

Piper, L. (2008) Positive reflections. *Nursing Standard* 22(44): 61.

Pothier, D., Monteiro, P., Mooktiar, M. and Shaw, A. (2005) Pilot study to show the loss of important data in nursing handover. *British Journal of Nursing* 14(20): 1090-1093.

Pullen, R. (2007) Tips for communicating with a patient from another culture. *Nursing* 37(10), 48-49.

Richards, S. (2007) How to address sensitive issues. *Practice Nurse* 33(2): 31-33.

Rowe, M. and Sherlock, H. (2005) Stress and verbal abuse in nursing: do burned out nurses eat their young? *Journal of Nursing Management* 13: 242-248.

Seed, J. (2006) Reflection on action: communication is the key. *JPP* 16(12): 581-584.

Smith, J. and Liles, C. (2007) Information needs before hospital discharge of myocardial infarction patients: a comparative, descriptive study. *Journal of Clinical Nursing* 16: 662-671.

Stickley, T. and Freshwater, D. (2006) The art of listening in the therapeutic relationship. *Mental Health Practice* 9(5): 12-18.

Stott, K. (2007) Better with people. *Nursing Standard* 22(3): 67-68.

Sullivan, F. and Wyatt, J. (2005) ABC of health informatics. Is a consultation needed? *BMJ* 331: 625-627.

Trevithick, P. (2005) *Social Work Skills: A Practice Handbook*, 2nd ed. Maidenhead: Open University Press. Cited in Moss, B. (2008) *Communication Skills for Health and Social Care*. London: Sage Publications.

Voulsden, M. (2000) Communication matters. *Journal of Wound Care* 9(10): 453.

Watson, A. (2003) Poor record keeping may indicate lack of care. *Nursing Times* 99(14): 33.

West, E. (2003) Computers: do they help or hinder? *Nursing Forum* 38(1): 29-31.

Chapter 6

Eating and Drinking: Fluid and Nutritional Care in Practice

Jane Say

Learning opportunities

This chapter will help you to:

1. Describe those nursing activities that help to assess and monitor a patient's nutritional status
2. Consider factors within clinical practice that may have a detrimental effect on a patient's nutritional intake
3. Describe a range of interventions that can be used to ensure a patient receives the most appropriate nutritional care
4. Explain the importance of maintaining a patient's fluid balance and correct hydration
5. Describe a range of nursing activities that can be carried out to ensure a patient has the correct fluid intake
6. Outline the unique role and function of the nurse when helping people to meet their nutritional needs

Pre-chapter quiz

1. What do you understand by body mass index?
2. List some of the factors associated with obesity
3. True or false – those with neurological and gastrointestinal diseases have higher rates of malnutrition than those with cardiovascular or musculoskeletal conditions
4. Why is it important to weigh clients upon admission?
5. How often should clients be weighed in a clinical setting?
6. What do you understand by the *Protected Mealtimes* initiative?
7. Why is it important to adopt a multidisciplinary team approach when caring for a client's fluid and nutritional needs?

8. Who are the members of the multidisciplinary team?
9. Describe the unique role and function of the nurse in relation to client's fluid and nutritional needs
10. Eating and drinking are normally sociable activities; how can the nurse help to ensure eating and drinking remain a sociable activity when caring for clients in hospital?

Introduction

This chapter will address particular nursing issues that arise in relation to eating and drinking within adult health care. It will consider how to assess your clients in relation to their nutritional and fluid needs. It will also explore strategies that can be used to ensure that your clients are receiving the most appropriate nutritional care. The key methods of replacing and maintaining fluid within the body will also be explored.

Nutritional issues and clinical practice

Within clinical practice, clients will present with a number of nutritionally related problems and issues. Serious health problems can arise due to inadequate food intake, dietary imbalance or nutrient deficiencies or over-nutrition due to excess consumption.

Obesity

Obesity can be defined as a body mass index (BMI) over 30 kg/m^2, whereas overweight can be defined as a BMI over 25 kg/m^2 (a further discussion on BMI and its significance is discussed later). Those defined as overweight or obese would normally have an excess of body fat stores.

If calorific intakes exceed energy expenditure (i.e. the total amount of energy used by the body to function metabolically, generate heat, synthesise new tissue and perform physical activity) the body will store increasing amounts of fat (as triglycerides) in the adipose tissue.

The reasons for the development of obesity are complex. Many social, personal and genetic factors are involved. However, within the UK two key factors related to our modern living have contributed to this epidemic. These are a lack of physical activity and poor nutrition associated with excessive eating in the form of fast or junk foods.

The Health Survey for England (Craig and Shelton, 2007) found that 65% of men and 56% of women were either overweight or obese, with a greater proportion of men than women being overweight. However, the proportion of men and women who were obese was the same at 24%.

Obesity is now seen as a major epidemic and can lead to complications such as type 2 diabetes mellitus, heart disease and hypertension. Type 2 diabetes mellitus is normally seen in ageing adults with a weight problem. However, the increase in obesity in children means that it is now been diagnosed in children as young as 13 years (Dyer, 2002). Diabetes at any age carries a risk of further complications such as renal failure and blindness. However, the longer a person has the condition, the more likely he or she is to develop complications. The economic cost of the health problems caused by obesity has been estimated at £6.6–7.4 billion per year (House of Commons Health Committee, 2004).

The government has now developed a cross-government strategy that aims to tackle this issue (Department of Health [DH], 2008). It hopes that individuals, communities, the NHS and other aspects of the public sector, local government, the voluntary and community sector, the food industry, employers and the media will all contribute to find reasonable solutions to this growing health problem. Nurses have a role in this strategy to promote healthy eating and lifestyle choices with their clients.

Undernutrition

The problems associated with hospital undernutrition (commonly termed malnutrition within clinical practice) have been widely recognised for many years and a number of studies have identified the extent of undernutrition within hospital clients. Recently, the British Association for Parenteral and Enteral Nutrition (BAPEN, 2008) undertook the largest nutrition screening survey to assess the nutritional status of patients during the first 3 days of their admission to hospital and of residents in care homes, who had been admitted during the previous 6 months. The figures from this survey suggest that in hospitals 28% were malnourished and in care homes the figure rose to 30%. Interestingly, the study found that those who were admitted from their own home to a hospital or a care home had a lower prevalence of malnutrition than those who were admitted from other institutions (i.e. other wards, care homes and hospitals).

Malnutrition increases the risk of minor and major complications, therefore increasing rates of morbidity and mortality; it extends the length of hospital stay and, as might be expected, increases the cost of treatment (Reilly et al., 1988; Sullivan et al., 1999).

Research into this area has demonstrated that maintaining a client's nutritional status is vital in aiding recovery and rehabilitation (National Institute for Health and Clinical Excellence (NICE) 2006; Veteran's Administration Trial, 1991).

Furthermore, the nature and provision of food and drink has been found to be an important indicator of the overall quality of care that patients and residents receive in hospitals and care homes (Age Concern, 2006; Commission for Social Care Inspection (CSCI), 2006).

The causes of undernutrition are complex but are usually related to the disease process. However, other non-disease-related factors can also affect the clients' nutritional status.

Disease-related factors

The nature of the disease can adversely affect appetite and this will lead to a reduction in food intake. The BAPEN (2008) survey found that patients and residents with certain diagnostic categories were more likely to be malnourished than others. Those with neurological and gastrointestinal diseases had higher rates of malnutrition than those with cardiovascular or musculoskeletal conditions.

Specific disabilities, which are associated with changes in mobility or sensation (e.g. arthritis, multiple sclerosis, cerebrovascular accidents or coma), may affect how the client can eat. Such disabilities can also lead to a need for assistance during mealtimes. Physical factors such as poor oral hygiene/dentition, dysphagia and pain on eating can also influence nutritional intake. Changes in gastrointestinal tract function can have a very serious effect on food absorption and may cause nausea, vomiting and diarrhoea. In many illnesses, there are changes in metabolic activity that can lead to increased requirements for protein and energy. Clients with severe burns or sepsis are known to have increased nutrient requirements. If such requirements are not met by the client's diet then deficiencies and undernutrition will occur. If the metabolic demands are very high, the client can become undernourished very quickly. Any alterations in the client's psychological welfare, which includes conditions causing chronic pain and depression, can also affect appetite and nutritional intake. A number of treatments including multiple medication and aggressive drug therapies such as chemotherapy may also induce nutritional deficiencies (McLaren, 2003).

Non-disease-related factors

Several organisations have highlighted the detrimental affect that hospital/clinical routines and practices can have on clients' mealtimes (Age Concern, 2006; Association of Community Health Council (ACHC), 1997; CSCI, 2006). Particular issues include problems with ordering and choice of food, communication, the quality and quantity of food, positioning of clients and assistance with meals, the eating environment and the availability of utensils to assist those with physical disabilities.

The need for appropriate nutritional assessment and monitoring has been highlighted as a fundamental aspect of care within health and social services settings (DH, 2007; NICE, 2006). Although this has been recognised for some time, BAPEN (2008) found that not all patients in their survey of malnutrition had been routinely weighed. As such, it is likely that malnutrition continues to be under-recognised and yet simple screening of clients will help to identify those requiring help and support with nutrition and facilitate the most appropriate treatment.

Within the community, social and economic factors can influence the way in which clients buy, choose and prepare their food when at home. The BAPEN (2008) survey also highlighted the community as the area where much malnutrition arises and recommends that consideration be given to prevent and treat such malnutrition.

Providing nutritional care in practice

Within clinical practice, nutritional care is an essential element of nursing care. To raise awareness the Council of Europe Alliance (UK) has drawn together *10 key characteristics of good nutritional care in hospitals*. This work is now being promoted by the DH (2007) and can be viewed at the websites of its partner organisations, these include a wide range of government and non-government stakeholders, and their addresses can be found at the end of this chapter.

Each of these ten characteristics identifies different aspects of care that are needed to maintain nutritional requirements of clients. Box 6.1 details the 10 characteristics.

Box 6.1 Ten key characteristics of good nutritional care in hospitals.

1. All patients are screened on admission to identify the patients who are malnourished or at risk of becoming malnourished. All patients are re-screened weekly
2. All patients have a care plan which identifies their nutritional care needs and how they are to be met
3. The hospital includes specific guidance on food services and nutritional care in its clinical governance arrangements
4. Patients are involved in the planning and monitoring arrangements for food service provision
5. The ward implements *Protected Mealtimes* to provide an environment conducive to patients enjoying and being able to eat their food
6. All staff have the appropriate skills and competencies needed to ensure that patients' nutritional needs are met. All staff receive regular training on nutritional care and management
7. Hospital facilities are designed to be flexible and patient centred with the aim of providing and delivering an excellent experience of food service and nutritional care 24 hours a day, everyday
8. The hospital has a policy of food service and nutritional care which is patient centred and performance managed in line with home country governance frameworks
9. Food service and nutritional care is delivered to the patient safely
10. The hospital supports a multidisciplinary approach to nutritional care and values the contribution of all staff groups working in partnership with patients and users

Screening/assessment to identify patients'/clients' nutritional needs

The requirement for all clients to receive nutritional screening on admission or at their first clinic appointment is viewed as vital if appropriate nutritional care is to be provided (DH, 2007; NICE, 2006).

Nutritional screening is a relatively quick and simple method of identifying those clients who may be malnourished or 'at risk' of becoming malnourished while they are in hospital or receiving treatment. A follow-up and more in-depth assessment can then ensure that those clients who require and would most benefit from nutritional support are identified and appropriately treated. To continue monitoring of the client's nutritional status, the screening should then be performed at weekly intervals. Health care professionals who perform screening should have received the necessary education and training (NICE, 2006). For clients who require a full nutritional assessment a more detailed process is required. A registered practitioner who has the necessary education and training and has been assessed as competent must perform this. Within clinical practice this is likely to be a registered nurse (and may include a nutrition nurse specialist) or a dietician. To facilitate the screening process a number of screening tools have been developed that aim to determine the nutritional 'risk' status of the client (BAPEN, 2003; Reilly et al., 1995; Robshaw and Marbrow, 1995; Royal College of Nursing (RCN), 1993)

An adapted version of Reilly et al.'s (1995) *Nutrition Risk Score* is shown in Figure 6.1. These tools are based on factors that have been identified as significant in the development of malnutrition.

Body mass index

Measurement of the client's BMI is viewed as an important indicator of nutritional status. This measurement is determined from the weight and the height of the client and can be calculated as follows:

$$\text{BMI} = \frac{\text{Weight in kg}}{(\text{Height in m})^2}$$

The significance of the BMI measurement is given in Table 6.1. This measurement closely correlates with body fat (Revicki and Israel, 1986). However it is important that the correct height (without shoes) and weight are obtained. In older people the measurement is less accurate since it does not account for the loss of height and muscle mass that can occur in this group (Bowling, 2004).

Weight loss

The percentage of recent weight loss is also viewed as an important method of determining nutritional status (NICE, 2006). Based on the evidence available, NICE (2006) states that an unintentional weight loss greater than 10% within the last 3–6 months or a patient with a BMI less than 20 kg/m^2 and unintentional weight loss greater than 5% within the last 3–6 months should be classed as malnourished.

In order to determine weight loss over a 3–6-month period, the following calculation is needed:

$$\text{Percentage weight loss} = \frac{\text{Usual weight in kg} - \text{actual weight in kg}}{\text{Usual weight in kg}} \times 100$$

Patient's name: ....

Hospital number: .... Ward: ....

Date: .... Time: ....

Weight: .... Height/Length: ....Signature: ....

Please circle relevant score. Select only one score from each section.
Select the highest score that applies.

		Score
1.	ADULTS (>18 years)	
	WEIGHT LOSS IN LAST 3 MONTHS (Unintentional)	
	No weight loss	0
	0–3 kg weight loss	1
	>3–6 kg weight loss	2
	6 kg or more	3
2.	BMI (Body mass index)	
	20 or more	0
	18 or 19	1
	15–17	2
	Less than 15	3
3.	APPETITE	
	• Good appetite, manages most of three meals/day (or equivalent)	0
	• Poor appetite, poor intake – leaving more than half of meals provided (or equivalent)	2
	• Appetite nil or virtually nil, unable to eat, NBM (for >4 meals)	3
4.	ABILITY TO EAT/RETAIN FOOD	
	• No difficulties in eating, able to eat independently. No diarrhoea or vomiting.	0
	• Problems in handling food, e.g. needs special cutlery. Vomiting/frequent regurgitation (or possetting)/mild diarrhoea.	1
	• Difficulty in swallowing, requiring modified consistency. Problems with dentures, affecting food intake. Problems with chewing, affecting food intake. Slow to feed. Moderate vomiting and/or diarrhoea (1–2/day for children). Needs help with feeding (e.g. physical handicap).	2
	• Unable to take food orally. Unable to swallow (complete dysphagia). Severe vomiting and/or diarrhoea (>2/day for children). Malabsorption	3
5.	STRESS FACTOR	
	• No stress factor (includes admission for investigation only)	0
	• Mild Minor surgery, minor infection	1
	• Moderate Chronic disease, major surgery, infections, fractures, pressure sores/ulcers, CVA, inflammatory bowel disease, Other gastrointestinal disease	2
	• Severe multiple injuries, multiple fractures/burns, multiple deep pressure sores/ulcers, severe sepsis, carcinoma/malignant disease	3

Document subsequent scores on the back of this sheet.

TOTAL:

Figure 6.1 Nutrition risk score chart. (Adapted from Reilly et al., 1995.)

DOCUMENTATION OF NUTRITION RISK SCORE

Date and Time	Signature	Weight	Score	Comments

Action for nutritional risk assessment score

Complete on admission and then weekly for all patients

Score	Risk Status	Nutritional action plan
0–3	LOW	• Check and record weight weekly. Monitor using Nutrition Risk Score (NRS)
4–5	MEDIUM	• Perform further assessment. Devise and implement a plan of care
6–15	HIGH	• Perform further assessment. Devise and implement a plan of care and refer to the dietician

Also refer to the dietetic department (via medical staff) if the patient needs specific advice about a special diet or education regarding a therapeutic diet.

Figure 6.1 *(Continued)*

Table 6.1 Body mass index and its significance.

Body mass index (kg/m^2)	Significance
<18.5	Underweight/malnourished
18.5–20	Underweight/malnourishment probable
20–25	Desirable weight, chronic malnutrition unlikely
25–30	Overweight and increased complications associated with chronic over-nutrition
30–35	Moderately obese and increased complications associated with chronic over-nutrition
35–40	Highly obese and at risk of complications associated with chronic over-nutrition
>40	Highly obese and at high risk of complications associated with chronic over-nutrition

Source: Adapted from Bowling (2004).

Table 6.2 Weight loss interpretations.

Percentage weight change over 3-6 months	Interpretation
<5	Within normal variations
5-10	More than normal individual variation - early indicator of undernutrition risk
>10	Clinically significant - requires nutritional support

If a client has ascites or oedema then allowances for the fluid weight must be made within the calculations (see Table 6.2). Often these clients will mask their true weight loss.

Recent dietary intakes

The client's current and recent intakes should also be determined by questioning the client or their carer. Talking to the client about their recent dietary intake and how this may have changed requires the nurse to consider a range of issues relating to the everyday life of the client. For each person, his or her circumstances and details will vary dramatically. However it is important that the nurse focus on the most relevant information and this should include details on the following:

- Any recent decrease in food intake
- Changes in their appetite
- Any difficulties with swallowing (also called dysphagia)
- Signs of recent weight loss including clothes or rings becoming loose fitting
- Any particular social or economic factors that may affect eating including their ability to afford their particular dietary requirements, their ability to shop and prepare their own food and any other support that they require to ensure adequate nutrition
- The details of any psychological or physical disabilities that may have contributed to a change in their nutritional status. This could include many differing factors from poor dentition and a need for new dentures to chronic depression as a result of a severe illness
- Any specialist dietary requirement. This may include a particular diet related to their medical condition or may be specific to their religious or cultural beliefs

Stress factors/nature of current illness

During illness the nutritional requirements of the body can alter significantly. Metabolic activity can alter in response to the physical stress experienced by the body. This can mean that the resting energy requirements of the body may increase and in clients with severe burns or sepsis this can be as much as 60% (Kinney, 1995). Many of the screening tools have a section that acknowledges the impact of specific illnesses on nutritional status and the scoring in the tool is weighted to demonstrate this.

For some patients, the nature of their condition may mean that they eat little or nothing for some time. NICE (2006) recommends that those who have eaten little or nothing for more than 5 days and/or are likely to eat little or nothing for the next 5 days or longer should be classed as at risk of malnutrition. Patients with poor absorptive capacity and/or high nutrient losses and/or increased nutritional needs from causes such as catabolism should also be classed as at risk of malnutrition (NICE, 2006).

For some clients a specific deficiency may be found (such as iron-deficiency anaemia). This may not lead to serious undernutrition but the subsequent care and treatment that the client receives should reflect their increased requirements for iron.

Further action, assessment and referral

The screening tools often include an action plan which details the steps to be taken next. For those clients who are identified as *high risk* or malnourished, the next step is usually referral to the dietician and a more in-depth assessment is carried out. This assessment can then fully identify the specific nutritional care that the client is likely to require and may involve further referrals or the implementation of a specialist feeding regime and an appropriate plan of care.

For those identified as at *medium risk* or at *risk*, further assessment should be performed by a qualified practitioner and a care plan devised. Nutritional monitoring should be continued on a weekly basis.

For those identified as *low risk*, the possibility of deterioration should be considered and as such these clients should be monitored on a regular basis. The timing of such monitoring will vary according to the nature of the client's condition and the type of care setting. The screening tool can also be used as a convenient means of monitoring.

Planning, implementation and evaluation of nutritional care

As recommended by the Council of Europe Alliance (UK), all patients should have a care plan which identifies their nutritional care needs and how they will be met. The details of the plan of care will differ from client to client. However, it may involve a number of health care professionals and include details of the specific nutritional support that is required by the client.

The methods and timing of evaluation are also important if the care is to be properly monitored and its effectiveness assessed. Later in this chapter a number of different methods of nutritional support and the associated care will be addressed.

Monitoring and re-screening

The need for continued nutritional monitoring and screening of clients during hospital stays has also been recognised as necessary to ensure a client's nutritional care (NICE, 2006; RCN, 2007; The Council of Europe Alliance). As previously discussed the organisation of hospital care, the nature of medical treatment and sudden changes in a client's condition can all lead to a decline in nutritional status. Therefore, it is important to monitor the nutritional intake of clients and to re-screen or re-assess them throughout their stay. Normally re-screening or re-assessment would be performed on a weekly basis. However, monitoring food intake needs to be performed and action taken if there is any cause for concern (DH, 2001a). Previous work has found that there may be a lack of documentation of nutritional care and no clear strategy for nutritional care (including monitoring) (BAPEN, 2008).

- Clients should be re-screened or where appropriate re-assessed on a weekly basis. This will include re-weighing the client and re-calculating BMI.
- Identified staff should be trained to monitor and record the fluid and nutritional intakes of their clients. If appropriate, carers may also be involved in this if they have been shown how to complete the proper records.
- A recognised form/record should be used. This will detail the type and amount of food taken at each meal or snack. This needs to be completed accurately and checked by a registered health care professional.
- The organisation of this monitoring must be coordinated with the staff involved in distributing and collecting the meals.
- Guidelines are needed to determine the best course of action when a client is not receiving adequate nutrition.
- An immediate referral to the dietician should also be undertaken by a registered nurse if there are concerns about nutritional intakes.

Factors that affect nutritional care: the hospital and care environment

The environment in which clients eat can have a real effect on the whole experience of eating and drinking and can influence client intakes (ACHC, 1997; Age Concern, 2006; CSCI, 2006; Eberhardie, 2000).

Food is more likely to be enjoyed if it is well cooked and presented and is of a good quality. Also if a client has particular requirements or follows a special diet (e.g. vegetarian) then for the client to enjoy and appreciate the meal these factors must be met. Eating and drinking are normally sociable activities and the experience of a meal can be greatly improved if there is a social element to it.

In hospitals or residential care there may be very unpleasant sights, sounds and smells occurring during meal times. A client may be using a bedpan while others continue with their meal in the same room. The alarms on equipment in the area may be constantly ringing while nurses and doctors are busy dealing with a sick client in the next bed. The client may not have been given the opportunity to wash their hands and the table and utensils may be dirty. All these factors will discourage clients to eat and can affect nutritional intakes.

The *Protected Mealtimes* initiative has been introduced to promote an environment conducive to eating and to ensure that the ward team can prepare clients and assist them with their meals. It is being promoted as an important measure to enhance care (RCN, 2007).

Within a clinical area the registered nurse will have ultimate responsibility for the overall environment and organisation of the area. However other staff including health care assistants, students, orderlies and housekeepers may be given the responsibility, where it is thought appropriate, to carry out these activities. For all members of staff the issues of ownership and accountability for this area of practice will need to be clear (DH, 2001a). As recommended by the Council of Europe Alliance (UK), all staff should have the appropriate skills to ensure that nutritional needs are met, and all aspects of food provision should be patient centred.

- Ensure that the environment is clean including any tables, tablemats and cooking utensils
- Wash your hands and remove dirty aprons before serving food
- Give clients the opportunity to wash their hands
- Where facilities allow, encourage eating at a communal table with other/clients
- Where possible, encourage clients to eliminate before the meal begins
- If a client requires the commode/toilet during mealtime, take them to the bathroom.
- Ensure that the area is well ventilated to minimise bad odours and to remove old and stale cooking smells after the meal
- Minimise unnecessary activity during mealtimes. If possible, introduce a dedicated mealtime approach where disruptions, visits, ward rounds and investigations are actively discouraged when the clients are eating
- If the client wishes, encourage the involvement of their next of kin or carer during the mealtime period

Assistance with eating and drinking

Many clients in hospital or residential care need extra assistance to eat their meals and without such help malnutrition can occur. This can be a particular issue with elderly clients and those with dementia. These groups of clients may have complex illnesses, previous malnutrition and increasing dependence (Mc Gillivray and Marland, 1999; RCN, 1993). Clients and their families have commented on problems with appropriate positioning at meal times, lack of assistance with their meals and the lack of appropriate utensils (ACHC, 1997; Age Concern, 2006). In other work, clients have felt that nurses do not always recognise the impact of motor and physical disabilities on their eating behaviour (Sidenvall and Ek, 1993).

As part of the initial screening and assessment process, those clients requiring extra help should be clearly identified. For some clients, simple strategies may be sufficient to ensure that they can manage to feed themselves. This may include the provision of special crockery or cutlery. Other clients may need one-to-one assistance at each mealtime and without such assistance they would not be able to eat. For all clients, independence should be promoted. This may be achieved through further education of the client and their carers. The involvement of other members of the multidisciplinary team may also be required particularly if specialist equipment is needed. Clients who have difficulty in swallowing (dysphagia) *must* be referred to a speech and language therapist (SALT) for further assessment.

A dedicated number of carers should be involved in assisting a client to eat. This aids continuity and allows a relationship to develop that will help to promote eating and drinking. Furthermore, regular helpers will begin to recognise important non-verbal cues in those patients where communication is difficult (Mc Gillivray and Marland, 1999).

Here are a number of key actions that will assist the client in their eating and drinking:

- Where possible, sit or support the client in an upright chair with easy access to the table and food
- Clients in bed should be sitting/supported upright with easy access to their table and food
- Ensure that those clients who need dentures have them
- Ensure that the mouth is clean
- Assess for pain or nausea well before mealtimes so that appropriate action can be taken in time for the meal
- Ensure that the appropriate member of staff gives any particular drug therapies due before mealtimes (e.g. insulin therapy)
- Ensure that any specialist utensils, fresh water, a hot drink and condiments are available
- Ensure that the client receives the meal of their choice that is suitable for their specialist dietary, religious or cultural requirements
- Be sensitive to the client's needs and any embarrassment they may have about eating
- Where necessary, protect the client's clothes with a napkin.
- Help the client with difficult packaging and rearrange the tray/plate to ensure that the client can reach its contents
- Ensure that hot food or drinks are not likely to spill and injure the client
- Explain to those clients who are confused or disorientated that it is mealtime
- When helping a client to eat sit at the same level so that you can reach them comfortably and make eye contact
- Communicate with your client as you feed them
- Give $\frac{1}{2}$ to 1 teaspoonful per mouthful and place on the stronger side of the mouth if the client has hemiplegia (paralysis on one side of the body) or hemiparesis (weakness on one side of the body)
- Allow the client time to chew and swallow twice before giving the next mouthful
- Ask the client to clear their throat between each mouthful to ensure that the airway is clear
- Ask the client to cough during and at the end of the meal. This will also clear the airway
- If the client shows any signs of distress, uncontrolled coughing or has a gurgly-sounding voice, *stop feeding immediately* and seek qualified assistance. This could be a sign of aspiration (food entering the respiratory tract)
- At the end of the meal check the mouth for retained food and offer a drink or a mouthwash where necessary
- To aid digestion, allow the client to remain upright for at least $\frac{1}{2}$ hour after the meal.
- For those patients requiring regular assistance, try to ensure that the same personnel are involved. If the client agrees and where appropriate, encourage the next of kin or carer to help with their feeding.

Other members of the ward team will often perform these activities. However, it is important that staff have been appropriately trained and educated in providing this care and that they recognise their roles and responsibilities in carrying out these activities.

Food provision

The *NHS Standards for Better Health* (DH, 2004b) requires health care providers to ensure there is a choice of food that is safely prepared and is balanced. It also emphasises the need for individual requirements to be met, help with feeding to be given and clients to have access to food throughout the 24-hour period.

To ensure a minimum standard for hospital meals, *Better Hospital Food Programme* (DH, 2001b) was initiated. Meals consist of breakfast, light lunch, two-course evening dinner, drinks and snacks on at least two occasions and the provision of a 24-hour catering service. There are still a number of concerns that clients are not receiving their meals or the most appropriate assistance and that proper regard is not given to their dignity when providing nutritional care (Healthcare Commission, 2006).

Some key activities that are needed to ensure that clients receive the most appropriate menu choice are now noted

- Ensure that the client and their carers understand the nature of the menu, and how to complete it.
- Particular requirements (medical, cultural and religious) and how they can be met should be discussed with the client and their carers
- On admission, inform catering and the dietician of specialist dietary requirements (the previous two points may well form part of the initial screening/assessment process and registered nurse or clearly identified health care professional should be responsible for this)
- An identified person should assist clients who have difficulty completing their menu choices
- Regular staff should be designated to serve food and drinks to the clients
- While serving meals, ward staff should check that the client is receiving the correct meal at the right temperature
- Clients who miss a meal should be offered a suitable alternative via the 24-hour service that is available
- Preparation of food and food storage in the area (including the client's own food) must follow health and hygiene standards

Completing menus and serving food may be designated to a number of other staff within the ward team (including health care assistants, students, orderlies and house-keepers). However, it is important that staff have been appropriately trained in providing this care and that they recognise their roles and responsibilities in carrying out these activities.

Nutritional support

It is important to remember that oral feeding is always the preferred method of meeting a client's nutritional needs. However, for some clients it will not be possible to follow a normal healthy diet and extra nutritional support may be necessary. Initially a full nutritional assessment of the client will be needed and the dietician will then determine the most appropriate method of nutritional support.

Specialist means of support such as nasogastric feeding or parenteral feeding may be required to meet a patient's needs. However, much simpler approaches such as the use of nutritional supplements can improve oral intakes. In practice, the nurses, dieticians and medical team will all consider the most appropriate form of feeding.

When starting or stopping any nutrition support, it is vital to obtain patient consent to act in the best interest of the patient (Nursing and Midwifery Council, 2008). There may be times where provision of nutrition is *not* appropriate and treatment may be withdrawn or withheld. However, any such decision must follow ethical and legal considerations (NICE, 2006).

Figure 6.2 shows a diagram to aid in this decision-making process.

Improving oral intakes

Where possible this is always the first mode of treatment. Remember from the previous discussions that changes in the hospital menu, alongside the availability of food and how it is presented and served, are all aimed at improving patient's oral intakes (DH, 2001a, 2001b).

Food can be supplemented or fortified by adding cream or cheese. This increases the protein and energy content of the food. It is important that nurses ensure that (if appropriate) clients choose and receive high-protein/high-energy meals and are given extra high-energy/high-protein snacks.

As previously stressed, it is essential that those patients who demonstrate signs of dysphagia have their swallowing reflex checked by a SALT to prevent potential aspiration. Patients with dysphagia may require a modified diet or enteral feeding.

Oral supplements

These should be used for clients who cannot maintain their nutritional intakes from everyday food and drink. Although supplements have been proven to have real benefits (Delmi et al., 1990), it is important that they are used appropriately since they are often wasted. There are a number of supplements available in liquid, semi-solid or powder form. Some are nutritionally complete, whereas others will only 'supplement' the usual oral diet. A dietician would normally assess the need for supplements and would decide the most appropriate supplement for the client. Within the clinical setting, it will be part of the nurses' role to ensure that clients receive and take the supplement. This activity should be monitored and recorded so that a proper evaluation can be performed. Other staff may be supervised by registered nurses to help with this activity.

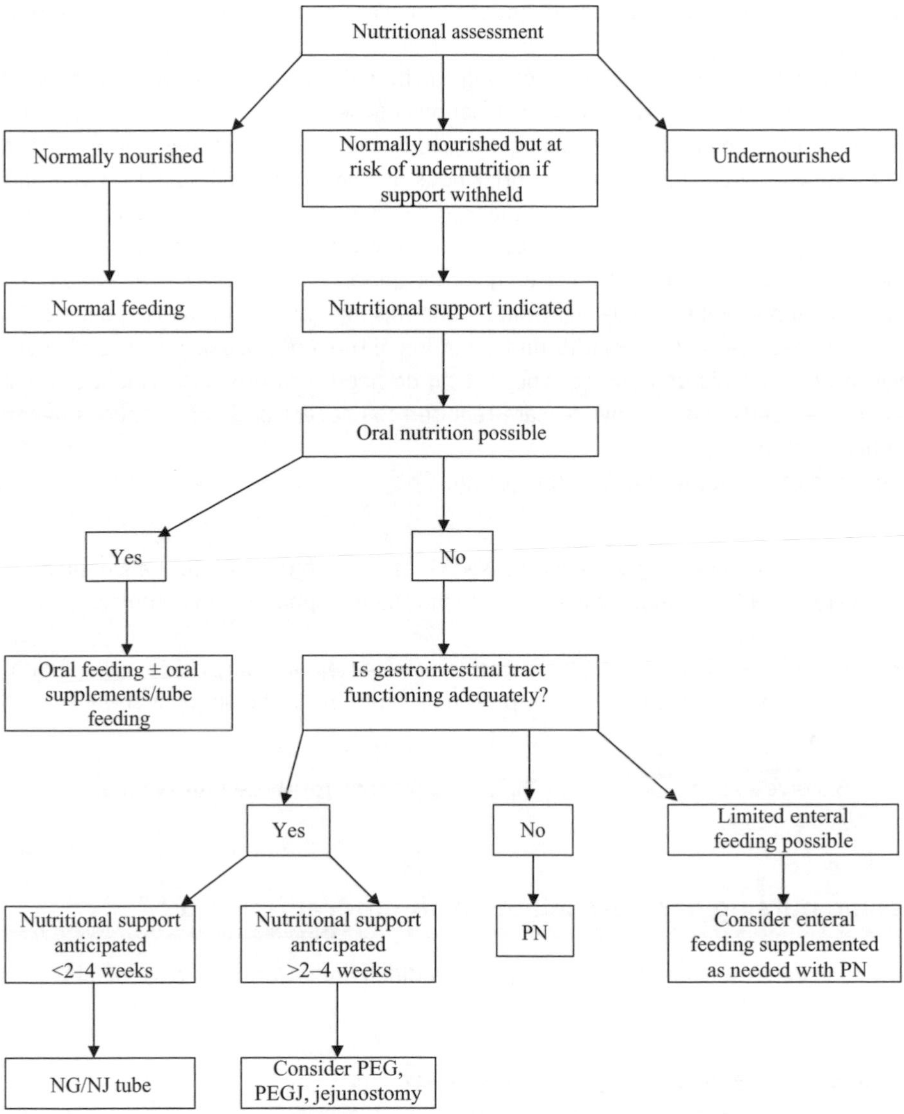

Figure 6.2 Choices for nutritional support: a decision-making process. NG, nasogastric; NJ, nasojejunal; PEG, percutaneous endoscopic gastrostomy; PEGJ, percutaneous endoscopic gastrojejunostomy; PN, parenteral nutrition. (Adapted from Bowling, 2004.)

Enteral (or tube) feeding

This method of feeding delivers a liquid feed via a tube directly into the gastrointestinal tract. Clients can receive all their nutritional needs in this way or it may be used as a means of supplementing oral intakes. The type of feed used will depend on the clients' requirements, their current dietary intake, the function of the gastrointestinal tract and their clinical condition (certain conditions such as liver and renal disease may require a specialised diet).

Clients (and their carers) who are receiving nutritional support in this way may be anxious and may need re-assurance and explanations of the treatment involved. Questions from the client or their carers should be directed to the appropriate member of staff. It must be remembered that eating and drinking is usually a pleasant social activity and receiving a tube feed can reduce these pleasurable aspects of eating. As such the client may need psychological and social support while receiving this type of feed.

Another aspect of care that must be given attention is the client's oral hygiene or mouthcare. Some clients will be nil by mouth and this may cause problems in the mouth such as dryness, cracking, stomatitis (inflammation of the mouth), pain, ulcers and infection. Therefore clients undergoing tube feeding do need a careful assessment of their oral hygiene needs and the specific care required to prevent oral complications needs to be highlighted.

There are three methods of enteral feeding:

1. Nasogastric (NG) feeding. A tube is passed via the nasopharynx into the stomach
2. Nasojejunal (NJ) feeding. A tube is passed via the nasopharynx and stomach and on into the jejunum
3. Percutaneous endoscopically placed gastrostomy or jejunostomy (PEG/PEJ) feeding. A tube is inserted directly into the stomach or jejunum via the abdominal wall

Table 6.3 gives a summary of the main considerations for these types of feed.

Specific nursing care associated with enteral feeding

The nursing care associated with this type of feeding can be considered as follows.

Nasogastric feeding/nasojejunal feeding

Nasogastric insertion/ensuring the correct position

- *NG tube insertion*: This is normally performed by a registered nurse, dietician or doctor. Within the clinical area, policies and guidelines should be used to advise on the exact procedures for insertion and checking of the tube position. These should be based on the guidance provided by the National Patient Safety Agency (NPSA, 2005).
- *NG tube position*: This should be done at the following times (NICE, 2006; NPSA, 2005) on initial placement, before a feed, before giving medication (if the tube is being used), following vomiting or coughing, after tube dislodgement, and if the patient complains of discomfort.

For a very comprehensive step-by-step account of how to insert and check an NG tube, refer to local policies and procedures.

Table 6.3 The types of enteral feed and their specific considerations.

Type of feed	Indication	Contraindication	Practical considerations
NG feed	• Short-term use for clients with use of stomach and no vomiting or aspiration • Also, impaired swallowing (e.g. stroke), altered consciousness, ventilated clients, dysphagia • For supplementation of inadequate oral intakes • Psychological requirements, e.g. anorexia nervosa	• Obstruction preventing passage of tube • Impaired stomach emptying due to obstruction • Intestinal obstruction • Intestinal perforation or nearby gastrointestinal fistula • Severe facial injury	• Two main types of tubes may be used: Fine bore or wide bore (e.g. Ryles). Normally a fine bore tube is used • Care of the NG tube. To include: Passing the tube Ensuring correct position Regular checking of tube position Feed administration • Complications. These include removal by the patient due to confusion or on purpose as a means of withdrawing consent. Ulceration/narrowing/strictures of the oesophagus. This is unusual when fine bore tubes are used. Diarrhoea
NJ feed	• Short-term use for clients whose stomach needs to be bypassed and where there is no vomiting • In clients with a high risk of aspiration • Pancreatitis	• As per NG feeding (see above)	• Two main types of tubes may be used: Single lumen (can be placed with or without an endoscope) or double lumen (needs specialist placement) • Care of the NJ tube. To include: Passing the tube (normally done endoscopically) Ensuring correct position (normally done under X ray) Regular checking of tube position Feed administration • Complications. As per NG feeding (see above)

(*Continued*)

Table 6.3 (*Continued*)

Type of feed	Indication	Contraindication	Practical considerations
PEG/PEJ feeds	• For longer term feeding more than 4 weeks. • Used particularly in cerebrovascular accidents (stroke), head injury, multiple sclerosis, motor neurone disease, severe physical and learning disabilities	• Ascites, severe obesity, blood clotting abnormalities, oesophageal or gastric varices (varicose veins in the gastrointestinal tract), gastric ulceration or malignancy.	• Care of the PEG/PEJ tube. To include: Insertion of the tube (performed endoscopically) Checking and management of insertion site Feed administration • Complications. Peritonitis, aspiration, infection of the site, haemorrhage, tube blockage, death of tissue (necrosis) around the site due to pressure from the tube limiting the local blood supply.

NG, nasogastric; NJ, nasojejunal; PEJ/PEG, percutaneous endoscopically placed gastrostomy or jejunostomy.

Nasojejunal insertion/ensuring the correct position

- *NJ tube insertion*: This is normally performed by staff using endoscopy and can be checked using X-ray.
- *NJ tube position*: To avoid the displacement of the tube, it must be securely fixed to the nose or cheek. A permanent mark should be made at the point where the tube leaves the nose. The position should be checked before commencing a feed. If there are signs that the tube may have moved, report this to the appropriate registered practitioner (registered nurse, dietician, doctor or nutritional nurse specialist). *Do not* commence a feed until the position is confirmed.

NG/NJ feed administration

A registered nurse will have ultimate responsibility for the management of the feed. However, other staff may provide aspects of care after receiving the appropriate training.

The guidelines below outline how to deliver an NG or NJ feed and have been adapted from Bowling (2004), NICE (2006) and NPSA (2005). However, always refer to local policies and procedures when delivering this type of care.

- Before any feed commences the position of the tube must be checked according to policy and procedures (see above). *Do not* commence a feed until the position of the tube is confirmed. Remember there is a significant risk of pulmonary aspiration (feed entering the lungs) if the tube is misplaced.
- Wash hands thoroughly and use a clean apron before beginning the procedure. Hygiene is extremely important when dealing with these feeds. Nasojejunal feeds carry a greater risk of infection since the acid environment of the stomach is bypassed. This acid environment would normally act as a barrier to infection.
- Position the client at a 30–45° upright angle unless their medical condition does not allow this (e.g. spinal injury). Keep upright for 1 hour after the feed to avoid aspiration due to reflux.
- For NG feeding, two methods of feeding may be used: *Pump feeding*, where an infusion pump continuously delivers the feed at a rate of approximately 100 mL/hour (this is determined by the dietician); or gravity feeding, where a 50–60-mL syringe containing feed is attached to the giving set. This is held higher than the client and allowed to drain into the NG tube.
- For NJ feeding, a pump feed will be used. The initial rate will be slower since the small intestine cannot hold as much fluid and it will be increased slowly over time
- Feeding duration will vary according to the method of delivery and the requirements of the client. Normally, a break in feeding is given to clients on NG feeds. However, NJ feeds can continue over the full 24 hours.
- Administer the feed as prescribed and documented by the dietician. Ensure that the correct feed is given at the correct time and rate of delivery.
- To prevent blockage the NG tube should be flushed with 50 mL cooled, boiled (at home) or sterile water (in the acute setting) pre- and post-feeds and medication. The NJ tube should be flushed every 6 hours with 30 mL sterile water using a 50-mL syringe.
- Record the amount of feed given.
- Report and record any complications immediately.
- Continue nutritional monitoring and screening to help evaluate the effectiveness of the feeding regime.

Percutaneous endoscopically placed gastrostomy or jejunostomy feeding

This type of feeding is used with clients who require enteral feeding for more than 4 weeks. The tube requires surgical placement using endoscopy. As with the other types of enteral feeding, the responsibility for the client's care will remain with the registered nurse. However other staff who have been properly trained may be involved in some aspects of care.

Care following a PEG/PEJ insertion

Initial care following insertion is based on monitoring the client's physiological status following an invasive surgical procedure. Any changes in the client's condition can then be quickly acted upon and further complications prevented.

- Following the procedure, monitor and record temperature, pulse, respirations and blood pressure half hourly for 4 hours and then hourly for 2 hours. Immediately report to the Registered nurse any changes in the client's observations.
- Report any signs or complaints of pain to the registered nurse. Analgesia can then be given.
- The client will remain nil by mouth and nil by tube for 4 hours post-procedure.
- Inspect the insertion site for blood or serous fluid leakage. Immediately report any leakage or continuous bleeding to a registered nurse or doctor since a further dressing or suturing may be required.
- After 4 hours the tube may be flushed with sterile water.
- The dietician will determine the full feeding regimen (course of treatment).

PEG/PEJ feed administration

The principles of care related to this type of feeding are similar to those related to NG and NJ feeding. However particular care is needed of the insertion site to prevent infection. If the site requires cleaning, full aseptic technique must be used. After 5–6 weeks (when a fibrous tract develops through the abdominal wall) the original tube may be removed and a more compact skin level gastrostomy 'button' tube is inserted. This offers a neat, easily managed tube for longer term feeding. When this type of feeding is no longer needed, the tube is removed via endoscopy.

The ongoing care of PEG and PEJ feeding is more specialised than that of nasogastric and nasojejunal feeding. To examine these in more depth, please refer to local policies and procedures.

Parenteral nutrition

Parenteral nutrition is a very specialised and invasive method of feeding. It is the administration of nutrient solutions via a central or peripheral vein. Several members of the multidisciplinary team including registered nurses, doctors, dieticians and pharmacists manage this type of feeding. It is normally used with clients whose gastrointestinal tract is not working or is not accessible. To carry out this type of feed, a dedicated feeding line is established. To do this a catheter is passed either centrally (via the subclavian or jugular veins) or peripherally (via the basilar or cephalic veins of the arm). Pharmacy then prepares the sterile infusion of nutrients. This is based on the particular nutrient requirements of the client as determined by the dietician and medical team. As you may be aware the care for this type of feed is highly specialised and is beyond the remit of this chapter.

Fluid management in clinical practice

Within clinical practice the maintenance of a client's hydration is a fundamental aspect of care. Water is essential for health and evidence has demonstrated that poor hydration can contribute to the following: pressure sores, constipation, urinary tract infections, kidney and gallstones, heart disease, hypotension, diabetes mellitus, changes in cognition, falls, increased length of hospital stay and increased mortality (American Geriatrics Society and other groups, 2001; Anti et al., 1998; Burge et al., 2001; Casimiro et al., 2002; Chan et al., 2002; Eckford et al., 1995; Kleiner, 1999; Math et al., 1986; Thomas et al., 2004).

The elderly have water requirements similar to those of younger people, and adequate hydration can help maintain health as they become more susceptible to disease. In hospitals and residential care a client's condition or particular clinical interventions may alter their ability to maintain their fluid balance.

In 2007, the RCN and the NPSA launched a campaign and published an online toolkit (available from Water UK, Water for health, http://www.water.org.uk) to promote best practice regarding patient hydration.

There are many reasons for clients not being able to manage their own fluid balance. Overall there are three main causes of fluid imbalance:

1. Excessive losses, e.g. vomiting and diarrhoea.
2. Reduced intake, e.g. *loss of thirst mechanism* which can occur in altered levels of consciousness/confused states; *lack of access to water* which can occur in clients who are bed bound or again in those with altered levels of consciousness/confused states; *inappropriate/inadequate intake* due to improper intravenous (IV) fluid regimens. Both excessive losses and reduced intakes will lead to a client becoming dehydrated.
3. Fluid retention, e.g. heart or kidney failure and excessive fluid replacement can lead to fluid overload where the body has an excess of fluids.

In order to determine any potential or actual fluid imbalance, it is important to first assess the client's fluid status.

Clinical assessment of fluid balance

A history of the client's recent fluid input and output along with any particular difficulties related to their fluid balance needs to be obtained. This must recognise planned and future interventions that will affect intakes. For example when a client is nil by mouth for surgery and certain procedures, they will not be able to eat and drink. Treatments such as chemotherapy or extensive head and neck surgery will obviously impact on their fluid intakes. Interventions will therefore be needed to overcome any potential fluid imbalance that may occur. There are a number of vital signs that can be used to assess and monitor a client's fluid balance. These include the monitoring of fluid input and output alongside laboratory findings and weight.

Table 6.4 summarises the key means of determining a client's fluid status.

Fluid input and output charts

This is a common means of monitoring fluid balance and can act as an important part of the assessment and monitoring process.

The following details how a fluid balance chart should be maintained:

- The registered nurse or other registered practitioner to determine the need for a fluid balance chart. All clients receiving IV fluids should be given a fluid balance chart.
- Inform the client, their carers and all other staff involved in the care about the fluid balance chart.
- Measure intake from all sources, i.e. oral fluids, IV fluids, enteral feeds (including water used to flush the tube), fluid medication and liquid food (e.g. soup).
- Accurately measure output from all sources, i.e. urine output (bedpan, urinal or catheter), nasogastric drainage, drainage tubes, diarrhoea, wound drainage and vomit.
- Record input and output on the chart.
- At the end of each 24-hour period, total the client's input and output values. Higher input values compared to output values indicate a positive fluid balance, whereas lower input values compared to output values indicate a negative fluid balance.
- Weigh the patient daily at the same time and in the same clothes. Sudden and acute weight changes are indicative of fluid gains/losses. One litre of water weighs 1 kg. These changes can then be assessed against the fluid balance record from each day.
- Significant changes in the client's input and output need to be reported to the registered nurse and doctor in case further monitoring or intervention is required.

Urine output that falls below 30 mL/hour over two consecutive hours can be indicative of renal failure, internal bleeding or dehydration. Further investigations and treatment would be urgently started if this occurs.

Maintaining fluid intakes

Fluid balance in adults normally comprises of an input of 2400 mL and an output of 2400 mL; however, this can vary from day to day.

Oral intakes

After assessing and determining a client's needs the most obvious method of ensuring their fluid intake is to give adequate amounts of oral fluids. Many of the issues that relate to ensuring adequate nutritional intakes in practice will also apply to maintaining oral

Table 6.4 Assessment of fluid status.

Observation	Fluid excess	Dehydration
History of recent fluid balance[a]	Reduced urine output (oliguria) No urine output (anuria) Excessive urine output (polyuria) NB: Oliguria/anuria can occur in conditions such as renal failure and will cause an excess of fluid in the body	Reduced urine output (oliguria) No urine output (anuria) Excessive urine output (polyuria) Diarrhoea Vomiting Polydipsia (excessive thirst) Excessive faecal fistula losses Unable to eat or drink normally NB: Oliguria/anuria will normally occur in dehydrated clients. However conditions such as diabetes mellitus can lead to polyuria and that can cause dehydration if intake is not maintained A faecal fistula can occur when a tract develops from the bowel to the abdominal surface where it oozes faecal fluid. This may occur after bowel surgery or in certain cancers
Physical assessment[a]	Firm, protruding eyeballs Oedema Ascites Bounding pulse Taut shiny skin	Sunken eyeballs Dry and flaky skin Dry cracked mouth Weak thready pulse

(*Continued*)

Table 6.4 (*Continued*)

Observation	Fluid excess	Dehydration
Vital signs[b]		
Blood pressure	Increased	Decreased (especially on standing)
Pulse	Increased	Increased
Temperature	Unchanged	Elevated
Respirations	Increased rate	Unchanged or increased
Key laboratory findings[b]		
Urine-specific gravity	Decreased (around 1.003)	Increased (around 1.025 or more)
Serum sodium	Less than 135 mmol/L	Greater than 145 mmol/L
Hourly urine output[b]	More than 60 mL/hour NB: normally hydrated individuals can have an output above 60 mL/hour	Less than 30–50 mL/hour NB: this may not be the case if the client has polyuria due to diabetes mellitus
Weight[b] This must be assessed in the context of a client's nutritional status. Acute losses and increases (over hours/a few days) are usually associated with fluid movement	A 5% gain	A loss of 2–6% may indicate dehydration

[a] These observations are based on a subjective or personal view of the client's presentation and as such may not always be accurate.
[b] These observations are based on more objective measurements and offer a more accurate means of determining fluid status.

fluid intakes. The RCN and NPSA (2007) have jointly detailed a number of practical tips to encourage water consumption in the clinical areas.

The following are a summary of these tips:

- Develop a policy on water provision and monitoring for patients
- Free fresh water should be available for patients and staff throughout the day
- Use picture reminders for the nursing staff to encourage water intakes
- Use a positive approach with patients to promote them to drink more
- Serve fresh and chilled water. The use of water coolers may be an option and a slice of citrus fruit may help improve vitamin C consumption
- Try a little and often offer water at mealtimes and also between meals. Offer larger volumes of water when giving medication and encourage patients to drink from early in the morning
- Offer water alongside tea and coffee. Hot water with a piece of fruit can appeal to those wanting a hot drink
- Remember older people and those who are sick can lose their thirst response
- Encourage carers and family to promote hydration with the client
- As the weather gets warmer, increase the availability of water and encourage greater intakes
- Identify those at risk of dehydration and those requiring assistance with drinking. Use strategies for confused patients to help them consume water
- Monitor and record fluid intake
- Keep trying – sometimes it takes times and patience

Intravenous therapy

For some clients it will not be possible to maintain an adequate oral intake. In this case IV therapy will be an important means of ensuring adequate fluid intakes. The choice of fluid will be determined by the client's condition and must be prescribed. There are a variety of IV fluids that are used to maintain electrolyte and fluid balance. *Normal saline* contains water and the electrolytes sodium and chloride. In this solution, there is specifically 0.9 g of sodium chloride per 100 mL of water. Other solutions contain glucose and water only (sometimes called a dextrose solution since dextrose is another term for glucose). A 5% glucose solution contains 5 g of glucose in 100 mL of water. There are also other forms of IV fluids that have combinations of glucose and saline and some that contain sodium lactate or sodium bicarbonate. The choice and amount of IV fluid for fluid replacement is dependent on the patient's condition and will be influenced by their blood results.

There are specific management issues related to IV infusions that are beyond the scope of this chapter.

Conclusion

This chapter has examined how to adequately maintain clients' nutrition and hydration while they are in hospital or residential care. The importance of nutritional and fluid assessment and screening has been addressed. The specific components that need to be considered when carrying out such assessments have also been discussed. A wide range of interventions have been considered to ensure that clients receive the most appropriate nutritional and fluid balance care.

Glossary

Accountability	A term used to mean to be counted on or to being able to be counted
Catabolism	The metabolic breakdown of complex molecules
Calories	Units of energy
Dementia	A progressive decline in cognitive function
Dysphagia	Difficulty in swallowing
Governance	A framework whereby NHS organisations are accountable for continuously improving quality
Haemorrhage	Bleeding, loss of blood
Insulin	A hormone that has an effect on metabolism and other body systems
Intravenous	The giving of liquid directly into a vein
Metabolism	Chemical reactions that occur in living organisms
Risk	The potential negative impact of something
Sepsis	Whole body inflammation
Stricture	Narrowing of a blood vessel or tubular organ

Post-chapter quiz

1. Why is it important to measure fluid intake and output?
2. What cultural influences may affect a person's nutritional status?
3. What signs could indicate a person has lost weight?
4. What is the role and function of the speech and language therapist?
5. List the key actions that will assist the client in their eating and drinking
6. Describe three specialist means of support that can be provided to clients to promote their nutritional status
7. Why is it important to monitor a client's nutritional status?
8. What impact might sepsis have on a client's nutrition?
9. What does NaCl 0.9% w/v mean?

References

Age Concern (2006) *Hungry to be Heard*. London: Age Concern.

American Geriatrics Society, British Geriatrics Society and American Academy of Orthopaedic Surgeons Panel on Falls Prevention (2001) Guidelines for the prevention of falls in older persons. *Journal of the American Geriatrics Society* 49: 664-672.

Anti, M., Pignataro, G., Armuzzi, A., Valenti, A., Iascone, E., Marmo, R., Lamaszza, A., Pretaroli, A.R., Pace, V., Leo, P., Castelli, A. and Gasbarrini, G. (1998) Water supplementation enhances the effect of high-fibre diet on stool frequency and laxative consumption in adult patients with function constipation. *Hepato-Gastroenterology* 45: 727–732.

Association of Community Health Councils (1997) *Health News Briefing: Hungry in Hospital.* London: Association of Community Health Councils.

Bowling, T. (ed) (2004) *Nutritional Support for Adults and Children: A Handbook for Hospital Practice.* Oxford: Radcliffe Medical Press.

British Association for Parenteral and Enteral Nutrition (2003) *Screening Tool for Adults at Risk of Malnutrition.* Maidenhead: BAPEN.

British Association for Parenteral and Enteral Nutrition (2008) *Nutrition Screening Survey in the UK in 2007: A Report by BAPEN.* Maidenhead: British Association of Parenteral and Enteral Nutrition.

Burge, M.R., Garcia, N., Qualis, C.R. and Schade, D.S. (2001) Differential effects of fasting and dehydration in the pathogenesis of diabetic ketoacidosis. *Metabolism* 50: 171–177.

Casimiro, C., Garcia-de-Lorenzo, A. and Usan, L. (2002) Prevalence of decubitus ulcer and associated risk factors in an institutionalzed Spanish elderly population. *Nutrition* 18: 408–414.

Chan, J., Knutsen, S.F., Blix, G.G., Lee, J.W. and Fraser, G.E. (2002) Water, other fluids, and fatal coronary heart disease. *American Journal of Epidemiology* 155: 827–833.

Commission for Social Care Inspection (CSCI) (2006) *Highlight of the day? Improving Meals for Older People in Care Homes.* London: CSCI.

Craig, R. and Shelton, N. (eds) (2007) *Health Survey for England.* Leeds: The NHS Information Centre.

Delmi, M., Rapin, C.H., Bengoa, J.M., Delmas, P.D., Vasey, P. and Bonjour, J.P. (1990) Dietary supplementation in elderly patients with fractured neck of femur. *The Lancet* 335: 1013–1016.

Department of Health (2001a) *The Essence of Care: Patient Focussed Benchmarking for Health Professionals.* London: HMSO.

Department of Health (2001b) *Better Hospital Food Programme.* Press Release 21.9.01. London: DH.

Department of Health (2004b) *NHS Standards for Better health.* London: TSO.

Department of Health (2007) *Improving Nutritional Care. A Joint Action Plan from the Department of Health and Nutrition Summit Stakeholders.* London: COI.

Department of Health (2008) *Healthy Weight, Healthy Lives: A Cross Government Strategy for England.* London: TSO.

Dyer, O. (2002) News: first case of type 2 diabetes found in white UK teenagers. *British Medical Journal* 324: 506.

Eberhardie, C. (2000) *Practical Eating and Feeding Skills. NT Clinical Monograph.* London: Nursing Times Books.

Eckford, S.D., Keane, D.P., Lamond, E., Jackson, S.R. and Abrams, P. (1995) Hydration monitoring in the prevention of idiopathic urinary tract infections in premenopausal women. *British Journal of Urology* 76: 90–93.

Healthcare Commission (2006) Caring for dignity. *A National Report on Dignity in Care for Older People in Hospital.* London: Healthcare Commission.

House of Commons Health Committee (2004) *Obesity – Volume 1. HCP 23-I, Third Report of Session 2003–04. Report, together with Formal Minutes.* London: TSO

Kinney, J.M. (1995) Metabolic response to starvation, injury and sepsis. In: Payne-James, J., Grimble, G. and Silk, D. (eds). *Artificial Nutrition Support in Clinical Practice.* London: Edward Arnold.

Kleiner, S.M. (1999) Water: an essential but overlooked nutrient. *Journal of the American Dietetic Association* 99: 201–207.

Math, M.V., Rampal, P.M., Faure, X.R. and Delmont, J.P. (1986) Gallbladder emptying after drinking water and its possible role in prevention of gallstone formation. *Singapore Medical Journal* 27: 531–532.

McGillivray, T. and Marland, G. (1999) Assisting demented patients with feeding: problems in a ward environment. A review of the literature. *Journal of Advanced Nursing* 29(3): 608–614.

McLaren, S. (2003) Disease related malnutrition. In: *The Nursing Times: Nutrition a Practical Guide*. London: Emap.

National Institute for Clinical Excellence (2006) *Nutrition Support for Adults Oral Nutrition Support, Enteral Tube Feeding and Parenteral Nutrition*. London: National Collaborating Centre for Acute Care, Royal College of Surgeons.

National Patient Safety Agency (NPSA) (2005) *Patient and Carer Briefing: Checking the Position of Naso-gastric Feeding Tubes*. Patient Briefing 05, NPSA.

Nursing and Midwifery Council (NMC) (2008) *The Code: Standards of Conduct, Performance and Ethics for Nurses and Midwives*. London: NMC.

Reilly, H.M., Martineau, J.K., Moran, A. and Kennedy, H. (1995) Nutritional screening – evaluation and implementation of a simple nutrition risk score. *Clinical Nutrition* 14: 269–273.

Reilly, J.J., Hull, S.F., Albert, N., Waller, A. and Bringardener, S. (1988) Economic impact of malnutrition: a model system for hospitalised patients. *Journal of Parenteral and Enteral Nutrition* 12: 371–376.

Revicki, D.A. and Israel, R.G. (1986) Relationship between body mass indices and measure of body adiposity. *American Journal of Public Health* 76: 992–994.

Robshaw, V. and Marbrow, S. (1995) Raising awareness of patients' nutritional state. *Professional Nurse* 11(1): 41–42.

Royal College of Nursing (1993) *Nutrition Standards and the Older Adult*. RCN Dynamic Quality Improvement Programme. London: Royal College of Nursing.

Royal College of Nursing (2007) *Enhancing Nutritional Care: Nutrition Now*. London: Royal College of Nursing.

Royal College of Nursing and National Patient Safety Agency (2007) Water for Health: Hydration Best Practice Toolkit for Hospitals and Healthcare. Available at http://www.waterforhealth.org.uk/. Accessed 18 December 2008.

Sidenvall, B. and Ek, A.C. (1993) Long term care patients and their dietary intake related to eating ability and nutritional needs: nursing staff interventions. *Journal of Advanced Nursing* 18: 565–573.

Sullivan, D.H., Sun, S. and Walls, R.C. (1999) Protein energy undernutrition among elderly hospitalised patients. *Journal of the American Medical Association* 281(21): 2013–2019.

Thomas, D.R., Tariq, S.H., Makhdomm, S., Haddad, R. and Moinuddin, A. (2004) Physician misdiagnosis of dehydration in older adults. *Journal of the American Medical Directors Association* 5: S31–S34.

Veterans Affairs Total Parenteral Nutrition Study Group (1991) Perioperative total parenteral nutrition in surgical patients. *New England Journal of Medicine* 325: 525–532.

Chapter 7
Elimination – Alimentary and Urinary Tract

Muralitharan Nair

Learning opportunities

This chapter will help you:

1. Identify the organs associated with the gastrointestinal tract
2. List the accessory organs of digestion and the functions of the stomach
3. Discuss mechanical and chemical digestion
4. Describe the care of patients with gastrointestinal disorders
5. List the functions of the kidneys
6. Describe the care of patients with common renal disorders

Pre-chapter quiz

1. List the functions of the gastrointestinal tract
2. What is the difference between mechanical and chemical digestion?
3. List the functions of the liver
4. Describe the endocrine and exocrine functions of the pancreas
5. List the structures associated with the renal system and describe their function
6. Describe the differences between the male and female urinary tracts
7. Discuss the causes of retention of urine
8. Discuss the nursing care of patients with renal disorders
9. List the equipment needed to insert a urinary catheter
10. What are the principles of care associated with safe and effective catheter care?

Introduction

The alimentary tract, also known as the digestive system, is composed of the gastrointestinal tract and the accessory organs of digestion. It involves the mouth, the salivary glands, pharynx, oesophagus, stomach, intestines, liver, pancreas and the gallbladder (Tortora and Derrickson, 2007). The main function of the alimentary tract is to provide nutrients, water and electrolytes for the body. These are obtained from food and fluids

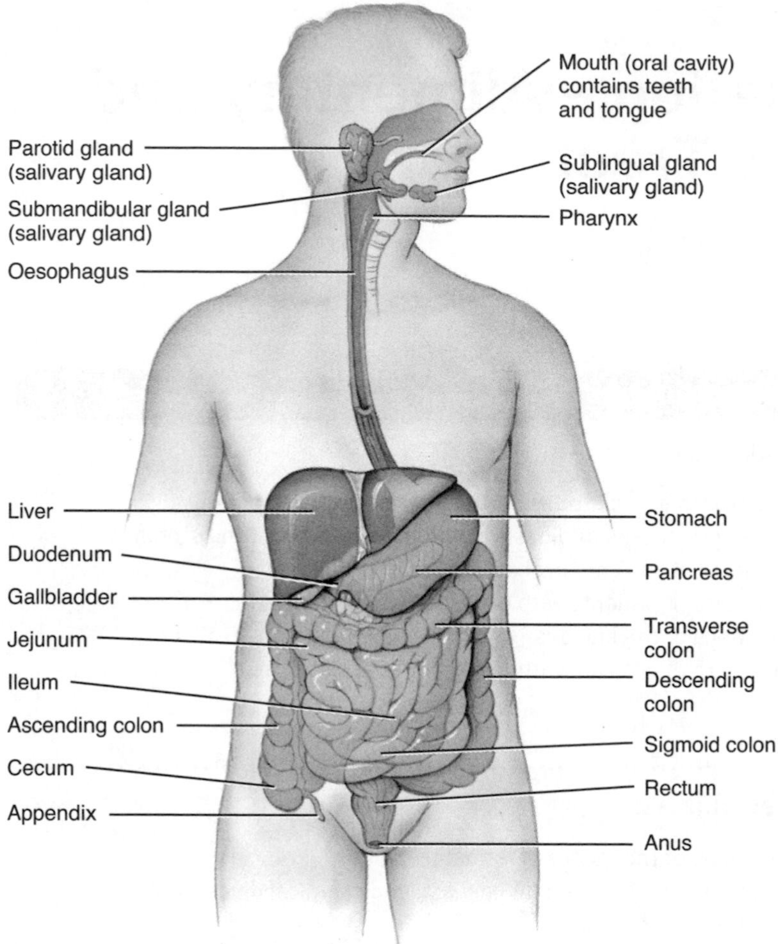

Figure 7.1 The alimentary tract. (Reproduced from Nair and Peate, 2009, with permission of Wiley-Blackwell.)

drunk; in order to carry out this function the gastrointestinal tract performs roles of digestion, absorption and the elimination of unwanted materials (see Figure 7.1).

The breaking down of food and making it soluble is called digestion (Clancy and McVicar, 2002). This involves two processes: mechanical and chemical. Mechanical processes break down large pieces of food into smaller food substances, while chemical processes break the food substances into simpler substances. The soluble substances are then absorbed to provide nutrients for the cells of body tissue. Any undigested food, water, bacteria and dead cells of the lining of the digestive tract are then eliminated.

The alimentary tract is a continuous tract and is approximately 10 m long from the mouth to the anus. The small intestine is around 6 m long and the large intestine is in the region of 1.5 m long (Mader, 2005). The accessory organs of digestion lie outside the tract and they secrete various chemicals that aid digestion. The accessory organs are the salivary glands, liver, pancreas and the gallbladder. They produce various enzymes which help the breakdown of foodstuffs. For example, salivary amylase (ptyalin) will act on sugars and starch in the diet, while pepsin will act on proteins. Other accessory organs include the lips, teeth, tongue and the palate. Thus the action of the digestive tract includes:

- Mastication of foodstuff eaten
- Involuntary movement called peristalsis along the digestive tract
- Conversion of large nutrient molecules into smaller molecules (digestion)
- Absorption of nutrients
- Elimination of any undigested and unwanted material

This chapter is concerned with a brief anatomy and physiology of the gastrointestinal tract, some of the common problems associated with this system and the nursing management related to it.

The oral cavity

Mouth

The mouth is the beginning of the alimentary canal. It receives food and the mechanical breakdown of food particles begins here. The broken-down food particles are mixed with saliva (Shier et al., 2004), which is a watery and tasteless fluid. The function of saliva is to lubricate food, keep the mouth clean and help the breakdown of carbohydrate with the aid of the enzyme salivary amylase. The activity of breaking down foodstuff and mixing it with saliva is called mastication. This broken-down foodstuff is then swallowed where it enters the stomach via the oesophagus. The mouth is also surrounded by lips, gums, teeth, cheeks, tongue and the palate. The space between the tongue and the palate is the cavity of the mouth and the space between the lips, gums, teeth and the cheeks is called the vestibule.

Lips

The lips form the orifice of the mouth. They form fleshy folds, which contain skeletal muscles and sensory receptors (Shier et al., 2004). These structures help in assessing the temperature and texture of foods eaten. The reddish colour of the lips is a result of numerous blood vessels. The junction between the upper and the lower lips forms the angle of the mouth.

Cheeks

The cheeks form the fleshy sides of the face and they run from the corner of the mouth to the side of the nose. Subcutaneous fat, muscles and mucous membranes line the cheeks. They assist in the chewing of food.

Palate

The palate is divided into two – the hard and the soft palate – and they both form the roof of the mouth while the tongue lies at the bottom of the oral cavity and forms the floor of the mouth. Both the hard and the soft palates are covered by mucous membranes.

Tongue

The tongue is a thick muscular organ composed of skeletal muscles and mucous membranes. It contains approximately 10 000 taste buds (Silverthorn, 1998), which tell us about the taste of the food we eat, for example whether the food is sweet or sour. The tongue detects four basic tastes: sweet, salt, bitter and sour (Marieb and Hoehn, 2007). Silverthorn (1998) identified a fifth taste called umami. This word is derived from the Japanese word meaning 'deliciousness'. This taste is associated with glutamate and some nucleotides. Hence in some Asian countries sometimes monosodium glutamate (MSG) is used to enhance flavour when cooking (Silverthorn, 1998).

The tongue is an accessory organ which forms the floor of the mouth; it helps to blend food when chewing and helps to push food particles to the back of the mouth when swallowing. Tongue movement can alter the volume of the oral cavity and also forms an important role in speech.

Teeth

Humans develop two sets of teeth: these are milk teeth and permanent teeth. There are approximately 20 milk teeth and they begin to develop usually, from the age of 6 months. Often one pair of milk teeth grows per month and they usually fall out between the ages of 6 and 12 years. Once the milk teeth fall out, they are replaced by permanent teeth. Usually there are 32 permanent teeth and they have the potential to last our lifetime. However permanent molars do not replace milk teeth. The first permanent molars appear at the age of 6 years, the second at the age of 12 years and the third may develop after the age of 13 years.

Pharynx

The pharynx lies behind the nose, mouth and the larynx. It is about 12 cm in length and is divided into three sections: the nasopharynx, the oral pharynx and the laryngeal pharynx. There are seven openings into the pharynx (Mader, 2005). These include the mouth, larynx, oesophagus, two small nasal cavities and two Eustachian tubes. When a person swallows food, the soft palate closes the nasal passages and the epiglottis moves over the glottis to close the larynx and the trachea. This allows the foodstuff to move down the oesophagus and not the respiratory tract.

Oesophagus

The oesophagus is a muscular tube approximately 25 cm long, running from the pharynx to the stomach. It lies posterior to the trachea and in front of the spinal column (backbone). The oesophagus is sometimes known as the food pipe (Mader, 2005). This is a collapsible muscular tube that channels food into the stomach. The movement of food down the oesophagus occurs due to peristaltic action. It is not possible for a person to both swallow and breathe at the same time; this part of swallowing is a reflex action.

Stomach

Stomach is a 'J' shaped muscular organ situated below the diaphragm. It consists of four regions: the upper portion is called the cardiac region, an elevated part called the fundus, a middle section called the body and a pyloric region (Marieb and Hoehn, 2007) (see Figure 7.2). The stomach expands and stores food. While the food is in the stomach it churns and mixes the food with various digestive juices. Approximately 2–3 L of digestive juices are produced per day by the stomach.

Normally the walls of the stomach are protected by thick mucous membranes. However, when hydrochloric acid (HCl) penetrates the wall, an ulcer can develop which can cause severe problems for the individual.

The stomach normally empties its contents in 2–6 hours. The contents emptied from the stomach are thick, pasty, semi-solid and acidic, this substance is called chyme. Chyme leaves the stomach by way of the pyloric sphincter and enters the small intestine.

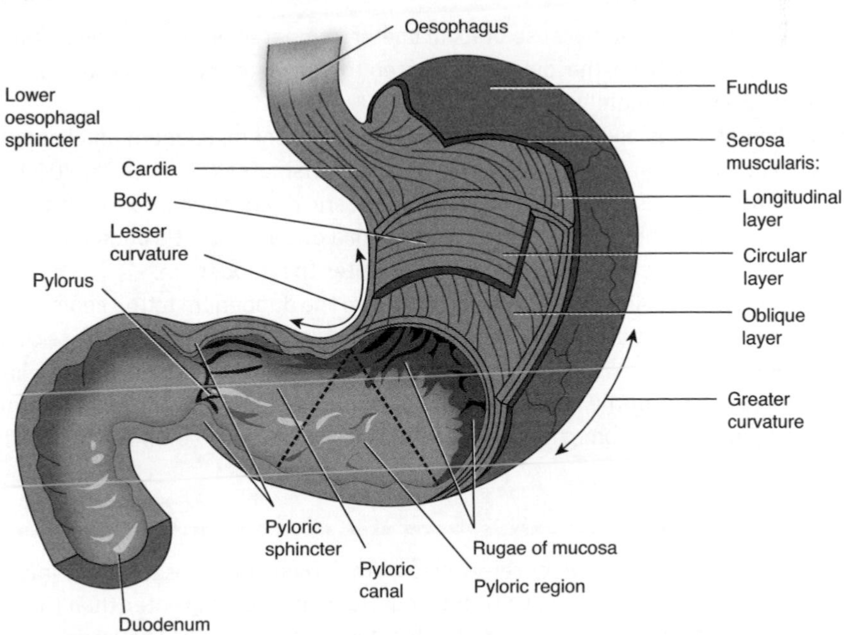

Figure 7.2 The regions of the stomach. (Reproduced from Nair and Peate, 2009, with permission of Wiley-Blackwell.)

Digestion

Digestion can be divided into physical and chemical digestion. The food entering the stomach does not leave straight away. It must be broken down and only a small quantity at a time is passed via the pylorus. The stomach with its unique action churns food. This action is the result of the three muscle layers in the stomach: longitudinal, circular and oblique muscles. This movement of the stomach is called the physical action of the stomach.

While in the stomach, various digestive enzymes also help to break down the food, thus helping in chemical digestion. During chemical digestion, semi-solid food particles are rendered into a semi-liquid form. Enzymes like pepsin, for example, act on proteins and then convert them to peptones, gastric lipase begins the digestion of fats and rennin converts the soluble protein of milk into an insoluble form.

Summary of the functions of the stomach

- Reservoir for food
- All food is liquefied, broken down and mixed with HCl
- Proteins are converted into peptones
- Milk is curdled and casein is set free
- Digestion of fats begins in the stomach
- Chyme is passed into the duodenum via the pylorus
- Anti-anaemic factor called vitamin B_{12} is formed in the stomach

Small intestine

Small intestine is so named because of its diameter compared with the large intestine's diameter. It extends from the pyloric sphincter to the ileocaecal valve of the large intestine and is approximately 3 m in length.

The small intestine is divided into three sections: duodenum, jejunum and ileum. The duodenum is approximately 20 cm long and 5 cm in diameter (Shier et al., 2004) and is said to be horseshoe shaped. The bile and pancreatic ducts open into the duodenum, approximately 10 cm from the pylorus, via the ampulla of Vater. It is through this channel that bile from the liver and the pancreatic juices enter the duodenum.

The jejunum is almost 2.5 m long and extends from the duodenum to the ileum (Marieb and Hoehn, 2007). It occupies two-fifths of the small intestine and the ileum occupies the last three-fifths. There is no distinct separation between the jejunum and the ileum. However, the diameter of the jejunum is greater, the wall of the jejunum is thicker, more vascular and more active compared to the ileum. See Table 7.1 for summary of digestion.

Large intestine

The large intestine is also known or referred to as the colon. It frames the small intestine and extends from the ileocecal valve to the anus. Its diameter is greater than the small intestine but is shorter in length, 1.5 m (Marieb and Hoehn, 2007). The large intestine consists of the caecum, to which the vermiform appendix is attached, colon, rectum and the anal canal. The colon is divided into the ascending, transverse, descending and sigmoid colon.

Table 7.1 Summary of organs and digestion.

Organ	Digestive fluid	pH	Enzymes	Function of enzymes
Mouth	Saliva	Slightly acidic	Salivary amylase	Commences the breakdown of starch
Stomach	Gastric juice	Acidic	(a) Rennin	Converts caseinogens into casein
			(b) Pepsin	Converts proteins into peptose
			(c) Gastric lipase	Begins hydrolysis of fats
Duodenum	Bile	Alkaline		Emulsifies fats
	Pancreatic juice	Alkaline	(a) Trypsin	Reduces proteins and peptones into polypeptides and amino acids
			(b) Pancreatic amylase	Converts sugars and starches into maltose
			(c) Lipase	Reduces fats into glycerine and fatty acids
Small intestine	Intestinal juice	Alkaline	(a) Enteropeptidase	Activates trypsinogen
			(b) Erepsin	Converts proteins into amino acids
			(c) Maltase, lactase	Converts carbohydrates into monosaccharides

Summary of the functions of the colon

- Absorption of water, glucose and electrolytes
- Secretion of mucin by the glands of the inner coat
- Preparation of cellulose which is a carbohydrate present in plants, fruits and vegetables
- Defecation

The accessory organs

Salivary glands

These glands secrete saliva, which helps moisten food particles, binds them together and begins chemical digestion of carbohydrates. Saliva is watery and it helps to maintain the pH in the mouth, which is alkaline, and to keep the mouth clean.

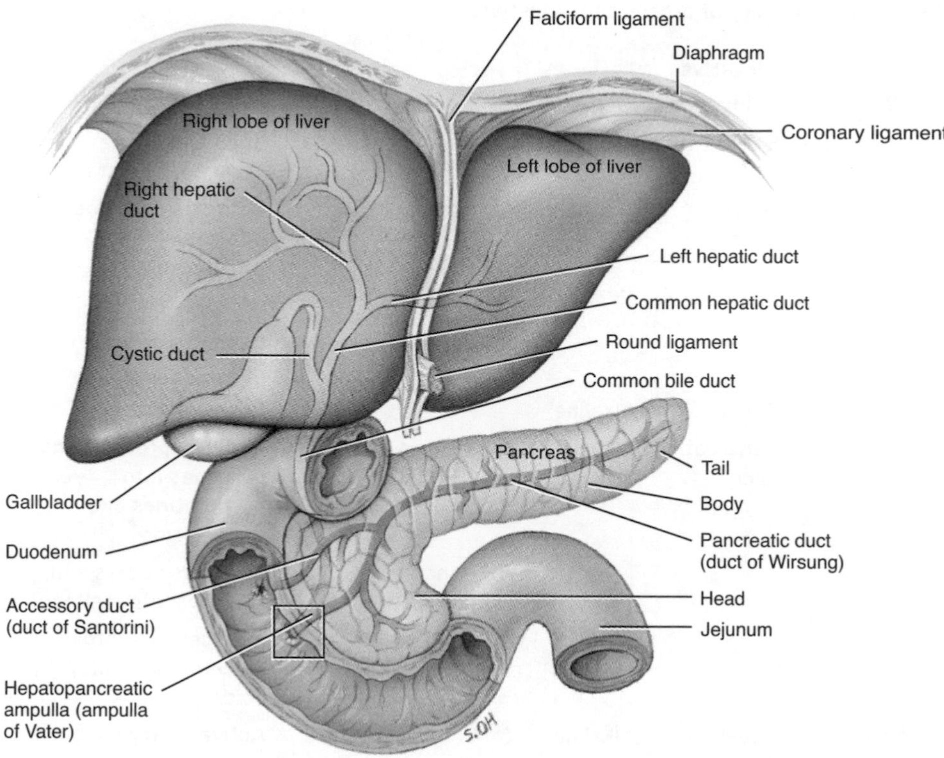

Figure 7.3 The liver, pancreas and the gallbladder. (Reproduced from Nair and Peate, 2009, with permission of Wiley-Blackwell.)

Liver

The liver is the largest gland in the body (see Figure 7.3). It is situated in the upper right quadrant of the abdominal cavity beneath the diaphragm. It is partially protected by the ribs. The liver is reddish brown in colour and is a vascular organ. In an adult it weighs about 1.5 kg.

Some functions of the liver

- Concerned with the metabolism of the body through chemical reactions from the absorbed nutrients
- Modifies waste products and toxic substances, i.e. drugs such as paracetamol, aspirin and alcohol
- Produces and stores glycogen
- Maintains blood sugar levels
- Produces bile, which emulsifies fats in the diet for absorption
- Forms urea, which is a waste product
- Forms red blood cells in fetal life
- Plays a part in the destruction of red blood cells
- Stores iron and vitamins A, D and B_{12}
- Manufactures plasma proteins

- Produces prothrombins
- Produces anticoagulants

Gallbladder

The gallbladder is a pear-shaped muscular sac, which lies underneath the liver (see Figure 7.3). It is divided into the fundus, the body and the neck. The gallbladder is around 7–9 cm in length and its main function is to store and concentrate bile. Bile is an alkaline fluid produced by the liver and its function is to *emulsify* fats.

Pancreas

The pancreas is a triangular-shaped organ. It is more or less 12–15 cm in length and about 2.5 cm thick. It is divided into three parts: the head, the body and the tail (see Figure 7.3). The head of the pancreas lies in the loop of the duodenum and the tail touches the spleen (Marieb and Hoehn, 2007). It has dual functions: *exocrine* and *endocrine*.

Exocrine functions

- Production of pancreatic juices
- Production of digestive enzymes, i.e. pancreatic amylase for the digestion of starch trypsin for the digestion of proteins and lipase for the digestion of fats

Endocrine functions

- Production of the hormone glucagon by the alpha cells
- Production of the hormone insulin by the beta cells
- Production of hormone somatostatin by the delta cells

Care of patients with gastrointestinal disorders

This aspect of the chapter provides the reader with insight concerning some common disorders of the gastrointestinal tract and outlines the nursing care of patients with gastrointestinal disorders.

Gingivitis

Gingivitis is also known as the inflammation of the gums and may lead to ulceration and necrosis of the gums. Gingivitis may be caused by plaque. Plaque is a sticky substance deposited on the exposed portions of the teeth, consisting of bacteria, food particles and mucous (Kozier et al., 2008). Other possible causes of gingivitis could be the vigorous brushing and flossing of the teeth. Some individuals who suffer from diabetes mellitus and certain women who are pregnant can develop gingivitis, which may be due to hormonal changes.

Predisposing factors

These may be due to poor oral hygiene whereby bacteria infect the gums, and the toxins produced by the bacteria may cause gingivitis. Long-term plaque deposits may also cause inflammation of the gums. Dental plaques are a type of sticky material on the teeth made up of mucin and colloid materials found in the saliva. Plaques can mineralise into hard deposits called tartar and accumulate at the base of the teeth. Thus poor dental hygiene is also one of the causes of gingivitis. Certain drugs, such as phenytoin, some birth control pills and ingestion of heavy metals, such as lead and bismuth, may cause inflammation of the gums. Bad-fitting orthodontic appliances, i.e. dentures, bridges and crowns, can irritate the gums and cause inflammation leading to gingivitis.

Clinical symptoms

- Swollen and painful gums, tender when touched
- Bleeding from the gums and blood may be visible on the toothbrush even with gentle brushing
- Excessive salivation
- Bad breath (halitosis)
- Gums may appear shiny and/or bright red

Treatment

A dentist should always be consulted when signs of gingivitis are suspected. The dentist may use dental instruments to remove the plaques and to clean the teeth. Meticulous oral hygiene is essential after visiting the dentist. The dentist or the dental hygienist will demonstrate the correct method of brushing and flossing the teeth. The mouth should be rinsed using copious amounts of water after brushing and flossing.

The nurse should encourage those people who are at risk of contracting gingivitis to brush and floss their teeth after each meal. This will help to remove any food particles that may become lodged between teeth. When people are unable to do this for themselves, the nurse must do this for them.

Sialolithiasis

Sialolithiasis are stones in the salivary gland and is the most common disease of the salivary gland (Iro et al., 1992). According to Cawson and Odell (1998), males are likely to be more affected than females and children are rarely affected. Sialolithiasis generally occurs within the submaxillary gland. The stones are often composed of calcium oxalate and are irregular in shape, whilst those in the ducts are small and oval in shape.

Predisposing factors

The exact aetiology and pathogenesis of sialolithiasis is unknown. They are thought to occur when stagnated in calcium-rich saliva in the salivary glands (Siddiqui, 2002). The stagnation may be due to:

- Glandular infection
- Inflammation of the ducts
- Trauma to the ducts

Clinical signs and symptoms

This condition is asymptomatic unless there is evidence of infection. The glands may be swollen and tender to touch. Pain may occur at mealtimes when the salivary glands secrete saliva to lubricate the food for mastication and swallowing and in response to other salivary stimuli. Other symptoms include palpable stones in the submandibular glands, excess salivation and the visibility of stones on X-ray (Siddiqui, 2002).

Treatment

Patients presenting with sialolithiasis may benefit from conservative treatment especially when the stones are small. If the condition is due to bacterial infection, a suitable antibiotic such as penicillin may be necessary as prescribed.

If the stones are large then they need to be removed surgically and in some cases when the condition reoccurs the affected gland may need to be removed. As Siddiqui (2002) suggests, the pain and swelling may be treated conservatively with medications such as non-steroidal anti-inflammatory drugs, i.e. ibuprofen.

Constipation

Constipation is the passing of hard and dry stools in small quantities. The frequency of the motion can be less than three times per week (Lemone and Burke, 2008). The causes of constipation are many and varied. Constipation may be due to a particular life style, organic diseases or functional disorders of the colon.

Predisposing factors

Poor dietary habits can lead to constipation when the diet is highly refined, with very little fibre and inadequate fluid intake (Dougherty and Lister, 2008). Fibre in the diet helps to form faecal bulk and water helps to keep the stool soft. Diseases of the large bowel, i.e. tumours, adhesions, diverticular disease and anal strictures, are some of the pathological problems that could cause constipation. Opioid drugs, i.e. morphine, may cause constipation (Lemone and Burke, 2008). Therefore, patients should be advised of the potential side effects and what they might do to avoid constipation. Other factors associated with constipation include:

- Poor fluid intake
- Lack of exercise
- Neurological disorders such as multiple sclerosis
- Psychological problems, i.e. depression

Clinical signs and symptoms

- Abdominal pain
- Abdominal distension
- Loss of appetite
- Complaints of nausea and vomiting
- Hard and dry faecal matter (if produced)

Nursing care

The patient must be assessed carefully by the nurses in order to ascertain likes and dislikes of food. If it is a dietary problem causing constipation then food high in fibre should be recommended, unless contraindicated. Vegetables and fresh fruits are a good source of fibre and they should form part of the diet (Winney, 1998). Fibre helps to form bulk and draws water into the stool, which helps to soften the stool and make defaecation easier.

Peate (2003) states that bulk laxatives such as fybogel are the fist line of treatment when managing constipation. They help peristalsis of the colon and thus reduce the time for the faeces to move through the colon. However, McCuistion and Gutierrez (2002) state that bulk laxatives should not be given to patients with gastrointestinal disorders such as bowel obstruction, acute abdominal pain and to those who have had recent bowel surgery.

If necessary laxatives, i.e. lactulose, suppositories or phosphate enemas, are given to assist in bowel evacuation, these medications need to be prescribed, prior to administration. The patients should be encouraged by the nurse to drink at least 2000–3000 mL of fluid daily for normal faecal elimination (Kozier et al., 2008). This daily intake of fluid would increase the water content of chyme and move the chyme more quickly in the large intestine, which gives less time for fluid absorption to take place and as a result the stool may be soft (Kozier et al., 2008).

Mobilisation such as walking should be encouraged if this is not contraindicated or if this is not permissible. Chair-bound exercises such as stretching will help to strengthen abdominal muscles and aid *peristalsis* of the colon, which facilitates the elimination of stool (Winney, 1998).

Enema

Enema is the insertion of liquid into the colon or rectum. There are various types of enemata available. These include cleansing and retention enemas (Smith et al., 2004). An enema must be prescribed prior to administration and adherence to the Nursing and Midwifery Council's (2008a) *Standards for Medicine Management* is required.

Reasons for administering enemata

There are several reasons for the administration of an enema; one of these is to encourage bowel movements in patients who are constipated. Enemata are also given to patients prior to bowel surgery, such as the formation of colostomy and certain investigations, for example sigmoidoscopy.

Nursing care

The nurse must always explain the procedure to the patient in order to ascertain that they understand what is to be done and the reason why it is necessary for administration of the enema. The bed should be screened in order to ensure privacy. If possible, you, the nurse, should ask the patient to empty their bladder as this may reduce discomfort during the procedure. Read the pharmacological information provided by the manufacturer fully and follow their instructions. Warm the fluid to body temperature between 36.5°C to 37°C in a bowel of warm water. Lie the patient on the left side in the Sims' position. This is a position in which the patient lies on the left side with the right knee and thigh drawn upward towards the chest. This facilitates easy insertion of fluid into the rectum and the flow of fluid by gravity into the sigmoid and descending colon (Kozier et al., 2008). Place a protective sheet under the patient's buttocks to protect the bed linen from any spillage.

Wash hands, don gloves and observe infection control procedures as suggested in local procedure and policy. Lubricate the tip of the enema with lubricant and squeeze the enema to expel the air in the bag. Introducing air into the rectum during the procedure may cause discomfort to the patient.

Gently insert the enema into the rectum and squeeze the bag to insert the fluid. Observe the patient for discomfort and pain at all times during the procedure. On completion, gently remove the enema from the rectum while at the same time keep the bag squeezed or rolled up when removing from the rectum. This prevents the liquid flowing back into the bag. Wipe the patient's anal area with tissue and encourage the patient to retain the enema for the appropriate amount of time, for example 5–10 minutes for cleansing enemas and 30 minutes for retention enemas (Kozier et al., 2008).

Ensure that the patient is comfortable, and then dispose of equipment safely and wash your hands. When the patient is ready to defaecate, assist the patient to the toilet, if possible, or give a bedpan or a bedside commode. Document the outcome of the procedure in the nursing care plan. Nurses need to be aware that in undertaking this procedure they are accountable for their actions and that documentation is in accord with the Code of Professional Conduct (NMC, 2008b) and Guidelines for Records and Record Keeping (NMC, 2005).

Suppositories

Reasons for inserting suppositories

Administering medications into the rectum is a common practice (Kozier et al., 2008). Suppositories are given to patients who are constipated to induce bowel movement, to evacuate the bowel prior to surgery and to administer medications such as antibiotics or analgesics (Jamieson et al., 2002) and to patients who are vomiting and therefore cannot take oral medications or those who may have difficulty in swallowing.

Nursing care

Explain the procedure to the patient to gain consent and cooperation for inserting the suppository. The bed should be screened in order to provide privacy; this may also encourage the patient to relax. Place a protective sheet under the patient's buttocks, in case of soiling by stool at the time of insertion of the suppository (Jamieson et al., 2002). Put a glove on the hand used to insert the suppository. Check the prescription chart to ensure that the suppository has been prescribed and that the correct patient is receiving the suppository and that the dose is also what has been prescribed.

Ask the patient to lie on the left side and then gently insert the suppository about 6 cm into the rectum. Moppett (2000) suggests that the blunt end of the suppository should be inserted first as this will help retention of the suppository as the muscles of the anal sphincter close tightly around the pointed end thus helping it to move up into the rectum.

Remove your finger after insertion and wipe the patient's anal region with a tissue. Ask the patient to retain the suppository for at least 30 minutes, or according to the manufacturer's recommendations, before evacuating the contents of the rectum. Dispose of used equipment safely and wash your hands. When the need arises to evacuate the patient's rectum, assist the patient to the toilet or offer a bedpan or a commode, ensuring privacy at all times. Document the outcome in the nursing care plan.

Colostomy

Colostomy is a surgical procedure where an artificial opening (stoma) is created on the abdomen to allow the drainage of stool from the colon. It could be either temporary or permanent. The stoma serves as an artificial anus through which the colon can empty the waste products of digestion. A stoma bag is applied to the colostomy where faecal matter can be collected (Smith et al., 2004) (Box 7.1).

Box 7.1 Sites to be avoided when siting a stoma.

- Umbilical region
- Hip bones
- Old scar/surgical incisions
- Waistline

Reasons for colostomy formation

- When the colon, rectum or the anus does not function normally, for example in cancer of the large bowel, ulcerative colitis and Crohn's disease.
- When the colon, rectum or the anus needs to rest for a period of time. This may be due to inflammation or oedema of the large intestine.
- In certain conditions such as Hirschsprung's disease – a condition in which the nerves controlling bowel function are abnormal or in imperforate anus – an absence of anal opening.
- In severe abdominal injuries, i.e. after road traffic accident and in patients who have had radiation therapy.

Nursing care

A full preoperative assessment is essential to ensure that the patient clearly understands the nature of the surgery and for any questions that the patient may want answered. Helping patients to adjust to altered body image can lead to uneventful recovery post-operatively.

Postoperatively, it is essential to observe the stoma site for bleeding, infection of the stoma site or any other problems such as retraction of the stoma. It is common to find some blood in the ostomy bag in the early postoperative days (Lemone and Burke, 2008). The stoma should appear pink and moist. The nurse must maintain skin integrity by ensuring that the stoma appliance fits well on to the stoma without any leakage, ensure that the skin surrounding the stoma site is clean and dry and provide skin barrier cream if necessary.

The contents of the bag should be observed and any changes such as retraction of the stoma reported to the nurse incharge. Patient education in the care of stoma such as the emptying of the bag when necessary, applying the pouch clamp and changing the stoma bag aids acceptance of the stoma and promotion of independence in the patient (Finlay, 2002). Whether the stoma is temporary or permanent, ultimately, the patient will be responsible for stoma management when discharged.

Changes in dietary habit are not necessary after the formation of a colostomy. If the patient is concerned about an offensive stool and the build-up of gases in the bag then some dietary advice from the dietician may help to alleviate their fear (Marjoram, 1999).

Any changes must be documented accordingly and nursing care plans should be updated as necessary; it is the nurse's responsibility to ensure that all records are accurate and up-to-date (NMC, 2005).

Discharge planning

- Discuss with both patient and relatives (if appropriate) about coping with a colostomy
- Arrange home visits by the stoma care nurse/clinical nurse specialist/nurse consultant
- Provide details about relevant agencies/voluntary agencies
- Give dietary advice, if necessary
- Provide letter for general practitioner and district nurse
- Give outpatient appointment
- Prescribe medications to take home, if necessary
- Ensure a good supply of stoma appliances
- Encourage patient education/health education on stoma care

Renal system

The renal system consists of the kidneys, ureters, bladder and the urethra. These structures ensure that a stable internal environment is maintained for the survival of cells and tissues in the body – homeostasis.

There are two kidneys, one on each side of the spinal column. They are approximately 11 cm long, 5–6 cm wide and 3–4 cm thick (Marieb and Hoehn, 2007). They are said to be 'bean'-shaped organs where the outer border is convex and the inner border is known as the hilum. It is here the renal arteries enter the kidneys. The functional units of the kidneys are called the nephrons and there are about 1.2 million nephrons in each kidney. The kidneys produce urine by filtering blood, which is then channelled into the bladder by the ureters (Marieb and Hoehn, 2007) (see Figure 7.4).

The bladder, a pear-shaped organ, lies in the pelvic cavity. It contains smooth muscle fibres, which stretch as the bladder fills with urine. The position of the bladder varies with age. In infants and younger children the bladder is slightly raised, while in adults it lies in the pelvis. In males, it is anterior to the rectum and in females it is anterior to the vagina and inferior to the uterus. The bladder has a good supply of blood vessels, hence it bleeds heavily in trauma and in bladder surgery. Urine is conveyed from the bladder to the exterior by the urethra (Box 7.2).

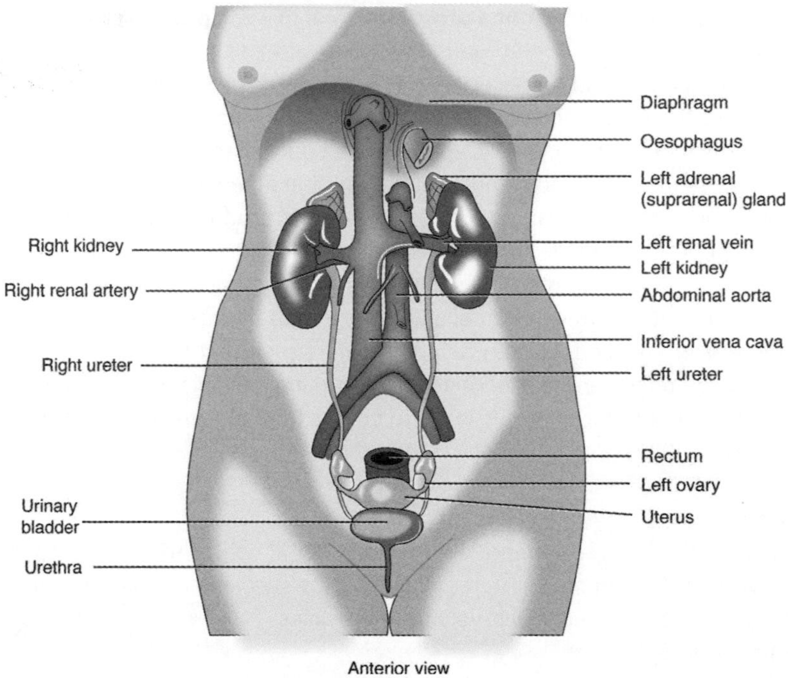

Figure 7.4 The renal system. (Reproduced from Nair and Peate, 2009, with permission of Wiley-Blackwell.)

Box 7.2 Summary of the functions of the kidney.

- Excretes urine and waste products such as urea, uric acid and creatinine
- Regulates fluid balance
- Regulates electrolyte balance
- Maintains pH of blood
- Secrets renin, which helps to regulate blood pressure
- Secretes erythropoietin, which stimulates the production of red blood cells

The prostate gland

Although the prostate gland is not part of the renal system, it does play a part in issues related to elimination of the bladder, hence the reason why the prostate gland is discussed in this section. The prostate resembles the size of a walnut. It lies below the bladder, surrounding the urethra. The prostate gland is very vascular and plays a major role in the male reproductive system. It secretes a thin, milky, alkaline substance which contains two enzymes, namely fibrinolysin and acid phosphatase (Clancy and McVicar, 2002). These enzymes help in the motility of the sperm. Enlargement of this gland, whether malignant or benign, can cause retention of urine.

Care of patients with urological disorders

This aspect of the chapter considers the care of people with urological disorders. Some of the common disorders of the renal system are discussed. The nursing care of those who have a renal disorder is outlined.

Retention of urine

Retention of urine is the inability to pass urine despite the desire to urinate. If untreated, in the long term, urinary retention can cause bladder enlargement and severe cases can affect the ureters and the kidneys, for example hydroureter and hyrdonephrosis (Lemone and Burke, 2008). There are many reasons why individuals cannot void urine.

Causes of retention of urine

- Enlarged prostate gland causing stricture of the urethra
- Urethral stricture due to trauma, urinary tract infection and bladder calculi
- Certain drugs, i.e. antihistamines, antidepressants or antipsychotics
- Some surgery adjacent to the urethra, i.e. abdomino perineal resection
- Neurogenic bladder due to disruption of the nerves to the bladder, multiple sclerosis and faecal impaction

Signs and symptoms

Patients may complain of nocturia, i.e. getting up two or more times during the night to pass urine. They may have difficulty in passing urine (dysuria) and may find that they cannot empty their bladder fully (Kumar and Clark, 2005). The patient may complain of 'dribbling' leading to urine-stained clothing. Incomplete emptying of the bladder can lead to over distention causing loss of muscle tone to the bladder. Haematuria may be present in the urine due to stricture of the urethra (Fickenscher, 1999).

Nursing care

The nurse must undertake a full assessment of the patient and establish when he or she last passed urine. The nurse should obtain a full nursing history in order to establish the cause of retention prior to treating the patient. If urinary retention was not due to mechanical obstructions such as an enlarged prostate or stricture of the urethra, the nurse may attempt to try to make the patient relaxed. If necessary the nurse may need to assist the patient to the toilet so that he or she can have privacy when attempting to void urine. For some patients the sound of running water from a tap may encourage them to pass urine.

Some patients may find it difficult to pass urine postoperatively. This may be due to pain from the surgical incision or they may find it difficult to pass urine when they are lying down in bed. The nurse should determine if the patient is in any pain and if so provide the prescribed analgesia in order to attempt to relax the patient.

If the above measures fail then the patient may need to be catheterised in order to artificially empty his or her bladder. The nurse should observe strict aseptic technique when catheterising a patient and must adhere to local policy and procedures related to the catheterisation of a patient. When the catheter is in situ, the patient should be encouraged to drink at least 2.5 L of fluid per day providing that the patient is not suffering from other physiological problems such as congestive cardiac failure (Wilson, 2001). An accurate record of all fluid intake and urine output must be maintained and recorded on a fluid balance chart; all those involved in caring for the patient should be made aware of the importance of maintaining an accurate fluid balance chart (Walsh, 2002).

Discharge planning

The patient may be discharged once the cause of the problem responsible for the retention of urine is resolved and the patient is able to void urine without the assistance of a urinary catheter. The patient should be encouraged to maintain his or her fluid intake of at least 2.5 L per day. This would promote constant urinary production, which may help to prevent urinary tract infection (Wilson, 2001). The patient should be encouraged to visit the toilet regularly to void and not to ignore the urge to micturate. This could prevent urinary tract infection and the development of an atonic bladder, which could in turn lead to retention of urine.

Bladder irrigation

Bladder irrigation is performed using a three-way urinary catheter. This procedure is undertaken in patients who have undergone, for example, transurethral resection of the prostate gland (TURP). The prostate gland becomes enlarged because of a malignancy or for benign reasons. Patients with an enlarged prostate gland may experience difficulty in voiding urine and can develop retention of urine. These patients may need to undergo TURP to alleviate the problem of urinary retention. Post-TURP patients usually return to the ward with bladder irrigation in situ, bladder irrigation is used postoperatively primarily to remove debris from the bladder (Walsh, 2002).

Nursing care

The nurse should check to ensure that the irrigating fluid is running as prescribed. The drip rate of the irrigating fluid can be adjusted by the roller clamp on the giving set tubing. The rate should be adjusted according to the colour of urine in the catheter bag (Smith et al., 2004). The nurse should increase the rate of fluid if urinary output is dark red and contains blood clots and to decrease the flow rate if the output is pink and clear of clots. The irrigation system must be a closed continuous system and the nurse must ensure that there is no leaking occurring at the connections. The patient is assessed every hour by the nurse to ensure that he or she is not in any discomfort as a result of retention of urine or pain related to surgery.

The drainage systems should be checked half hourly for the first 36–48 hours for patency (Walsh, 2002). The colour, consistency or sediment in drainage should be noted. The urine will be bloodstained for at least for the first 24 hours and gradually become less bloodstained. The nurse must empty the catheter bag as often as is necessary (Dougherty and Lister, 2008) and maintain a strict fluid balance chart. It is important to observe that the volume drained is the same as the volume used for irrigation plus any urine that may be produced. If the volume drained is less than the volume instilled, the nurse incharge must be informed immediately. The rationale for the reduced drainage may be due to obstruction of the drainage tube by a blood clot, which could lead to retention of urine and discomfort for the patient.

Once the patient is fully conscious and is able to tolerate fluids, unless contraindicated the nurse should encourage him or her to drink and gradually increase fluid intake to at least 2-2.5 L of fluid per day. Once the patient is tolerating fluids, bladder irrigation should be discontinued if the urine output is free of blood clots and the urine is draining freely into the urinary drainage bag. Catheter care, as described below, should be provided daily to prevent the possibility of an infection.

Discharge planning

- Encourage the patient to continue taking 2.5 L of fluid daily to ensure that the urine output is clear
- Ask the patient to observe the colour of the urine. If bleeding is observed, he or she should consult his doctor immediately
- Avoid becoming constipated as straining during defaecation could put pressure on the urethral passage and cause bleeding (Walsh, 2002)
- Some would suggest that patients should avoid sex (including masturbation) for about 3 weeks

Catheter hygiene

Urinary catheters are used to remove urine from the bladder or to instil fluid or drugs into the bladder. Urinary catheters come in various sizes and there are different types of catheter made from different types of materials. When catheterising a patient, nurses should ensure that they use the correct size catheter, i.e. 12-4 Fr (Ch) (Marjoram, 1999). A catheter between 10 and 12 Fr (Ch) is recommended for women and between 12 and 14 Fr (Ch) for men. An incorrect catheter size may result in damage to the urethra during insertion and can cause urethral scarring and stricture.

Reasons for catheterisation

- Acute or chronic urinary retention
- Preoperatively and postoperatively in abdominal, rectal and pelvic surgeries
- For administration of drug treatments, for example cytotoxic drugs
- To irrigate the bladder to remove blood clots or sediment

Teflon-coated catheters reduce urethral irritation and may be used for patients who need short- to medium-term catheterisation. This type of catheter may remain in situ for up to 1 month. Silicone catheters have a longer life span compared to Teflon-coated catheters, which may remain in situ for approximately up to 3 months. The hydrogel catheters absorb water and cause less friction when catheterising a patient. These catheters may last in situ for up to 4 months (Marjoram, 1999) (Table 7.2).

Nursing care

Patients with a urinary catheter in situ should be encouraged to drink at least 2.5 L of fluid per day, provided they do not have other physiological problems such as cardiac

Table 7.2 Some types of catheters.

Types	Description
Teflon	The rubber is Teflon coated
	Short- to medium-term use
Silicone-coated latex	Soft and causes less irritation
	Catheter may be left in situ for up to 3 months
Hydrogel-coated latex	Absorbs water and are easy to insert
	Last up to 12 weeks in situ

failure. Approximately 2–2.5 L of fluid normally results in an increase in urine production, which in turn will help to prevent urinary tract infection. It is important that the nurse maintains an accurate fluid balance chart for monitoring input and output.

If necessary, daily meatal hygiene should be undertaken to ensure that the patient does not develop urinary tract infection. Routine personal hygiene is all that is needed to maintain meatal hygiene (Pratt et al., 2001). For uncircumcised males, gently retract the foreskin over the head of the penis away from the catheter. Using soap and clean water, cleanse around the meatus. Gently apply tortion to the catheter and clean away from the tip of the penis where the catheter enters the penis, wiping 7–10 cm down the tubing towards the catheter bag (Smith et al., 2004).

When cleaning the meatus of the penis, the nurse must ensure not to introduce any infection into the bladder. Ensure that the catheter bag is not lying on the floor and that it is attached to a catheter bag stand. Furthermore, make certain that there are no kinks in the catheter drainage system that might prevent the urine from flowing unimpeded into the bag (Smith et al., 2004). All care and outcomes must be documented accordingly to ensure that the care provided is based on an individual assessment of the patient's needs.

Conclusions

The overall aim of this chapter was to provide the reader with insight into some of the problems associated with elimination and the care of a patient with certain disorders connected with the alimentary and eliminatory tracts. The content of this chapter included disorders of the gastrointestinal tract and the urinary system. It is not possible to include all the disorders related to these areas; some of the more common problems have been discussed in this chapter.

Attending to the patient's elimination needs is an important part of holistic care. Nurses are often involved in assisting or giving advice to patients who have elimination problems. These problems could affect the patient both psychologically and physically. The inability to defaecate and urinate may be caused by various disorders, for example carcinoma. These disorders may impinge on the patients' ability to perform their activities of living.

Some patients may need assistance with defaecation in the form of suppositories or enemata, whilst others may need a colostomy as a result of cancer of the colon.

Patients who are catheterised for urinary problems such as retention of urine or male patients who have had prostatectomy and have a catheter in situ will need catheter care in order to prevent urinary tract infection (Dougherty and Lister, 2008). The nurse must provide evidenced-based care resulting from individualised and holistic assessment.

Glossary

Accessory organs	Organs that contribute to digestion but are not part of the digestive tract
Cardiac region	Surrounds the cardiac orifice through which food enters the stomach
Chyme	Semisolid substance containing partially digested food and gastric juices found in the stomach
Electrolyte	Chemical substances such as salts, acids and bases found in the blood and other body fluids
Emulsify	The dispersion of large fat molecules into smaller molecules in the presence of bile
Endocrine	A ductless gland that secretes hormones into the blood stream
Enzymes	A substance that speeds chemical reaction
Exocrine	A gland that secretes hormones into ducts that carries the secretions to other sites
Homeostasis	A state of equilibrium of the internal and the external environment of the body
Mastication	Chewing process
Peristalsis	Wave-like movements of the intestinal tract that helps to move foodstuff down the intestine
Pyloric region	Funnel-shaped portion of the stomach where the pyloric sphincter is situated, which controls emptying of the stomach
Sensory receptors	Specialised neurons that detect changes or respond to a stimulus
Ulcer	An erosion or loss of continuity of a mucous membrane, which may lead to the formation of pus
Vestibule	Enlarged area at the beginning of a canal

Post-chapter quiz

1. List the digestive juices of the stomach
2. List the functions of the colon
3. Describe chemical and mechanical digestion
4. Is the gallbladder essential for the digestive process? Explain your answer
5. Which position will you ask the patient to lie in prior and during the administering of enema or suppositories? Explain your answer
6. Identify the reasons for the formation of a colostomy
7. What is the primary function of the urinary system?
8. Discuss the possible complications of bladder irrigation
9. What actions should the nurse take in attempting to reduce urinary tract infection in those patients with an indwelling urinary catheter?
10. List the roles and functions of the multidisciplinary team with specific reference to caring for people with elimination problems

References

Cawson, R.A. and Odell, E.W. (1998) *Essentials of Oral Pathology and Oral Medicine*, 6th ed. Edinburgh: Churchill Livingstone.

Clancy, J. and McVicar, A.J. (2002) *Physiology and Anatomy: A Homeostatic Approach*, 2nd ed. London: Edward Arnold.
Dougherty, L. and Lister, S. (eds) (2008) *The Royal Marsden Hospital Manual of Clinical Nursing Procedures*, 7th ed. Chichester: Wiley-Blackwell.
Fickenscher, L. (1999) Evaluation of adult haematuria. *Nurse Practitioner* 24(9): 58–64.
Finlay, T. (2002) Caring for the patient with a disorder of the gastrointestinal system. In: Walsh, M. (ed). *Watson's Clinical Nursing and Related Sciences*, 6th ed. London: Bailliere Tindall.
Iro, H., Schneider, H.T., Fodra, C., Waitz, G., Nitsche, N., Heinritz, H.H., Benninger, J. and Ell, C. (1992) Shockwave lithotripsy of salivary duct stones. *Lancet* 339: 1333–1336.
Jamieson, E.M., McCall, J.M. and Whyte, L.A. (2002) *Clinical Nursing Practice*, 4th ed. Edinburgh: Churchill Livingstone.
Kozier, B., Erb, G., Berman, A., Berman, A., Synder, S., Lake, R. and Harvey, S. (2008) *Fundamentals of Nursing: Concepts, Process and Practice*. Harlow: Pearson Education.
Kumar, P. and Clark, M. (ed) (2005) *Clinical Medicine*, 5th ed. London: WB Saunders.
Lemone, P. and Burke, K. (2008) *Medical-Surgical Nursing – Critical Thinking in Client Care*, 4th ed. New Jersey: Pearson Prentice Hall.
Mader, S.S. (2005) *Understanding Human Anatomy & Physiology*, 5th ed. London: Wm.C. Brown Publishers.
Marieb, E.N. and Hoehn, K. (2007) *Human Anatomy & Physiology*, 7th ed. San Francisco: Pearson Benjamin Cummings.
Marjoram, B. (1999) Elimination. In: Hogston, R. and Simpson, P.M. (eds). *Foundations of Nursing Practice*. London: Macmillan.
McCuistion, L.E. and Gutierrez, K.J. (2002) *Pharmacology*. Philadelphia: WB Saunders.
Moppett, S. (2000) Which way is up for a suppository? *Nursing Times Plus* 96(19): 12–13.
Nair, M. and Peate, I. (2009) *Fundamentals of Applied Pathophysiology*. Chichester: Wiley-Blackwell.
Nursing and Midwifery Council (2005) *Guidelines for Records and Record Keeping*. London: NMC.
Nursing and Midwifery Council (2008a) *Standards for Medicine Management*. London: NMC.
Nursing and Midwifery Council (2008b) *The Code: Standards of Conduct, Performance and Ethics for Nurses and Midwives*. London: NMC.
Peate, I. (2003) Nursing role in the management of constipation: use of laxatives. *British Journal of Nursing* 12(19): 1130–1136.
Shier, D., Butler, J. and Lewis, R. (2004) *Hole's Human Anatomy and Physiology*, 10th ed. London: McGraw Hill.
Siddiqui, S.J. (2002) Sialolithiasis: an unusually large submandibular salivary stone. *British Dental Journal* 193(2): 89–91.
Silverthorn, D.U. (1998) *Human Physiology – An Integrated Approach*. New Jersey: Prentice Hall.
Smith, S.F., Duell, D.J. and Martin, B.C. (2004) *Clinical Nursing Skills – Basic to Advanced Skills*, 6th ed. New Jersey: Pearson Prentice Hall.
Tortora, G.J. and Derrickson, B. (2007) *Principles of Anatomy and Physiology*, 11th ed. New York: John Wiley and Sons.
Walsh, M. (2002) *Watson's Clinical Nursing and Related Sciences*, 6th ed. London: Bailliere Tindall.
Wilson, J. (2001) *Infection control in Clinical Practice*, 2nd ed. London: Bailliere Tindall.
Winney, J. (1998) Constipation. *Nursing Standard* 13(11): 49–53.

Chapter 8
Breathing

Sean Mallon

Learning opportunities

This chapter will help you to:

1. Understand the structure and function of the respiratory tract
2. Assess, measure and record respiration rates
3. Define common respiratory diseases
4. Understand the significance of cough and sputum
5. Discuss some of the ways the nurse can help treat breathlessness
6. Assess the effectiveness and efficacy of medications

Pre-chapter quiz

1. How many lobes are there in the lungs?
2. Where is the diaphragm?
3. When assessing the patient's respiratory status what should you consider?
4. What are the signs and symptoms of a chest infection?
5. List some other common respiratory diseases
6. What is a nebuliser?
7. What can you measure to assess the effectiveness of nursing interventions?
8. Define cyanosis
9. Describe what is meant by oxygen saturation measurement

Introduction

Breathing is essential to life; it occurs so that the bloodstream can transport oxygen to cells of the body. Jenkins (2003) points out that as a rule breathing is an independent activity occurring immediately after birth. Roper et al. (2000) state that breathing can be effortless and people are not usually consciously aware of this activity of living, until certain abnormal conditions force the individual to become consciously aware of it. Hilton (2005) defines breathing in two stages:

> *Inspiration*, inhaling (breathing in) air in order to extract the oxygen from the air, and *expiration*, exhaling (breathing out) in order to expel carbon dioxide.

Pryor and Prasad (2002) suggest that diseases associated with the respiratory tract account for the highest number of general practitioner consultations. The effects of respiratory tract disease impinge on all activities of living and the disease is also responsible for the highest number of days lost from work (Griffin and Potter, 2006).

To care effectively for patients who have diseases of the respiratory tract, the nurse will need to understand the role that the respiratory tract plays in the metabolism of the cells of the body (Cutler and Murch, 2003). The nurse's role in assessing a patient with a respiratory disease is outlined in this chapter. The complexities of breathing are only briefly addressed here and the reader is advised to refer to other texts on the subject in order to understand fully the physiological principles and resulting nursing care.

Structure and function of the respiratory tract

The respiratory tract extends from the nose to the alveoli of the lungs. The lungs and respiratory passages are shown in Figure 8.1.

Respiration

One of the key requirements of the cells in the human body is to receive oxygen (O_2). The bloodstream delivers O_2, protein, fats and glucose; these products enable the body to produce energy (known as catabolism). Carbon dioxide (CO_2), a poison in high concentrations produced by the cells along with water (H_2O; a process known as metabolism), is excreted through the process of respiration, which occurs via the lungs. Without this process, humans would die (Law and Watson, 2005).

Control of breathing

Regulation of respiration is complex and is essentially controlled by the brain in response to two factors: neural and chemical (Thibodeau and Patton, 2005). Normal breathing is known as eupnoea (Cutler and Murch, 2003).

Neural control

The respiratory centre is situated in the medulla oblongata in the brain. Along with the pons Varolii it produces nervous impulses that influence breathing (McGeown, 2002). During inhalation, when tension is reached on the walls of the bronchi, the vagus nerve (tenth cranial nerve) passes an impulse to the bronchi. The respiratory centre sends nerve impulses to the diaphragm and intercostal muscles to relax, and expiration occurs; this causes the thoracic cage to enlarge. These actions are involuntary and as such occur unconsciously. Voluntary actions are activities over which we have some degree of control; they include coughing or sneezing when stimulated by irritating substances.

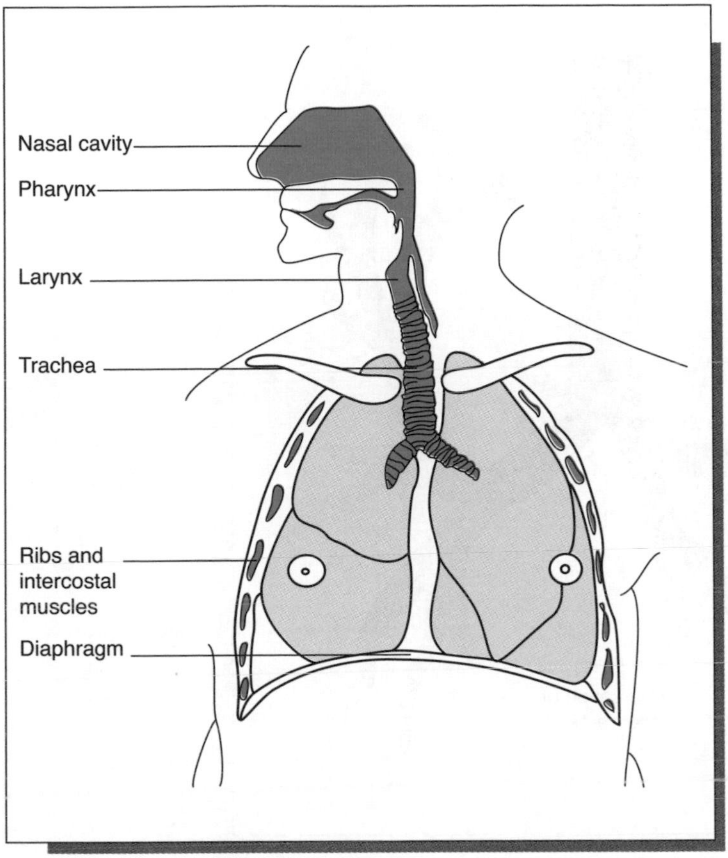

Figure 8.1 The respiratory tract.

Chemical control

Control of respiration by chemical stimulation is achieved by the actions of a specialised group of cells known as chemoreceptors, which are situated in the walls of the aorta and the carotid arteries. In addition, the carotid sinus of the carotid artery is sensitive to an excess of CO_2 and a deficiency of O_2. The resultant changes associated with either high or low levels of O_2 or CO_2 (partial pressures) can send nerve impulses to the respiratory centre to alter the rate and depth of breathing (Hogston and Simpson, 2002).

The bronchi

Air passes into the lungs from the trachea and bronchi. Initially air is filtered, saturated with water vapour and warmed by the nose. It then passes through the pharynx and larynx and down into the trachea and bronchi (Figure 8.2). There are two bronchi; they start at the bifurcation of the trachea and each bronchus leads to a lung, either right or left (Whittaker, 2004). The right bronchus is more vertical and shorter than the left; the left bronchus is slightly smaller and narrower than the right as a result of the

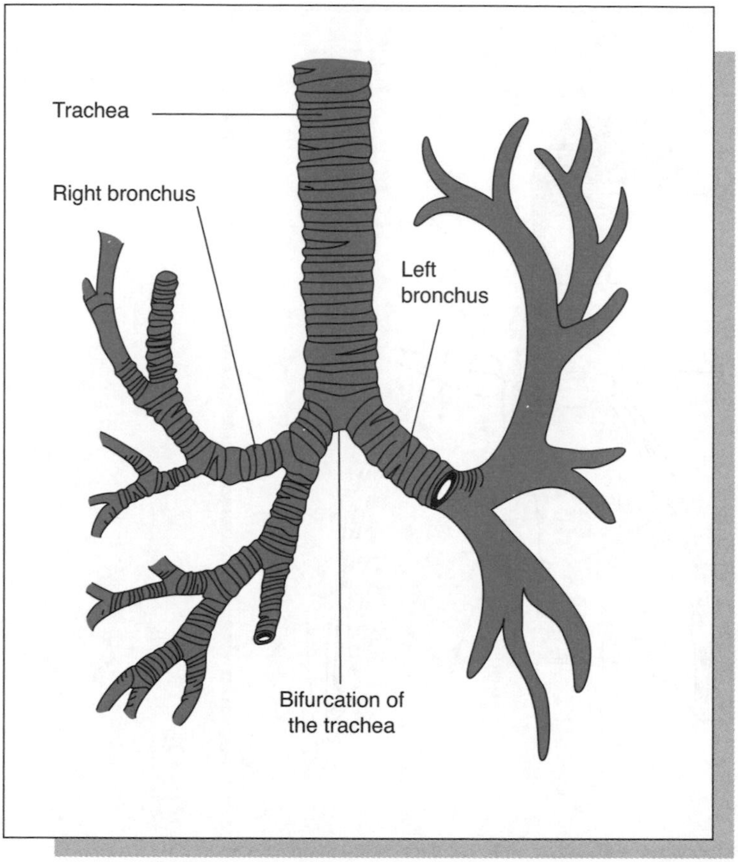

Figure 8.2 The trachea and associated structures.

position of the heart within the mediastinum. Each of the bronchi divides into branches corresponding to each of the lobes of the lung.

Lining of the respiratory system

The trachea is lined with small cells called columnar epithelial cells. These cells have small hair-like projections called cilia, which are covered with mucus (produced by the bronchial glands); they trap foreign or dirt particles, which if causing irritation can usually be coughed up by the individual.

The diaphragm

This muscle is shaped like a dome that separates the thorax from the abdomen. This sheet of muscle fibres connects to fibrous tissue known as the central tendon. Phrenic nerves on either side of the diaphragm cause the diaphragm to contract, and the respiratory centre, situated in the brain (the medulla oblongata), controls this action.

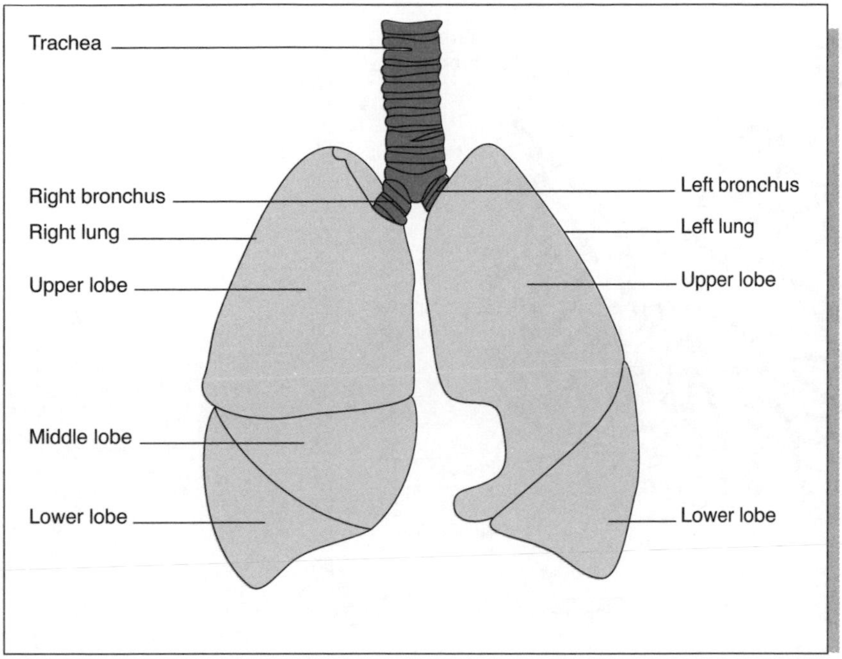

Figure 8.3 The lungs.

Accessory muscles

Anterior to the wall of the chest is the pectoralis major muscle, around the lateral wall is the serratus anterior muscle and the sternomastoid muscle passes from the back of the skull to the clavicle. Although the main function of these muscles is for movement of the head, arms and scapulae, they may also assist when breathing becomes difficult. This group of muscles helps respiration by moving the ribcage (Law and Watson, 2005).

The lungs

There are two lungs, and it should be noted that the right lung has three lobes - upper, middle and lower lobes - whereas the left lung is made up of two lobes - upper and lower lobes. Both lungs are conical in shape, with the base on the diaphragm and the apex reaching up towards the clavicle (Figure 8.3).

Each lung is surrounded by the pleura, which is a continuous membrane that folds back on itself. At the root of the lung is the parietal pleura, covering the interior of the chest, the mediastinum and the diaphragm. The inner layer is the visceral pleura, which covers the lungs; between both these layers is a potential space - the pleural space.

The alveoli

The alveoli are the terminal ends of the bronchioles (Figure 8.4). It is here that gaseous exchange takes place. These minute terminal bronchioles form tiny air passages known as alveolar ducts, which open into alveolar sacs (Whittaker, 2004). The walls of the

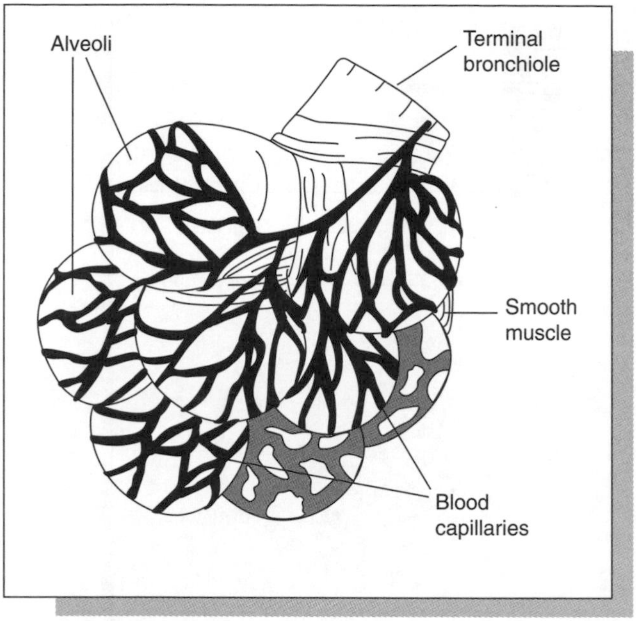

Figure 8.4 The alveoli.

alveoli are single-thickness, squamous epithelial cells (Thibodeau and Patton, 2005). Externally, the alveoli are surrounded by a very thin pulmonary capillary network. There are millions of alveoli providing a large surface area which is greatly increased by the alveolar walls. Air and blood are separated by two layers of cells and a layer of moisture: the alveolus wall and the capillary wall; together they form the respiratory membrane. On one side of this membrane there are gases and on the other side there is a fast-flowing bloodstream-enabling gases to move rapidly between air and blood. Simple diffusion allows gas exchange to occur. Deoxygenated blood enters the capillary network via the pulmonary artery and as this occurs (by simple diffusion) oxygenated blood leaves the network entering the pulmonary veins. There are millions of gas-filled alveoli in the lungs, which allow for massive amounts of gas to be exchanged (Marieb, 2004).

Assessment of respiration

Respiratory assessment involves observation of the patient, collecting information, including the measurement of respiratory function and physical examination. The nurse will need to speak to the patient to obtain a history; however, caution must be taken because the patient may be so short of breath that encouraging him or her to speak may be detrimental to their health. Secondary data (data collected from a variety of sources other than the patient) may have to suffice if the nurse is unable to gain primary data (data given to the nurse by the patient).

Data may be given to the nurse by other health care professionals or significant others, or taken from the patient's nursing/medical notes. Chapter 3 describes the assessment process generally; this section concentrates on how to assess the patient's respiratory needs, confidently and competently, in order to gain insight into this complex activity of living.

Breathing should normally be effortless. Breathlessness may be accompanied by the use of the accessory muscles, so distress may be visual, the nurse can learn much from the patient by accurate observation. The rate, depth and rhythm of respiration must be noted, and the nurse should observe the chest wall to see whether it moves equally on both sides. The skill of listening is also required and the nurse must be alert to any noises that are made during inspiration and expiration.

Jenkins (2003) makes it clear that to assess breathing effectively the nurse must give due consideration to aspects of Roper et al.'s (1996) model of nursing:

- Lifespan: consider effect of age on breathing
- Dependency: linked to lifespan and ill health
- Independence: linked to health
- Factors affecting breathing

  Biological:
  - Degree of physical activity
  - Body's physiological responses to stressors
  - Intact respiratory system to enable effective internal and external respiration
  - Intact circulatory system and nervous system
  - Noted by observation of normal breathing
  - Note any abnormal breathing, i.e. wheeze, sputum production

  Psychological: effect of emotional state on breathing, i.e. anxiety, panic, fear

  Sociocultural: expectoration of sputum and coughing habits

  Environmental:
  - Exposure to microorganisms
  - Exposure to air pollutants at home or at work

  Politicoeconomic: mechanisms to limit smoking-related diseases and air pollutant diseases. The law banning smoking in public buildings and company vehicles

Measuring respiratory rate, depth and rhythm

When assessing the patient's respiratory status, the nurse must assess the rate, depth and pattern of respiration (rhythm). The normal resting respiratory rate in the adult is 12–18 breaths/minute, with expiration taking nearly twice as long as inspiration (Jamieson et al., 2007).

Respiratory assessment is carried out by the nurse to determine a baseline observation, which allows the nurse to make a comparison at a later date. The nurse may also use respiratory assessment to evaluate how the patient has responded to medications or treatments that have been given for a respiratory disease.

The nurse must be aware that the respiratory rate, depth and rhythm can be altered by a patient who is aware that the nurse is measuring this activity. The nurse should attempt to assess the patient's respiratory status without his or her knowledge.

Respiratory rate is the number of inspirations and expirations that the patient makes in 1 minute while at rest. It is therefore important that the respiratory rate is not assessed after the patient has undergone any form of exercise because an incorrect finding may be recorded.

Procedure for assessing the patient's respiratory status

- Explain the procedure to the patient, but do not inform him or her when you will be undertaking the activity
- A more accurate assessment of respiratory rate, depth and rhythm will occur if the nurse does not alert the patient to the fact that he or she is observing this activity. Some nurses may pretend to be taking the radial pulse when in fact they are counting and observing respiratory function
- Keep a watch with a second hand
- Observe movement of the chest wall and count the respirations for 60 seconds (do not be tempted to do this for 30 seconds and double your findings because this could be detrimental to the patient's health)
- Observe the rhythm and depth of respiratory effort. Depth of respiration is best assessed by observing the amount of movement made by the chest wall. The measurement of depth will relate to the amount of air being moved into and out of the lungs (Jamieson et al., 2007)

The nurse must document the observations in the patient's nursing notes according to the *Guidelines for Records and Record Keeping* (Nursing and Midwifery Council (NMC), 2007) and report any respiratory abnormalities. He or she may need to alter or adjust the frequency of observation as the patient's condition dictates. Respiratory effort can be categorised as follows:

- Rapid, shallow breathing - in excess of 20 breaths/minute is termed 'tachypnoea' and may be the result of an increase in activity, anxiety, fear, pain or pyrexia. This can be caused by the body's response to extra demands being made on it - a need for extra oxygen.
- A decrease in respiration to less than 12 breaths per minute is known as bradypnoea and may be caused by the effects of strong medications such as opiates (i.e. morphine), sleep, head injury, brain lesion or hypothermia. This type of breathing is slow but regular.
- Apnoea occurs when the patient fails to breathe for at least 10 seconds. Apnoea may precede or occur immediately after cardiac/respiratory arrest.
- Cheyne-Stokes breathing is characterised by a waxing and waning of respiratory depth over a minute or more. Respiratory depth may be deep and may become almost absent. This type of respiratory effort is often seen in patients who are terminally ill and may occur immediately before death (Hilton, 2005).

Respiratory sounds

In some instances when respiratory disease is present, the patient may make audible respiratory sounds; in 'normal' respiration, no sound is heard. The sounds made may

Table 8.1 Respiratory sounds and their potential meanings.

Name of sound	Potential meaning
Wheeze	Wheeze is a high-pitched whistling sound. It can occur in inspiration and expiration but is often loudest in expiration. It implies narrowing of the lower airway and is common in asthma.
Stridor	A harsh sound heard on inspiration and expiration can indicate obstruction of the larynx.
Snoring	Usually occurs during sleep and may indicate an obstruction of the airway. The obstruction may be nasal, oropharyngeal or laryngeal. Sleep apnoea may occur if snoring is severe and can lead to hypoxic episodes.
Crepitations	Heard when a stethoscope is placed on the chest wall and may indicate pulmonary oedema.

Source: Reproduced from Griffin and Potter (2006).

indicate or alert the nurse to specific type of illness so he or she must be aware of these sounds and their possible meanings. Table 8.1 outlines the names given to particular sounds that the patient may make when respiratory disease is present. Assessment of the patient with a respiratory disease includes the observation of the skin for signs of cyanosis. When tissue oxygenation is low or high, there may be some particular signs that will alert the nurse to this. When cyanosis (a bluish or purplish discoloration of the skin or mucous membranes) is present, this indicates a reduction in haemoglobin in the blood.

Central cyanosis (a bluish tinge to the mucous membranes of the mouth - buccal mucosa, the lips and conjunctivae) indicates serious lung and/or heart disease or any disease that prevents adequate oxygenation of the blood. Peripheral cyanosis involves the extremities, i.e. the hands and feet, although the tongue (as opposed to central cyanosis) remains a healthy pink colour (Evans-Smith, 2005).

Observation of cough and sputum

Cough

The characteristics of the cough, together with other symptoms, may give an indication of the cause. Cough is a result of irritation to the cough receptors in the pharynx, larynx and bronchi. The nurse should note the presence, frequency, depth, nature and sound of the cough. Furthermore, the nurse should note whether the cough has any effect on the patient's ability to carry out the activities of living, i.e. to communicate or sleep.

Cough may be caused by:

- Infection
- Physical and chemical stimuli
- Circulatory problems
- Cancer
- Habit

The cough may be productive, i.e. sputum is expectorated when the patient coughs, or non-productive or dry when little or no sputum is produced (Jamieson et al., 2007).

Sputum

It is usual for an adult to produce approximately 100 mL sputum/day (Walsh, 2002). There are many types of sputum and the amount produced can vary from 100 to 500 mL/day. The amount of sputum produced increases when the respiratory tract is irritated or inflamed. Patients may refer to sputum as phlegm; if this is the case, the nurse must use this word when questioning the patient. The patient should understand the importance of reporting any changes in respiratory function such as increased sputum (National Institute for Health and Clinical Excellence (NICE), 2004).

The nurse also needs to observe, note and report the type of sputum the patient is producing. The following should be noted and documented in the patient's nursing notes:

- Quantity
- Consistency
- Colour
- Odour

The clinical features of sputum are as follows (Law and Watson, 2005):

- White or grey
  - Smoking
  - Chronic bronchitis
  - Asthma
- Yellow or green
  - Acute bronchitis
  - Asthma
  - Bronchiectasis
  - Cystic fibrosis
- Frothy, blood stained
  - Pulmonary oedema
- Haemoptysis
  - Bright red secretions and froth may indicate that the patient has tuberculosis, carcinoma of the lung, trauma or pulmonary embolism

To determine the cause of sputum production and to aid with diagnosis, the nurse must ask the patient specific questions. The following are some useful questions to ask:

- What colour is the sputum (phlegm)?
- How often are you coughing it up?
- How much do you cough up?

- Do you have difficulty coughing it up?
- Do you use anything from the doctor or the chemist to help you with the sputum (phlegm)?

Although it is important to assess the type of sputum the patient produces and to ask pertinent questions such as those above, the nurse may need to obtain a sputum specimen in order to confirm or to make an accurate diagnosis.

Procedure for collecting a sputum specimen

The nurse is advised to adhere to local policy and procedure for collecting a sputum specimen for analysis. Outlined below are some points that should be considered when collecting a sputum specimen.

Equipment needed for the collection of sputum specimen

- Sterile, leak-proof container
- Specimen bag and request form with the laboratory tests required noted on it

The procedure

- Explain carefully in a way that the patient understands why the specimen is needed. Ensure privacy
- If the patient is to be commenced on prescribed antibacterial medication, the nurse should endeavour to collect the sputum before the course of antibiotics is started
- Before starting the collection of sputum, ask the patient to rinse the mouth with water because this will remove oral plaque and secretions that may contaminate the specimen
- Point out that the patient needs to provide a sputum specimen, not a specimen of saliva or mucus from the postnasal space
- Provide the patient with a sterile sputum pot for collection of the specimen if she or he is able to do this independently with tissues at hand
- Explain that contamination of the inside of the pot by the fingers should be avoided because this will interfere with an accurate analysis of sputum from the lung and may impede diagnosis and subsequent treatment
- Encourage the patient to breathe deeply to stimulate coughing expectoration and to loosen secretions
- In some cases the nurse may need to instigate, with the assistance of the physiotherapist, postural drainage to encourage the removal of secretions.
- The specimen should be refrigerated until processing takes place
- Document your actions and also record in the nursing notes the colour, smell and consistency of the sputum.

A sputum specimen may be easier to obtain from the patient if collected early in the morning. As the patient has been sleeping through the night and the respiratory rate is slower and the depth of breathing shallower, there may be more of a chance for secretions to have accumulated in the lung (Daniels, 2002).

Other methods of assessing respiratory function

Pulse oximetry

Pulse oximetry enables the nurse to measure the O_2 saturation of haemoglobin; this is a non-invasive technique and is represented by the following notation: SaO_2. The oximeter probe is attached to the finger, toe or ear lobe. The normal level is 95–99% (British National Formulary, 2006); if the SaO_2 falls below 85%, the reading becomes less reliable. It is important to note that the oximeter can take up to 30 seconds to detect a fall in O_2 concentration, which could be a critical time for instigating treatment or therapy. To obtain an accurate reading, the nurse should ensure that:

- The probe has been positioned correctly, ensuring a good flow of blood to the area
- There is no nail varnish on the finger or toe nails
- There is no direct overhead light
- The patient is not shivering
- There is no mechanical movement of the probe

The nurse must ensure that he or she has documented in the nursing notes the SaO_2 and whether the patient is receiving O_2 therapy. Any changes or abnormalities must be reported immediately (British Thoracic Society, 2004).

Peak expiratory flow rate

The peak expiratory flow rate (PEFR) allows the nurse to note objectively how much air the patient can empty from his or her lungs in litres per minute; it measures the individual's ability to exhale (Hilton, 2005). It is important that the nurse understands how to measure and record the PEFR because it is one of the most commonly used methods to assess the patient's respiratory status.

The PEFR is most often recorded to assess and monitor the effects of treatment. The British Thoracic Society (BTS, 2008a) guidelines state that patients with asthma often experience problems with lung capacity and variable obstruction of the airways. As a result, it is often (but not exclusively) the patient with asthma for whom the nurse will use the PEFR measurement. It is recommended that a PEFR be performed before and after treatments such as a nebuliser or inhaler to assess the effectiveness and efficacy of the medications. In this case, the PEFR should be recorded approximately 20 minutes after the medication has been given.

The procedure for measuring PEFR

Equipment needed

- Chart to record measurement
- Peak flowmeter
- Disposable mouthpiece

Procedure

- Explain the reason for the procedure and how you intend to carry it out
- PEFR is best measured if the patient is standing up. If the patient is unable to do this then he or she should be sitting in a chair or sitting upright in bed

- Attach disposable mouthpiece
- Set the peak flowmeter at zero
- Instruct the patient to inhale deeply, place the lips around the mouthpiece and, holding the meter horizontally, exhale forcibly
- Note the measurement
- Repeat twice
- Record the highest of the three measurements. The dial attached to the peak flowmeter should be returned to the lowest setting in between each attempt

The procedure may bring about coughing or wheezing. If this is the case the nurse should ask the patient to attempt the procedure only once and this should be noted on the chart.

Aerosols and nebulisers

Aerosolisation and nebulisation are two methods of drug administration that allow the inhalation of a variety of drugs with the aim of localised therapeutic effect (Rees and Kanabar, 2006). The most common types of drugs that are used via inhalation in the UK are bronchodilators and steroids (Francis, 2006).

Aerosols

Over 90% of people with asthma take the medications that they require by inhalation. There are a variety of inhaler devices available and the most common type is the metered dose inhaler. The patient needs a great deal of skill and the ability to coordinate for effective administration. The nurse has an educational role to play in teaching the patient or carer how to administer the inhaler correctly in order to ensure that the correct dose is delivered to the patient. The Asthma Training Centre (2007) estimates that one in five people do not use their inhaler correctly and that asthma costs the NHS over £900 million.

The main principles for using an aerosol are as follows:

- Ensure that the medication (the inhaler) is the correct medication prescribed for the patient.
- Remove the cover of the inhaler and shake the inhaler.
- Ask the patient to breathe out gently but not fully.
- When the patient's head is tilted slightly backwards, place the mouthpiece between the lips and ask the patient to breathe in as deeply as possible; activate the inhaler at the start of inspiration.
- Remove the inhaler from between the lips.
- The patient holds his or her breath for 10 seconds and then breathes out slowly.
- Repeat the procedure if necessary and as prescribed.
- The drug should be signed for on the drug administration sheet in the normal and accepted manner. The nurse must record the effect of the medication in the patient's notes.

Nebulisers

A nebuliser is attached to a flow of air or O_2 and converts a solution of the prescribed drug (with 2–3 mL physiological [0.9%] saline) into an aerosol for inhalation. Nebuliser therapy is usually administered three to four times a day and the administration of the nebuliser must be consistent with local policy and procedure.

Some common respiratory diseases

Asthma

Asthma is a chronic inflammatory condition of the airways. The term 'asthma' is derived from the Greek word meaning 'panting' (Bassett and Makin, 2000). The cause of this disease is still not completely understood (BTS, 2008a). It is characterised by spasm of the bronchial muscles and oedema of the bronchial mucosa, resulting in recurrent attacks of wheezing during expiration. Narrowing of the airways occurs as a response to stimuli such as infection, allergy or unknown cause. Bronchoconstriction occurs and breathing becomes difficult and laboured (dyspnoea). McEwing et al. (2003) suggest that asthma is a form of airway obstruction that is reversible.

The British Thoracic Society (2008b) suggests that 2000 deaths occur each year in the UK as a result of asthma, 70% of which could be prevented by long-term therapy, assessment skills, and appropriate nursing care and management. Thirty per cent of the patients who die as a result of asthma do so within 2 hours of the onset of an attack.

Altered physiology

Bronchospasm occurs as a result of contraction of the smooth muscle. Inflammation happens and this causes hypersensitivity of the airways, which narrow as the result of a wide range of stimuli. Inflammatory cells cause even more narrowing of the airways.

Predisposing factors (triggers)

There are certain factors that can trigger an asthmatic attack. Cutler and Murch (2003) suggest that asthma trigger factors include:

- Allergies, e.g. to pollen or house-dust mites
- I, e.g. colds or other viral infections
- Emotions, e.g. crying
- Environment, e.g. tobacco smoke, pollution

Signs and symptoms

- The patient may complain of a 'tight chest' or the feeling of suffocation
- Breathing starts to increase in rate; there is exaggeration of the accessory muscle of respiration, with an audible wheeze on expiration
- The patient may become distressed, wanting to sit upright
- Accessory muscles are used to force air out
- There is a tachycardia

- The chest becomes hyperexpanded with some evidence of peripheral cyanosis
- There will be a lower PEFR than the patient is 'normally' able to produce (if the patient can produce a PEFR)
- The inflammatory response may result in the production of thick mucoid sputum
- The event can last for 1 hour to several days, resulting in central cyanosis, exhaustion, dehydration and eventually respiratory failure

Diagnosis

Diagnosis is based on the patient's history of his or her present condition; the nurse must ensure that he or she does not exacerbate the patient's condition by asking questions that will make the patient's breathlessness worse. Data may need to be obtained from a significant other, another health care professional or the patient's notes. The nurse's questioning technique will have to be sensitive to the patient's condition.

The nurse must have acute observational skills for observing the patient's posture, verbal and non-verbal signs. A chest radiograph may demonstrate pulmonary consolidation. Respiratory effort will be decreased and SaO_2 may fall below 95%. The nurse must record observations in the patient's notes and report any abnormalities.

Nursing interventions

The nurse must show that he or she is calm and in control and act in a reassuring manner. The patient should be sat in the upright position or a position that he or she finds comfortable in order to increase thoracic capacity. Then the following interventions may be carried out:

- Administer all treatment as prescribed. Remove, if possible, the allergen, e.g. if the patient is allergic to feathers then ensure that the pillow is not made of feathers
- Oxygen therapy
- Salbutamol nebuliser
- Ipratropium bromide nebuliser
- Aminophylline (bronchodilator)
- Hydrocortisone (steroid with anti-inflammatory properties)
- Antibiotics
- Intravenous fluids

Patient education

Specifically, the patient will need to be made aware of the possible triggers that may cause an asthmatic attack. The nurse needs to ensure that the patient is using the correct inhaler technique. If, despite repeated attempts to teach the patient the correct technique, the performance does not improve, the nurse should consider another inhaler delivery system, e.g. a volumatic or breath-actuated device (Hilton, 2005). The patient will need to be told what to do if he or she experiences another asthma attack. It is important that the patient has an adequate supply of inhalers at home and at work in case he or she needs to use them in order to relieve symptoms.

Chronic obstructive pulmonary disease

Chronic obstructive pulmonary disease (COPD) is an umbrella term applied to diseases such as chronic bronchitis, emphysema and asthma, which may result in permanent airway restriction. According to the white paper Smoking Kills (Action on Smoking and Health [ASH], 2008), 99% of people who have COPD have smoked or are still smoking. Smoking costs the National Health Service £2.7 billion in 2006–2007 (ASH, 2008).

COPD is the world's fourth leading cause of disease-related death, killing three million people a year; it can mean a life of disability for the patient (BTS, 2008b). As a result of the permanent reduction in airflow, patients will become reliant on lower levels of O_2 and higher levels of CO_2 to stimulate breathing. This is known as a hypoxic drive. It is vital that care is taken when delivering prescribed O_2.

Altered physiology

The disease spectrum varies widely from total obstructive airway disease with bronchitis to severe emphysema without bronchitis. The pathophysiological processes that cause the changes associated with pulmonary disease are neither static nor necessarily progressive (BTS, 2004). The altered physiology therefore depends on the underlying disease process.

To treat the patient appropriately and successfully, the nurse must determine what the underlying pulmonary disease is that is causing the patient's individual COPD. Often COPD is divided into key areas, e.g. chronic bronchitis, emphysema and asthma.

Caring for a patient with asthma has been outlined earlier. The following subsections briefly outline the signs and symptoms, nursing interventions and related patient education associated with chronic bronchitis because the clinical manifestations for both chronic bronchitis and emphysema are similar.

Chronic bronchitis

Signs and symptoms

Chronic bronchitis is often associated with the inhalation of physical or chemical irritants; cigarette smoking is by far the major risk factor in chronic bronchitis (ASH, 2008). The effect of the irritants on the airways results in hypersecretion of mucus and inflammation. Exacerbations of chronic bronchitis are most likely to occur during the winter months. The symptoms are:

- Productive cough (especially on waking)
- Chest infection (pyrexia, tachycardia)
- Shortness of breath, dyspnoea
- Cyanosis (central/peripheral)

Diagnosis

To make a diagnosis of chronic bronchitis, the nurse needs to obtain a full history of the present condition; he or she also needs to include a family history and to ascertain whether the patient has been exposed to any environmental factors such as tobacco, air pollution or occupational exposure to hazardous airborne materials. An in-depth holistic assessment is required to gather both subjective and objective data. The following investigations are also needed to make a definitive diagnosis:

- Chest radiograph
- Arterial blood gas analysis
- Respiratory rate, rhythm and depth
- Temperature
- Pulse oximetry
- Pulmonary function studies
- Venous blood analysis
- Sputum studies for microscopy, culture and sensitivity

Nursing interventions

The key aim of nursing care is to try to keep the bronchioles open and functioning in order to prevent infection and remove secretions. The nurse must assist the patient to carry out the activities of living so as not to exacerbate the condition. Regular measurement of vital signs is imperative; these must be recorded and abnormalities reported. A multidisciplinary approach is advocated and the nurse should act as the pivot for such an approach. Observation of any sputum must be made by the nurse and he or she should note and report any change in colour, amount and tenacity.

- Nurse the patient upright (unless contraindicated); encourage the patient to rest to conserve energy
- Provide the patient with regular opportunities to clean the mouth because he or she may be mouth breathing; place tissues, sputum pot and a bag in which to put the used tissues, within easy reach
- Prevent cross-infection by restricting visits from people who have respiratory infections; encourage the patient to use tissues when dealing with his or her own secretions. Used tissues must be disposed of safely and in accordance with policy and procedure
- Administer and report the effectiveness of any prescribed bronchodilators
- Administer prescribed antibiotic therapy
- Administer prescribed steroid therapy
- Administer the prescribed amount of oxygen with humidification
- Ensure that the patient is appropriately hydrated with oral fluids or intravenous fluids (correct hydration will help to loosen secretions and encourage expectoration)
- The nurse must ensure that he or she explains about treatment and nursing care to the patient in a way that he or she will understand

Patient education

Every effort should be made by the nurse working in conjunction with the patient, the family and if need be the employer to prevent recurrence of the condition (BTS, 2004). Those who are prone to respiratory tract infections should be given information that will enable them to make the decision about taking the vaccine against influenza and *Streptococcus pneumoniae* (NICE, 2004). The patient should be encouraged to give up smoking and avoid respiratory irritants and infections. In some instances, the patient will need to undergo an occupational health assessment at his or her place of work.

The nurse may need to teach/reinforce the correct method of using nebulisers or inhalers at home. It is important that the patient understands the reasons for the prescribed medications. Instil in the patient, the signs that may necessitate seeking nursing/medical attention should another episode of illness occur, because often antimicrobial therapy should be started at the first sign of purulent sputum.

Conclusions

This chapter has provided the nurse with the underlying physiological, anatomical and nursing concepts to help the provision of high-quality care that is commensurate with the requirements laid down by the NMC (2008). It has also provided the nurse with the fundamental concepts and the reader is urged to delve further in order to improve on knowledge and thus nursing care.

Caring for a patient with a respiratory disorder requires skilled nursing care in order to assess, plan, implement and evaluate appropriate nursing interventions. The nurse must be an effective communicator in order to communicate with patients and family, who are often distressed, anxious and fearful. The nurse needs to have a good understanding of the anatomy and physiology of the respiratory tract, in order to make clinical decisions that are based on fact as opposed to hearsay or tradition. The assessment of respiratory function is complex. The maintenance of optimum oxygenation in patients with respiratory tract disorder is a key priority for nurses in both hospital and community settings. This chapter has briefly introduced the nurse to many key nursing skills, and the skills required to assess the patient's respiratory needs have been discussed in some detail. By understanding and using the information provided, the nurse will be able to perform in a more effective manner, respond appropriately and enhance the quality of care that he or she provides.

The nurse needs to be able to detect any abnormalities quickly and to act on his or her findings. It is advocated that the nurse should record and report any changes in the patient's condition (NMC, 2007). Ongoing assessment and evaluation of nursing interventions are vital in order to respond quickly to changing situations, which may have implications for patient outcomes.

Glossary

Aerobic	With oxygen
Apnoea	Absence of breathing
Asthmatic breathing	Audible wheeze on expiration, difficulty on expiration
Bradypnoea	Slow but regular breathing
Cheyne-Stokes breathing	Cycle of increased rate and depth followed by gradual decrease and may become absent. May occur immediately before death.
Cyanosis	A bluish discolouration of the skin or mucous membranes, caused by inadequate oxygen intake
Dyspnoea	Difficulty in breathing
Expiration	Breathing out
Haemoptysis	Blood in sputum

Hypoxia	A lack of oxygen
Inspiration	Breathing in
Stridor	A harsh sound heard on inspiration, may indicate an obstruction
Tachypnoea	Increased rate of breathing
Wheeze	A high-pitched whistling sound

Post-chapter quiz

1. Define the following terms:
   a. Apnoea
   b. Dyspnoea
   c. Hypoxia
   d. Haemoptysis
2. What is the normal respiration rate of an adult at rest?
3. Describe how you would calculate respiratory rate, depth and rhythm
4. Why and how would you obtain a sputum specimen?
5. How can you measure the effectiveness of oxygen therapy?
6. Name the most common side effect of salbutamol
7. Does oxygen need to be prescribed?
8. What is the normal level of oxygen saturation of haemoglobin in an adult?
9. List three common respiratory diseases
10. When should you record or report any changes in the patient's condition?

References

Action on Smoking and Health (2008) Smoking Kills. White Paper. Available at www.ash.org.uk/beyondsmokingkillssummary. Accessed December 2008.

Asthma Training Centre (2007) *The Asthma Training Centre Learning Package*. Stratford upon Avon: Asthma Training Centre.

Bassett, C. and Makin, L. (2000) *Caring for the Seriously Ill Patient*. London: Arnold.

British National Formulary (2006) *Oxygen*. London: British Medical Association and the Royal Pharmaceutical Society of Great Britain, London.

British Thoracic Society (2004) *British Guideline on the Management of Chronic Obstructive Pulmonary Disease: A National Clinical Guideline*. London: BTS.

British Thoracic Society (2008a) *British Guideline on the Management of Asthma: A National Clinical Guideline*. London: BTS.

British Thoracic Society (2008b) *British Guideline on the Management of Oxygen Therapy in Adult Patients*, Vol. 63. London: BTS.

Cutler, L. and Murch, P. (2003) The respiratory system. In: Bassett, C. (ed.) *Essentials of Nursing Care*. London: Whurr Publishers, pp. 47–92.

Daniels, R. (2002) *Delmar's Guide to Laboratory and Diagnostic Tests*. New York: Delmar.

Evans-Smith, P. (2005) *Taylors Clinical Nursing Skills – A Nursing Process Approach*. Philadelphia: Lippincott Williams and Wilkins.

Francis, C. (2006) *Respiratory Care*. Oxford: Blackwell Publishing.

Griffin, A. and Potter, P. (2006) *Clinical Nursing Skills and Techniques*. Mosby: Elsevier.

Hilton, A. (2005) *Fundamental Nursing Skills*. London: Whurr Publishers.

Hogston, R. and Simpson, P.M. (2002) *Foundations of Nursing Practice: Making a Difference*, 2nd ed. Basingstoke: Palgrave Macmillan.

Jamieson, E. Whyte, L.A. McCall, J.A. (2007) *Clinical Nursing Practices*. Edinburgh: Churchill Livingstone.

Jenkins, J. (2003) Breathing. In: Holland, K., Jenkins, J., Solomon, J. and Whittam, S. (eds). *Applying the Roper, Logan and Tierney Model in Practice*. Edinburgh: Churchill Livingstone, pp. 121–161.

Law, C. and Watson, R. (2005) Respiration. In: Montague, S., Hinchliff, S., Watson, R. and Herbert, R. (eds). *Physiology for Nursing Practice*. Edinburgh: Churchill Livingstone.

Marieb, E.N. (2004) *Human Anatomy and Physiology*, 6th ed. London: Pearson Benjamin Cummings.

McEwing, G., Kelsey, J., Richardson, J. and Glasper, A. (2003) Insights into child and family health. In: Grandis, S., Long, C., Glasper, A. and Jackson, P. (eds). *Foundation Studies for Nursing: Using Enquiry-Based Learning*. Basingstoke: Palgrave, pp. 48–114.

McGeown, J. (2002) *Physiology: A Clinical Core Text of Human Physiology with Self Assessment*. Edinburgh: Churchill Livingstone.

National Institute of Health Clinical Excellence (2004) *Management of Chronic Obstructive Pulmonary Disease in Adults in Primary and Secondary Care*. Clinical\guideline 12. London: NICE.

Nursing and Midwifery Council (2007) *Guidelines for Records and Record Keeping*. London: NMC.

Nursing and Midwifery Council (2008) *The Code of Conduct*. London: NMC.

Pryor, J. and Prasad, S. (2002) *Physiotherapy for Respiratory and Cardiac Problems*. London: Churchill Livingstone.

Rees, J. and Kanabar, D. (2006) *The ABC of Asthma*. Oxford: Blackwell.

Roper, N., Logan, W.W. and Tierney, A.J. (1996) *The Elements of Nursing: A Model for Nursing Based on a Model for Living*, 4th ed. Edinburgh: Churchill Livingstone.

Roper, N., Logan, W.W. and Tierney, A.J. (2000) *The Roper, Logan and Tierney Model of Nursing Based on Activities of Living*. Edinburgh: Churchill Livingstone.

Thibodeau, G. and Patton, K.T. (2005) *The Human Body in Health and Disease*. Philadelphia: Elsevier.

Walsh, M. (2002) *Watson's Clinical Nursing and Related Sciences*, 6th ed. London: Bailliere Tindall.

Whittaker, N. (2004) Chronic obstructive pulmonary disease (COPD). In: Whittaker, N. (ed.). *Disorders and Interventions*. London: Palgrave, pp. 201–232.

Chapter 9
Personal Cleansing and Dressing

Laureen Hemming

Learning opportunities

This chapter will help you to:

1. Identify the factors that affect the integrity of the skin and cause the protective barrier to break down
2. Understand the physiology of the skin, how it works to protect from infection and diseases and how it responds to chemicals used when washing
3. Reflect on the impact of being groomed and how this can affect a person's psychological and spiritual well-being
4. Consider the impact the rituals of washing and dressing have on our place in society
5. Understand that the embodiment of caring is bound inextricably with helping patients maintain their personal cleansing routines and rituals when they are unwell
6. Consider the unique role and function of the nurse when helping people with their personal cleansing and dressing needs

Pre-chapter quiz

1. List four functions of the skin
2. Explain how illness and medical treatments can affect the state and function of the skin
3. Describe how you feel when you have not been able to meet your own hygiene to your own satisfaction, noting the key points of annoyance
4. What factors make meeting a patient's hygiene needs difficult?
5. Explain how soap and hot water can damage the skin and put the patient at risk from acquiring infection
6. Describe the impact of having a sore mouth on a patient's nutritional status
7. What equipment will be needed to offer bed bath to a patient?

8. How can the nurse encourage independence with respect to personal cleansing and dressing?
9. Describe the observations made when bed bathing
10. How should the nurse wash a patient's hair when he or she is confined to bed?

Introduction

When people are ill, they may not be able to meet their own hygiene needs to their own satisfaction and will require help to complete their rituals and routines. The illness itself may affect the skin and require special nursing care to minimise these effects. Helping people meet their hygiene is often regarded as 'basic' care, rather than 'fundamental' care and often relinquished to the most junior members of the nursing team rather than being considered as an essential and fundamental act of caring. Recent government policies have considered changing the role of the nurse, reducing their numbers whilst increasing the role and numbers of 'assistant practitioners' who would then take on the more mundane tasks such as assisting patients with their personal hygiene (Williamson et al., 2008). However, Allen (2008) points out that assisting patients with their personal hygiene needs provides the nurse with the opportunity to assess and observe the patient, communicate and learn more about the patient and responding to the patient's concerns. Allen (2008) claims that it 'can be the most significant interaction of the day for the patient'.

When we are well, caring for personal hygiene is often an activity carried out in private and determined by personal preference; usually, the products used are a matter of individual choice and may be determined by what is affordable and available. Some people prefer showering to bathing; how often and when is a matter of personal choice. However, for some, these practices such as washing in running water and products used may be determined culturally or by personal beliefs; e.g. some vegetarians or vegans will not use soaps made from animal products containing tallow.

The NMC's (2008) Code states that people must be able to trust nurses with their health and well-being, and that nurses must respect a patient's individuality and maintain their dignity. This is essential when assisting with personal care, as it can be embarrassing for patients to undress and require help with intimate aspects of personal care such as washing or going to the toilet.

The skin is the largest organ of the body (Allen, 2008; Burr and Penzer, 2005), it forms a protective barrier and it can be harmed through neglect or exposure to the elements (Tortora and Derrickson, 2009). There are many factors affecting skin condition:

- State of health
- Age
- Diet
- Pollutants in the atmosphere
- Irritants that may be applied to the skin in the process of personal cleansing
- Weather – sun, wind, snow and ice

People in the Northern Hemisphere are more likely to experience dry skin in winter, especially when climatic temperatures fall below skin temperature. Ersser and Penzer

Table 9.1 Skin diseases in different parts of the world.

Skin diseases of developed countries	Skin diseases of developing countries
Chronic skin conditions	Infections
Inflammatory diseases	Infestations, e.g. lice
Eczema	Scabies
Psoriasis	Fungal infections
	Bacterial infections

Source: Reproduced from Ersser and Penzer (2000).

(2000) point out that various skin diseases are a problem all over the world, whilst their causes and outcomes may be very different in different countries; it is an area in which nurses are best placed to help in providing direct care, health education and support. They report that 70% of the population in developing countries suffer from skin disease and many cannot access the requirements for fundamental skin care.

The most common diseases are infestation and opportunist bacterial infections (see Table 9.1).

Ersser and Penzer (2000) write:

> The promotion of healthy skin is a fundamental concern of nursing in almost all speciality areas. By maintaining healthy skin to serve as a disease barrier, nurses not only help to manage acute and chronic skin disease but also help to prevent and manage pressure sores and wounds.

They believe that a great deal of suffering can be managed by appropriate nursing care because they require low-technology health care strategies to combat problems. Nurses can advise on skin hygiene, the use of moisturisers, measures to protect from sunburn and provide dietary advice.

Disease and illness can cause the patient to feel unclean and dirty; the desire to be cleansed extends beyond the mere washing of the skin. Patients with a cancer diagnosis may claim to feel contaminated and dirty; similarly people who are survivors of abuse may instinctively want to wash before they report the abuse perpetrated against them. Thus the ritual of washing takes on symbolic significance. Whilst washing the patient may not eliminate the disease or abuse, it does make them feel better. The act of assisting in personal cleansing works not only on the physical level but also on the psychological and spiritual levels (Collins and Hampton, 2003).

Anatomy and physiology of the skin

The skin or integumentary system is the largest organ of the body (Ersser et al., 2004), and the only visible one, comprising of the cutaneous membrane, which is the skin and the accessory structures – the hair and nails (Tortora and Derrickson, 2005).

The skin has several functions, it:

- Protects the internal tissues and organs
- Excretes water – approximately 500 mL is lost a day through the skin, taking with it salts and organic waste products, known as insensible loss

- Stores nutrients
- Is necessary for the synthesis of vitamin D when exposed to sunlight
- Detects sensations such as touch, pain, pressure and temperature
- Maintains body temperature

The skin consists of two layers: the dermis, the inner layer, and the epidermis, the outer layer. Under these two layers is a third layer called the subcutaneous membrane or sometimes referred to as the hypodermis or the superficial fascia.

The epidermis

The epidermis has mainly four layers of cells; on the soles of the feet and the palms of the hand, there is an additional layer of cells. The cell thickness of each layer varies with more exposed skin being thicker than unexposed skin (Clancy and McVicar, 2002).

The basal layer of the epidermis called the stratum germinativum or *stratum basale* is the layer, which produces the skin cells, which migrate outwards to form the outer layer of skin. These layers form genetically defined ridges, which are unique to each person, and are visible at the fingertips - hence the use of fingerprints to help solve crimes. Within this layer, Merkel cells are found which are sensitive to touch and pressure. This layer becomes thinner as we age, which is why the skin in older people becomes more delicate and more easily damaged and requires more care (Collins and Hampton, 2003). If the stratum basale is damaged, new skin cannot grow and the patient will require a skin graft (Tortora and Derrickson, 2005).

The next layer consists of eight to ten layers of cells called the stratum spinosum. The cells are characteristically prickly or spiny and are held together by desmosomes - a very strong intercellular cement type protein. Within this layer are Langerhans cells, which produce an immune response when the skin is damaged and protect the skin from microbes.

The stratum granulosum produces keratin, which is needed for the production of hair and nails. In the soles of the feet and the palms of the hand only, the next layer is the stratum lucidum; these are clear hard cells that are filled with keratin to give extra protection.

The final layer is the stratum corneum, believed by Tortora and Derrickson (2005) to be 25-30 layers deep. It takes the cells approximately 4 weeks to reach the outer layers and fall off. Brushing the skin with a soft bristle brush using short strokes removes the most outer layer of cells. The brushing is invigorating and stimulates the underlying blood circulation, thus improving tone and colour. It was believed that the cells in the stratum corneum are dead, but more recent research by Johnson (2004) suggests that these cells are not to be viewed as such. He claims that 'the stratum corneum is not an inert protective barrier, but a most elegantly designed and dynamic structure'.

The cells in the stratum corneum as they reach the surface become flatter and dryer, the dry surface prevents the growth of microorganisms; however, if this layer becomes too dry, other skin problems can occur. This protection from microorganisms is aided by the production of sebum from sebaceous glands in the dermis that open out onto the epidermis, which gives the skin surface an oily covering. The stratum corneum is water-resistant but not waterproof. When the skin is immersed in clean fresh water as in a bath, water enters the cells through the process of *osmosis*. The cells can absorb four times their normal volume.

After washing skin tightness

Using some kinds of soaps has the same effect on the skin as swimming in the sea, in that the lather produced by the soap whilst on the skin has a higher concentration and thus draws water out of the epidermis. This is referred to as trans-epidermal water loss (TEWL) (Lodén et al., 2003) or after wash tightness (AWT) (Ananthapadmanabhan et al., 2004). The very product that is used to promote cleanliness and clean the skin can have damaging effects on the skin and lead to the development of conditions such as acute dermatitis and eczema. Soaps affect the stratum corneum's protein balance and damage to the proteins affect the body's own natural moisturising factor. As the skin dries, the water loss from the stratum corneum is felt as tautness, and the skin looks shiny and tight. To combat this, manufacturers of soaps and other cleansing products are introducing moisturisers to soften and protect the skin. Whilst the skin is taut, it is more easily damaged; a supple skin is more resilient and less likely to be damaged (Collins and Hampton, 2003).

The dermis

The dermis has two layers next to the epidermis; the layer is papillary, that is, folds and follows the folds of the stratum germinativum, providing it with a blood supply as this layer contains blood capillaries. The layer is made up of loose connective tissue that contains sensory nerve fibres as well as the blood capillaries.

Under this, lies the reticular layer, which is made up of collagen fibres, elastin and connective tissue. The collagen and elastin fibres give skin its durability and elasticity. The collagen fibres run through the dermis into the epidermis and at the other end into the subcutaneous tissue. The collagen fibres form rough bundles, which flow in a given direction called lines of cleavage. If a surgeon cuts along the lines of cleavage, when the wound heals, there is little scarring. Cutting across the lines of cleavage inevitably leads to more pronounced scarring. Collagen and elastin in the dermis alters with age and is damaged by hormones and ultraviolet radiation, leaving the skin wrinkled and thinner (Malik, 1998; Rawlings, 2003).

Within the dermis there are hair follicles, glands, blood vessels and nerve fibres. The nerve fibres are sensitive to pressure, pain and temperature and they also adjust the secretions from the sweat glands. There are three types of glands in the skin: sebaceous, sweat and ceruminous glands. Sebaceous glands secrete sebum, an oily substance containing cholesterol, fatty acids proteins, salts and bactericidal chemicals. These glands lie close to the hair follicles. Sweat glands are either apocrine or eccrine. The apocrine glands are mainly in the axilla and the pubic region and their secretions contain pheromones – a scent that can be sexually stimulating. The eccrine glands secrete watery substance, which contains waste products. Ceruminous glands line the ear and produce wax, which has a protective function. If the secretions from the glands remain on the skin surface, they attract bacteria and this changes their composition and can cause odour, hence the need for washing and maintaining personal hygiene (Collins and Hampton, 2003).

Cultural perspectives

There are rituals involving cleansing that have a symbolic significance, the person is cleansed of their 'sin' through baptism, or they are cleansed as an act of purification. In some religions, the event as in Christian baptism may only occur once, but in other religions, such as Islam and Judaism, cleansing may form part of a daily ritual. Malik (1998) points out that the ancient civilisations of Greece, Rome and Egypt introduced hygiene and cleanliness, but these practices changed through the Middle Ages; particularly in Europe, where spiritual purity was considered more important than physical cleanliness, indeed washing could expose one to illness. Spiritual purity was achieved through other means such as being involved in good works. The use of hot water at this time was considered to open up the pores in the skin and leave one susceptible to infection. However, Ersser et al. (2004) point out that hot water can have a drying effect on the skin as it strips the skin of its natural oils and dry skin can crack, thus leaving the person exposed to the possibility of infection. Over time, practices have changed; where once houses in the UK were built without bathrooms, now most have more than one room allocated to washing and the master bedroom may have en suite facilities.

Islam is more than a religion; it is a way of life and Islamic teaching includes guidance on social behaviours, observances and practices, which assist the individual in developing a healthy lifestyle. Besides declaring their faith, engaging in prayer, fasting and making a pilgrimage to Mecca, Muslims are expected to engage in self-purification. Self-purification involves more than just personal cleanliness, it requires the setting aside a proportion of wealth for the needy. Fasting can also be a means of self-purification and good for health (Rassool, 2000).

Muslims are expected to maintain a high standard of personal hygiene not merely from a physical need but because this also has spiritual significance. The ritual of washing needs to be performed before any other act or behaviour, such as eating or praying. Cleanliness extends beyond keeping the body clean, to keeping the internal aspect of the body clean - this means not eating food considered to be unclean, e.g. pork or pork products, or drinking alcohol. Rassool (2000) explains that washing has a symbolic significance. Illness is perceived as a means whereby the sufferer can be cleansed on physical, emotional, spiritual and mental levels; it is a way in which one can atone for one's sins. This does not mean that a Muslim will not seek remedial therapies; however, they will abstain from medication that includes alcohol or pork products. The rituals around cleanliness are important and must be maintained. Thus when Muslims are patients they require access to running water for washing, and need to be able to wash as and when they desire. However, personal preferences are to be respected, the nurse may not assume that all of the above applies because a patient is Muslim. Nor should the nurse assume that the patients are also Muslim if they are of Asian or Arabic origin. Gerrish (2000) points out that frequently nurses do not ask patients what their preferences may be. She writes: 'Ethnic categories, however carefully defined do not correspond with cultural, linguistic, dietary or religious preferences and needs.'

Some cultures and social groups have strict guidelines on what clothing is worn. Malik (1998) and Rees (1997) both describe that total removal of all objects and items of clothing for cleansing purposes is not permitted in some religions. Most Sikhs have five items that are symbols of their religion; one of these is *kaccha*, a loose pair of underpants which are never fully removed, not even for washing. When changing from one pair of *kaccha* to a clean pair, the soiled ones are not removed totally, a leg remains inside one pair whilst the other leg is placed in the clean pair and then as the soiled pants are removed the second leg is inserted.

Martini et al. (2008) point out that those women who have to cover their skin totally, as is the custom for some religious groups, and are not exposed to sunlight may experience bone problems because they are unable to synthesise calcium from vitamin D using sunlight as the catalyst.

Nursing care

Routines and rituals associated with personal cleansing bring the nurse into intimate contact with the patient. That which may be perceived as basic or even menial care is in fact fundamental to the patient's sense of well-being, thus transforming the act of cleansing to an essential aspect of nursing care. Maintaining patient hygiene needs is a clinical skill whose importance ranks alongside other skills such as assessing vital signs, administering medication or redressing a wound aseptically. In Boxer and Kluge's (2000) research, 83% of respondents rated bathing of patients in bed as an essential clinical nursing skill. It is seen as fundamental to patient care, as it enhances patients' sense of well-being as well as being a functional necessity (Collins and Hampton, 2003).

How often patients wash is mainly a matter of personal preference; however, Abbas et al. (2004) report that European and North American women report washing their faces at least twice a day, and bathe or shower once a day. This may change to more frequently depending on the weather. Abbas et al. (2004) believe that faces are washed or cleansed more frequently because it is the part of the body that is permanently on view.

Patients prefer to meet their own hygiene needs (Collins and Hampton, 2003); however, they value nursing assistance when they are unable to do this for themselves (Ratcliffe, 1991). This is emphasised in a poem written and published by a patient, severely disabled by multiple sclerosis and unable to speak or hold a pen, about his nurse - Narinder.

> I have seen many certificates and diplomas
> many gilded trophies too
> but only in my mind.
>
> They're for Narinder Kaur
> the nurse with elegant hands
> and read embossed with truth:
>
> 'World record, established September 1990,
> for wet shaving, bathing (with hair wash)
> and application of gels to gums and teeth
>
> 27 minutes'. Signed by me.
> So fast were you there was no time for thanks,
> so please
> may I thank you now?

Ratcliffe (1991)

Helping patients meet their personal needs may be embarrassing for both the patient and the nurse, especially if they represent opposite sexes. Malik (1998) outlines the difficulty male nurses may have in helping female patients, believing that this kind of care is atypical. Female nurses caring for male patients are not perceived to have the same problems because the role is similar to 'mothering'. Junior or novice nurses may also find this kind of care embarrassing, and they may shy away from helping patients with their personal needs.

Assessment

Patients may need help in meeting all or some of their personal hygiene needs, and a great deal depends on their mobility and dexterity as well as their state of health and the prevailing disease. A nursing assessment needs to establish what patients usually do to maintain their personal hygiene, how often they like to wash and at what time of day and whether they require assistance getting in and out of the bath or shower. A full holistic assessment needs to address whether there are any special needs with regard to cultural observances, so that these practices are not infringed whilst the patient is in receipt of nursing care. The assessment will include a review of the patient's mobility, can they actually go to a bathroom or do facilities need to be brought to the patient (Allen, 2008).

The assessment should take into account the patient's skin condition, whether the skin is intact or damaged. Those patients who may suffer from either urinary or faecal incontinence or both may require more frequent care. Whilst cleansing the skin removes bacteria, dirt and oil and is essential and desirable for good skin care, the process could damage the skin barrier, depending on which cleansers are used. Subramanyan (2004) and Holloway and Jones (2005) list several factors, which can affect skin and lead to dryness and skin disorders such as atopic dermatitis and xerosis. Stress and anxiety can also affect the skin condition as it may lead to excessive sweating resulting in increased body odour, which patients may find extremely unpleasant as it can isolate them from close contact with others.

The development of a comprehensive care plan will mean that the patient does not have to repeat the information each time a nurse wishes to assist him or her in order to meet his or her hygiene needs.

Planning care

Whether the nurse is assisting the patient to meet their personal hygiene needs in a designated bathroom or in bed, the operation needs careful planning to ensure maximum privacy, minimum exposure and greatest comfort for the patient. Most patients have their own personal items such as flannels/face cloths, towels and toiletries with them. Some establishments have en suite facilities but sometimes there may only be one communal bathroom available. The nurse should ensure that it is available, warm and clean before ushering in the patient.

If the patient is too ill to leave the bed, then the patient's hygiene needs can be accommodated whilst in bed. Once again, forward planning is of the most importance to ensure maximum privacy and minimum exposure. Patients who are ill and confined to bed may well have an increased temperature (pyrexia) and the plastic protective coverings to the pillows and mattress may cause excessive sweating; they may also require washing more than once a day to maintain their comfort.

Bed bathing

Having ascertained that the patient has consented to being bathed in bed, the nurse needs to ensure that he or she has accumulated all the appropriate equipment - bowl, towels and toiletries. The nurse should make certain that there would be no interruptions during this procedure as it may leave the patients in a compromised situation that can threaten their dignity and their comfort. The physical environment requires preparation; open windows may cause draughts and chill the patient. Screens that offer sufficient privacy should also be placed around the area. The bed, if fitted with a variable height device, will need rising to the correct height so that the nurse is not bending over and risking back damage whilst assisting the patient (Aston and Wakefield, 1998).

The top layers of bedding are removed, leaving the top sheet covering the patient. Night attire or bedclothes are removed. Most patients will want to wash their own faces, but may require assistance in preparing the facecloth and rinsing it out in clean water before towelling dry. It is very difficult to dry someone else's face, the person being washed is the only one who can feel if their skin is dry or not; therefore, it is best to facilitate their achievement of this task rather than doing it for them.

The main aim for the nurse when washing a patient in bed is not to expose too much of the patient at any one time, and to wash section by section of the body so that it can be rinsed and dried quickly, in order that the patient does not get cold. The water in the bowl will require changing frequently, particularly if the cleansing product or soap lathers up excessively. If cleansing products are not removed adequately, the patient may experience itching and dry skin. Lodén et al. (2003) claim that mild soap has the potential to irritate and dry the skin if it is not adequately rinsed off. The soap barrier can build up over time, thus aggravating the situation.

It is usual to wash and dry the upper half of the body first before proceeding to the lower half, and it is usual to leave washing the genital area until last. If the patient is able, they will probably wish to wash this area themselves, as it may be embarrassing to have this area of the body washed by someone else. It is usual to use disposable cloths for this procedure, especially if patients have a urinary catheter in place.

After being washed and dried the patient may require assistance with applying deodorants, talcum powder, perfume, face creams and moisturisers or make-up before putting on fresh clothing. This is usually a matter of personal preference and the nurse should not assume that the patient wants or does not want to use these products. Extravagant use of a patient's products is considered poor practice, especially as some products may be very expensive to purchase.

The patient may be able to sit in a chair for a short period of time whilst the bed is remade with clean linen, but if this is not possible, the bed is made with the patient remaining in bed.

For those patients who have their hygiene needs met in bed, retain the bowl for future use; if this is not possible, then the bowl needs thorough cleaning to prevent cross-infection before returning it to the stock.

Cleansing products

Cleansing products used in washing are largely a matter of personal preference and available finances but may also be determined by beliefs and cultural practices. Abbas et al. (2004) point out that soap has been in use since 2500 BC and that Yardley, launched in 1770, is the oldest brand. However, whilst soaps are widely used, new cleansers have emerged on the market which cleanse whilst not damaging the skin. Some soap is unacceptable to vegans and vegetarians because they contain animal products such as tallow. These soaps are also often unacceptable in Indian and Middle Eastern countries. Where soaps do not contain tallow, they consist of vegetable oils. Most soaps, however – whether containing animal fats or vegetable oils – are drying and can cause skin irritation, dryness and after-wash tightness (AWT).

Most soaps are alkaline whilst the skin pH is slightly acidic; the alteration of the acidic balance may put the patient at risk of infection (Baranda et al., 2002). Abbas et al. (2004) and Holloway and Jones (2005) believe that synthetic detergents are significantly milder than soap. Much of the research seems to be driven by public demand for products that are cosmetically pleasing as well as functional. Baranda et al. (2002) discovered that the most highly priced soaps were not necessarily the best; the cheapest soap in the market used in their research was the least irritant to sensitive skins.

Some soaps are being replaced by body wash lotions, which contain emollients as well as perfumes such as aqueous cream (Holloway and Jones, 2005). These body washes, according to Abbas et al. (2004), are less drying and the emollients moisturise the skin. They leave fewer deposits on the skin after rinsing and as such do not alter the skin acidity balance.

'Soft towel' bed bathing

The 'soft towel' bed bath is a relatively new approach to maintaining patient hygiene that is being practised in some parts of Australia, and research suggests that patients find it more relaxing and pleasant than the traditional bed bath. It appears to take less time, and nurses find it less messy and more rewarding than the traditional method as reported by Hancock et al. (2000).

Three towels and two disposable cloths are placed in a plastic bag with 30 mL of proprietary cleansing lotion called 'Dermalux Soft Towel Lotion' specifically manufactured in Australia. Two litres of hot water are added and the contents are kneaded together so that most of the water is absorbed into the towels. Hancock et al. (2000) do not specify an exact temperature. Malik (1998) describes a similar procedure which stipulates that the water temperature should be 43°C.

The patient has one towel placed over the upper half of their body and a second towel is placed over their legs. The patient is offered one disposable cloth to wash their face; there is no need to rinse the solution off, and the warmth of the cloth means that there is no need for drying. The upper half of the body is massaged with the wet towel, followed by massage to the legs. The patient is offered the second cloth for cleansing the genitalia. The patient is turned onto their side and the third towel is used to massage the back, ending with the perianal area.

Hancock et al. (2000) report that patients preferred to meet their own hygiene needs; but as this were not always possible, they enjoyed being bathed in this manner and some reported that it was preferred to showering. The nurses involved in this research were also very enthusiastic about the method, as it was quicker, less messy and relatively uncomplicated. The patient satisfaction meant that nurses also experienced satisfaction in a procedure completed well.

Using 'BagBath'

Collins and Hampton (2003) outline a new product - BagBath, which is a packet of pre-packed rayon/polyester disposable cloths impregnated with a cleanser that does not require rinsing from the skin surface. The cloths are used once and disposed; there are eight cloths in a packet, so that individual parts of the body are washed a section at a time, maintaining patient privacy. Their evaluation suggests that it is a cost-effective method of providing patient hygiene as it reduces not only time taken to administer but also cross-infection. The use of a cleanser and emollient combined also reduces the risk of 'skin tear' occurring in elderly patients.

Bathing aids

Assisting patients with their hygiene needs may require the use of special aids such as hoists, which help raise the patient in and out of the bath. The hoist may be a frightening piece of equipment for patients particularly the elderly as when the hoist is raised, the patient finds themselves dangling in mid-air, with little below them as they are swung over and then lowered into the bath. It is important that whilst this is done, the patient remains covered with towels, and due attention is paid to maintaining their dignity and modesty. The towels may be removed once they are partially lowered into the warm water. It is important to check with the patient that the temperature of the water is to their liking before they are lowered into the bath, as this is a matter of personal preference (Switzer, 2001). Switzer (2001) advocates that the bath water temperature should not exceed 38°C, as older people may lose their ability to feel the heat of the water; however, allowing a person to test the temperature helps to maintain their sense of control.

There are some specially adapted baths, such as the Parker bath (Malik, 1998), with sides that are raised so that the patient can slide in to. This makes the hoist redundant. Some baths can be raised and lowered once the patient is in so that the nurse is not bending over and straining their backs. There are a number of different makes available on the market, and it is advisable to ensure familiarity with equipment prior to its use with patients.

Hair washing

Hair washing is part of the routine of maintaining personal cleanliness and is a matter of personal preference. Some people wash their hair daily, and this is easily managed in a shower. It is possible to wash a patient's hair whilst they remain in bed; this requires careful planning and is easily achievable if organised properly. Washing a patient's hair at home is also possible and the principles alluded to here can be adopted for home bathing also.

It is possible to remove the head of the bed on most hospital beds. The bed has to be raised so that the height is comfortable for the nurse to complete the operation without bending over and risking back strain.

There are specially designed bowls available on the market for use in bed, with a spout for drainage. The bed must be protected with plastic sheeting. The amount of warm water required for completion of hair washing depends largely on the thickness and length of hair and how much lather the shampoo produces.

The nurse needs to ensure patient comfort; the rim of the bowl can be softened with the use of towels and correct positioning is required before the procedure commences. Once the hair is washed and rinsed, it can be towel dried and then blown dry with a hairdryer if the hair is long (Allen, 2008).

Mouth care

The mouth is the central and most important part of the face; besides being used for feeding its main function is in communication. The importance of enabling patients to meet their oral hygiene needs was reinforced in the Department of Health's publication *Essence of Care* (DH, 2001). If the health of the oral cavity is compromised then both feeding and communication is severely affected (Henshaw and Calabrese, 2001; Rydholm and Strang, 2002). Poor oral care may mean that patients may experience problems with several activities of living; they may not drink or eat as they should and can become malnourished, they cannot communicate because of dryness (xerostomia), which impacts on their ability to socialise. Rydholm and Strang (2002) found that patients with xerostomia not only complained of the discomfort caused to them from having a dry mouth, but were also more prone to develop infections such as oral thrush and ulceration. They report that patients expressed feelings of shame, which led to social withdrawal as a direct result of this condition. Reduction of saliva results in difficulty with chewing food, swallowing and talking. Finally it makes kissing difficult, which may impact on their ability to express their sexuality. All of these reduce the patients' sense of themselves and they may recoil from the company of others, finding themselves isolated at a time when social support is most needed. Box 9.1 lists some drugs that may cause xerostomia.

Box 9.1 Some drugs that may cause xerostomia.

Medications that may cause xerostomia:

Antihypertensives
Anticholinergics
Antihistamines
Antipsychotics
Anorectics

Anticonvulsants
Cancer Chemotherapy drugs, cytotoxic drugs
Sympathomimetics
Antidepressants
Diuretics

Source: Adapted from McNeill (2000).

Ford (2008) states that ventilated patients who are not given adequate oral care are at risk of developing ventilator-associated pneumonia.

When people are healthy, oral care is a natural part of routine personal cleansing, and the majority of people brush their teeth at least once daily (Paulsson et al., 1999). When ill, there are several factors that compromise a healthy mouth, but generally these may be overlooked as more urgent needs are attended to and are given priority by nursing staff (Ford, 2008). Ford (2008) points out that when patients are ill, the normal bacteria in the mouth alters from being gram-positive flora to gram-negative flora and changes to the oral; mucous membranes allow bacteria to adhere to the surfaces in the oral cavity, which means that the mouth becomes a source of infection. Nosocomial pneumonia pathogens have been found on dental plaque and oral mucosa of patients in intensive therapy units. There are many other factors that affect the mouth in ill people, e.g. oxygen therapy, intubation, suction, reduced fluid intake and treatments such as radiotherapy and chemotherapy (Southern, 2007). Rydholm and Strang (2002) found that 70% of patients with cancer and 97% of those in the terminal stages of the disease had problems with xerostomia, predominantly caused by the opioids and other drugs used to control other symptoms. Patients with cancer who were interviewed by Rydholm and Strang (2002) stated that they found having a dry mouth woke them up during the night so their sleep pattern was disturbed and it affected their sense of taste which meant that they could not cook the meals they previously enjoyed making for friends; in fact, for many, it altered their lifestyle considerably.

Assessment

Dougherty and Lister (2008) point out that there are several assessment tools available and claim that the most used is the simple tool designed by Eiliers et al. (1988), which scores on six categories:

- Lips
- Tongue
- Saliva
- Mucous membranes
- Gingival
- Teeth

However, it is their belief that nurses have little confidence in their skills associated with oral hygiene.

Nursing care

Paulsson et al. (1999) report that providing oral care is difficult for nursing personnel because the mouth is one of the most intimate areas which individuals attempt to protect from abuse. A subject in Paulsson et al.'s (1999) research stated: 'One's whole health deteriorates if one doesn't have good oral health.'

If a patient is to recover from illness then a good nutritional status must be maintained and this is not possible if the mouth is sore due to poor oral hygiene and aggravated by medication. However, Paulsson et al. (1999) discovered that nurses who were repulsed at the thought of assisting patients' with mouth care were less likely to engage in this aspect of nursing care. They also found nurses cited lack of time as an important reason for not attending to patients needs in this regard. Whilst nurses claim that a healthy mouth is crucial to a patient's well-being and important for their self-esteem, there are those who do not give it the priority it deserves.

The best method of providing oral hygiene is to assist the patient in using a toothbrush. When the mouth is sore, a soft child's toothbrush is preferred, and the mouth may be rinsed with either water or simple mouthwashes such as 0.2% chlorhexidine, alternatively sponges dipped in antiseptic mouthwashes may be used. Petroleum jelly may be applied to the lips to prevent drying and cracking (Ford, 2008). The frequency of care is largely determined by the patient's condition; if they have a pyrexia, are breathing mainly through the mouth or have developed oral ulceration, then the care needs to be assessed two hourly.

Conclusions

This chapter has focused on the need for helping patients maintain their personal hygiene according to their own preferences, practices and cultural perspectives; this adheres to the NMC's requirements to respect personal preference and individual needs. Maintaining hygiene is vitally important for the physical, psychological, emotional and social well-being of the patient. It has been deemed as 'basic' care, but this undermines the significance and importance that it has for patients unable to meet their own hygiene needs. This aspect of nursing must receive the recognition it richly deserves as this is the core of what is deemed essential patient care.

Not attending to patients' hygiene needs or not doing it well compromises the patients' health status when they are already vulnerable because of ill health, and this is unacceptable when health care is a costly commodity.

Maintaining a patient's hygiene needs is not a luxury but a necessity if the patient's health status and well-being are to improve.

Glossary

Cutaneous	The skin or relating to the skin as in cutaneous membrane
Dermis	The layer of skin that lies under the epidermis
Dermatitis	An inflammation of the skin
Eczema	A skin condition

Epidermis	The outer layer of the skin and has four layers of cells that are shaped differently
Integumentary system	The name given to the skin, hair and nails and the sweat and oil glands that help the skin to function effectively as an organ
Langerhans cells	Cells that are part of the immune response
Merkel cells	Cells which are interspersed through the stratum basale and are sensitive to touch and pressure
Osmosis	The diffusion of particles or solvent from a more concentrated solution through a semi-permeable membrane in order to achieve a balance in the solution on either side of the membrane
Stratum basale	The base layer of the epidermis which replenishes the skin with new cells
Stratum corneum	The final outer layer of the epidermis, the cells are flattened and give a semi-waterproof barrier
Stratum granulosum	The outer layer of cells that produces keratin cells and contains the hair and nails
Stratum lucidum	The layer of cells found only on the feet and hands; it is a toughened layer of cells that offers protection against all the hard work that feet and hands do
Stratum spinosum	Cells in this section are spiny and prickly in shape locking into each other
Xerosis	An abnormal dryness of the skin which looks scaly
Xerostomia	Dry mouth where there is decreased saliva and the mouth feels like cotton wool

Post-chapter quiz

1. Which skin diseases are most prevalent in developing countries?
2. List the five layers of the epidermis.
3. Why does the skin feel tight after washing?
4. Why is skin brushing beneficial?
5. Why is it important to moisturise skin?
6. What are the potential problems that can result from washing in hot water and using soap?
7. Which treatments affect the mucosa of the mouth?
8. What factor affects the patient's nutritional status?
9. What is the most effective way of cleaning teeth and removing plaque?
10. How does helping a patient with their personal care impact on their sense of the spiritual?

References

Abbas, S., Weiss Goldberg, J. and Massaro, M. (2004) Personal cleanser technology and clinical performance. *Dermatologic Therapy* 17: 35–42.

Allen, K. (2008) Personal hygiene: skin care. In: Dougherty, L. and Lister, S. (eds). *The Royal Marsden Hospital Manual of Clinical Nursing Procedures Student Edition*, 7th ed. Oxford: Wiley Blackwell.

Ananthapadmanabhan, K.P., Moore, D.J., Subramanyan, K., Misra, M. and Meyer, F. (2004) Cleansing without compromise: the impact of cleansers on the skin barrier and the technology of mild cleansing. *Dermatological Therapy* 17: 16-25.

Aston, L. and Wakefield, J. (1998) Moving and handling. In: Malik, M., Hall, C. and Howard, D. (eds). *Nursing Knowledge and Practice*. London: Balliere Tindall.

Baranda, L., Gonzàlez-Amaro, R., Torres-Alvarez, B., Alvarez, C. and Ramírez, V. (2002) Correlation between pH and irritant effect of cleansers marketed for dry skin. *International Journal of Dermatology* 41: 494-499.

Boxer, E. and Kluge, B. (2000) Essential clinical skills for beginning registered nurses. *Nurse Education Today* 20: 327-335.

Burr, S. and Penzer, R. (2005) Promoting skin health. *Nursing Standard* 19(36): 57-65.

Clancy, J. and McVicar, A.J. (2002) *Physiology and Anatomy: A Homeostatic Approach*, 2nd ed. London: Arnold.

Collins, F. and Hampton, S. (2003) The cost-effective use of BagBath: a new concept in patient hygiene. *British Journal of Nursing* 12(16): 984-990.

Department of Health (2001) *The Essence of Care: Patient Focussed Benchmarking for Health Care Professionals*. London: HMSO.

Dougherty, L. and Lister, S. (2008) *The Royal Marsden Hospital Manual of Clinical Nursing Procedures Student Edition*, 7th ed. Oxford: Wiley Blackwell.

Eiliers, J., Berger, A.M. and Peterson, M.C. (1988) Development, testing and application of the oral assessment guide. *Oncology Nursing Forum* 15(3): 325-330.

Ersser, S. and Penzer, R. (2000) Meeting patients' skin care needs: harnessing nursing expertise at an international level. *International Nursing Review* 47: 167-173.

Ersser, S.J., Getliffe, K., Voegeli, D. and Regan, S. (2004) A critical review of the inter-relationship between skin vulnerability and urinary incontinence and related nursing intervention. *International Journal of Nursing Studies* 42(7): 823-835.

Ford, S.J. (2008) The importance and provision of oral hygiene in surgical patients. *International Journal of Surgery* 6: 418-419.

Gerrish, K. (2000) Researching ethnic diversity in the British NHS: methodological and practical concerns. *Journal of Advanced Nursing* 31(4): 918-925.

Hancock, I., Bowman, A. and Prater, D. (2000) 'The day of the soft towel?': comparison of the current bed-bathing method with the Soft Towel bed-bathing method. *International Journal of Nursing Practice* 6: 207-213.

Henshaw, M.M. and Calabrese, J.M. (2001) Oral health and nutrition in the elderly. *Nutritional Clinical Care* 4(1): 34-42.

Holloway, S. and Jones, V. (2005) The importance of skin care and assessment. *British Journal of Nursing* 14(22): 1172-1176.

Johnson, A. (2004) Overview: fundamental skin care - protecting the barrier. Dermatological Therapy 17: 1-5.

Lodén, M., Buraczewska, I. and Edlund, E. (2003) The irritation potential and reservoir effect of mild soaps. *Contact Dermatitis* 49: 91-96.

Malik, M. (1998) Hygiene. In: Malik, M., Hall, C. and Howard, D. (eds). *Nursing Knowledge and Practice*. London: Balliere Tindall.

Martini, F.H., Nath, J.L. and Bartholomew, E.L. (2008) *Fundamentals of Anatomy and Physiology*, 8th ed. New Jersey: Pearson Benjamin Cummings.

McNeill, H.E. (2000) Biting back at poor oral hygiene. *Intensive and Critical Care Nursing* 16: 367-372.

Nursing and Midwifery Council (2008) *Code of Professional Conduct*. London: NMC.

Paulsson, G., Nederfors, T. and Frdlund, B. (1999) Conceptions of oral health among nurse managers: a qualitative analysis. *Journal of Nursing Management* 7: 299–306.

Rassool, G.H. (2000) The crescent and Islam: healing, nursing and the spiritual dimension: some considerations towards an understanding of the Islamic perspectives on caring. *Journal of Advanced Nursing* 32(6): 1476–1484.

Ratcliffe, K. (1991) *An Echo of Reflections*. Bishops Waltham: Meon Valley Printers.

Rees, D. (1997) *Death and Bereavement: The Psychological, Religious and Cultural Interfaces*. London: Whurr Publishers Ltd.

Rydholm, M. and Strang, P. (2002) Physical and psychosocial impact of xerostomia in palliative cancer care: a qualitative interview study. *International Journal of Palliative Nursing* 8(7): 318–323.

Southern, H. (2007) Oral care in cancer nursing: nurses' knowledge and education. *Journal of Advanced Nursing* 57(6): 631–638.

Subramanyan, K. (2004) Role of mild cleansing in the management of patient skin. *Dermatological Therapy* 17: 26–34.

Switzer, J. (2001) How to supervise a general bath. *Nursing and Residential Care* 3(5): 226–228.

Tortora, G.J. and Derrickson, B.H. (2009) *Anatomy and Physiology*, 12th ed. New Jersey: John Wiley & Sons.

Williamson, C.R., Jenkins, T. and Proctor- Childs, T. (2008) *Nursing in Contemporary Healthcare Practice*. Poole: Learning Matters.

Chapter 10

An Ergonomic Approach to Safe Manual Handling

Kim Walter

Learning opportunities

This chapter will help you to:

1. Understand the principles of safe manual handling
2. Describe basic spinal anatomy and understand how back injury occurs
3. Begin to understand how risk assessment is used in the workplace to promote safe manual handling
4. Understand how ergonomics is used to promote safe systems of work
5. Identify and discuss controversial techniques and hazardous tasks
6. Begin to understand the challenges associated with manually handling a bariatric person

Pre-chapter quiz

1. List the nursing tasks you think would be classed as manual handling activities.
2. What do you understand by the term 'risk'?
3. What manual handling tasks do you think may cause injury to the back?
4. Where would you find the intervertebral discs?
5. Describe how ageing and levels of fitness affect a person's ability to perform manual handling tasks
6. Discuss why assessing the risks involved with manual handling tasks is important
7. What would you need to know about a patient before performing any manual handling tasks?
8. Discuss why it is important to assess the individuals who will be carrying out manual handling tasks.
9. List possible hazards in the environment where manual handling occurs
10. What are the main functions of the spine?

Introduction

Manual handling has been defined as any activity that involves exertion by a person to lift, lower, push, pull, carry, move or hold a person or object (Carrivick et al., 2001). Despite legislation to protect workers in the health and social care sector, the Health and Safety Executive (HSE) (2008) reports that musculoskeletal injuries account for 40% of all sickness in the National Health Service (NHS). Approximately 2500 injuries are reported each year as a direct result of patient handling and one in four nurses have at sometime taken time off work as a result of a back injury. The Royal College of Nursing (2002) produced guidance stating that 'hazardous manual handling should be eliminated in all but exceptional or life-threatening situations'. In addition to this, the HSE (1992) places a duty on employers to avoid hazardous manual handling operations as far as it is reasonably practicable. Where this cannot be avoided, the regulation requires an assessment to be undertaken and the risks of injury reduced to the lowest level possible.

As can be seen from the guidance and statutory requirements, nurses face a dilemma when they are required to manually handle patients. The risk of injury is high but they also owe a duty to patients to meet their nursing care needs which may only be possible by manual handling (Griffith and Stevens, 2004). As it is beyond the scope of this chapter to discuss individual manual handling techniques in any detail, the aim is to give an overview that equips the reader with a firm evidence base for the safe handling of patients and enables the reader to identify risk thereby promoting a problem-solving approach to manual handling.

Principles of safe handling and the biomechanics of back injury

To understand how back injury occurs from manual handling activities, a brief overview of spinal anatomy is required. The spine or vertebral column consists of 24 separate, movable, irregular bones called vertebrae plus the sacrum consisting of 5 fused bones and the coccyx consisting of 4 fused bones (Figure 10.1).

In effect, the vertebral column is a strong flexible rod that moves anteriorly, posteriorly and laterally and rotates. It encloses and protects the spinal cord, supports the head and serves as a point of attachment for the ribs and the muscles of the back. On the superior and inferior surfaces of the neural arch, there are two articular processes for articulation with the vertebra above and below. These are known as the facet joints or zygapophysial joints. The facet joints provide an important locking mechanism between consecutive lumbar vertebrae. They limit twisting movements and stop forward sliding of the vertebrae (Figure 10.2).

Between the vertebrae are openings called intervertebral foramina. The nerves that connect the spinal cord to other parts of the body pass through these openings. Between the vertebrae from the first vertebrae to the sacrum are fibrocartilaginous intervertebral discs. Each disc is composed of an outer fibrous ring consisting of fibrocartilage called the annulus fibrosis and an inner gel like, highly elastic structure called the nucleus pulposus. The discs form strong joints between the vertebrae, permit various movements of the vertebral column and absorb vertical shock. When viewed from the side, the vertebral

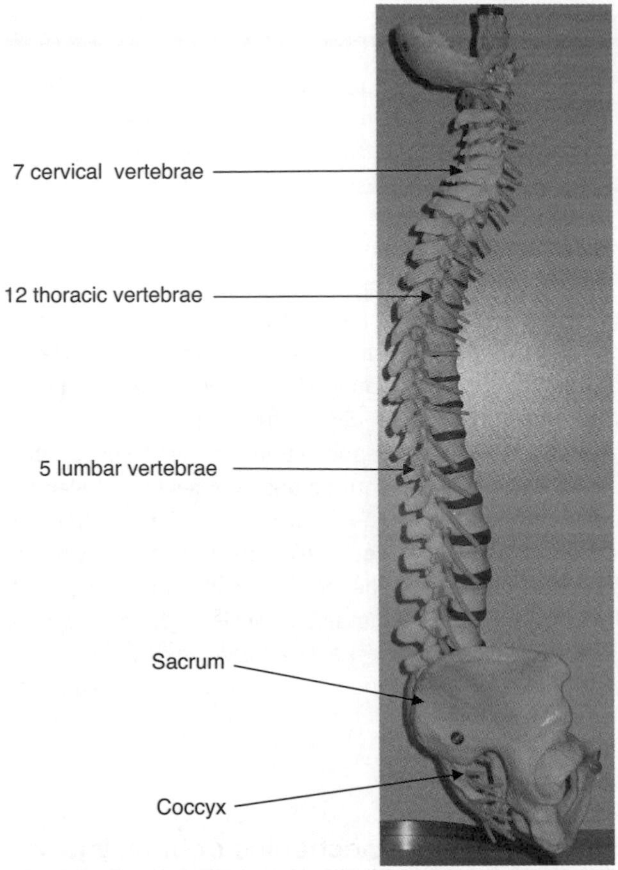

Figure 10.1 The spinal column.

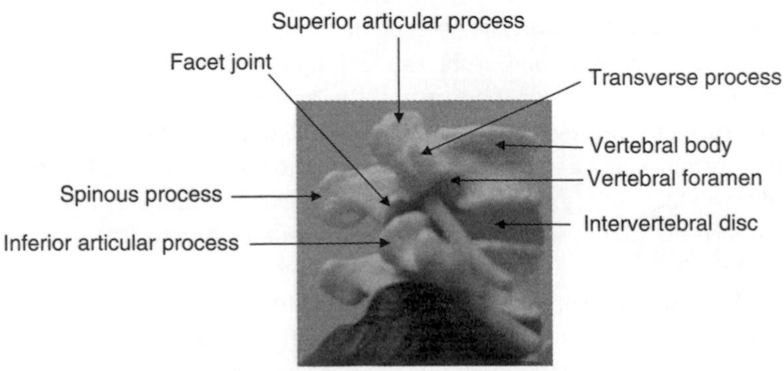

Figure 10.2 Vertebra.

column shows four normal curves, two of which are convex and two of which are concave. The curves of the spinal column like the curves of a long bone are important because they increase its strength. The curves also help maintain balance in the upright position, absorb shock from normal movements of the body and help protect the vertebral column from fracture.

As with all joints, the spine is supported by ligaments. Many of the structures in the spine referred to as ligaments are not true ligaments. This is because they are either too weak to serve as ligaments or do not connect bone to bone. The most important ligaments are the anterior longitudinal ligament, which supports the anterior aspect of the vertebral column, including the intervertebral discs and extends the length of the vertebral column; and the posterior longitudinal ligament, which provides posterior support to the vertebral bodies. It also forms the anterior wall of the vertebral canal and extends the length of the vertebral column: the ligamentum flavum, which passes between adjacent vertebrae. This ligament contains a large amount of elastic tissue and permits forward flexion of the spine. The joints and ligaments of the spine provide stability and a small amount of protection from excessive movement, but it is the skeletal muscles surrounding the vertebral column that are most important for movement. The muscles of the spine are numerous and complex as they have several origins and insertions with considerable overlapping among them. Skeletal muscle is designed for voluntary movement and is specialised for forceful contraction, which facilitates movement and maintain posture (Adams et al., 2002).

Acute back injury is rare and generally associated with trauma. The main culprits of back injury caused by manual handling are a combination of poor posture, lifting loads that are too heavy and repetition of tasks that involve the aforementioned. The injury is usually brought about by a cumulative effect as opposed to a single incident reflecting the often-repetitive nature of tasks associated with manual handling. When muscular work is performed repetitively with insufficient rest periods, microruptures of the muscle tissue can occur. If microruptures are sustained repeatedly, regeneration is impaired and an inflammatory response occurs which may also affect surrounding tissues and nerve endings (Wilson, 2002).

Poor posture occurs when the body moves away from its centre of gravity. Gravity is an invisible vertical force exerted down through each part of the body in direct proportion to its mass (Adams et al., 2002). The centre of gravity is at the geometric centre of a symmetrical body, and in a human, it is in the pelvic region. The line of gravity is the force exerted by gravity from the object's centre of gravity to the earth and must fall in the object's base of support to achieve stability. As the body bends forward and adopts a stooping posture, it moves away from the centre of gravity pushing the line of gravity outside the base of support. As a result the muscles of the back tense to prevent falling and to move and protect the spine.

The main cause of muscle fatigue and injury is muscle tension without sufficient time to recover. The degree of muscle tension is determined by the workload performed by the muscle (Wilson, 2002). The tension of the back muscles subjects the spine to high compressive forces and potential injury (Adams et al., 2002). If a twisted posture is added and a weight is lifted at the same time, this further increases the likelihood of injury occurring as the muscles and ligaments of the back are required to work even harder. Twisting and bending motions can also potentially damage the intervertebral discs and facet joints. It can be seen from this discussion why an important principle of safe handling is to avoid twisting, stooping and forward bending as far as possible. Instead of bending the back forward, the handler should always bend from the knees. Beds, cots and trolleys should be adjusted to a height that prevents stooping when carrying out nursing activities. It is also important for the handler to stand square on when supporting an object or a limb to avoid twisting the spine whilst holding a load.

Handling a load at arm's length increases what is referred to as the 'leverage effect'. For example, a relatively lightweight feels heavier when held away from the body's centre of gravity because the lever arm is increased. This underpins the principle of safe handling, which is to keep any load close to the body and preferably at waist height. The HSE (1992) guidance recommends that a female should lift no more than 17 kg at waist height and a male no more than 25 kg to prevent a significant risk of injury. These recommendations are only guidelines, however, and other factors need to be considered, for example the physical build of the handler or existing injuries. If a load is moved away from the body, for instance above the head, the weight of the object must be significantly reduced to prevent injury. Another principle of safe handling is to ensure that there is a stable and wide base of support. As the body's centre of gravity moves, the base of support should also move. The position of the handler's feet can also facilitate transference of weight, which allows the movement to be carried out more effectively and with less effort. The final principle is to carry out the movement smoothly. When moving a load, sudden jerky movements should be avoided as these will cause peaks of pressure, which place stress on the intervertebral discs.

It is important to note that a number of other factors affect the likelihood of injury. These include the individual's level of fitness. Regular exercise strengthens bones, muscles and ligaments, which in turn makes them less susceptible to injury. Ageing produces degenerative changes in soft tissues and joints making them more prone to injury. Underlying medical conditions may also play a part, for example thyroid disorders can affect muscular metabolism. A person's physical characteristics may also influence the risk of injury. Very tall people have longer leverages, which creates high joint forces (Wilson, 2002). It is also believed that some people are just more genetically prone to back injury than others (Adams and Dolan, 2005).

Ergonomics

Ergonomics is a science that focuses on the individual in relation to their work environment from both psychosocial and physiological perspectives (Wilson, 2002). It aims to improve the effectiveness of work and safety (Sanders and McCormick, 1992). An example of ergonomic design is a hoist. Hoists were designed to mechanise the lifting of loads so that people do not have to lift, which makes the task safer. Ergonomics has also been used more broadly in the health and social care setting; for example Owen and Staehler (2003) studied nursing activities in patients' homes to identify tasks that carers perceived as being the most physically demanding. Another study investigated the internal layout of UK ambulances, discovering that the layout was less than ideal for paramedic staff to work efficiently or safely. The study identified that there are many design implications to be taken into consideration and provides a foundation for future research (Hignett, 2005a). Other examples of the use of ergonomics in the health and social care setting are the development of postural analysis systems that are sensitive to musculoskeletal risks in a range of work-related tasks. The Rapid Entire Body Assessment (REBA) tool was developed by Hignett and McAtamney (2000) to assess the often-difficult working postures of health care staff and other service industries. A score is allocated following the assessment indicating the level of musculoskeletal risk and the urgency with which action should be taken (Hignett, 2005b).

Box 10.1 Case study.

Mrs Green with a suspected chest infection is admitted to the medical ward of her local NHS trust hospital. She has advanced multiple sclerosis and is unable to move at all. Despite her condition Mrs Green is able to communicate with staff and make her wishes known. She has an electric wheelchair which she would normally spend the day in while at home which she has brought into hospital with her. Her husband who is also her carer at home has been lifting her for all transfers. The couple had been supplied with a portable hoist when Mrs Green originally became immobile, but Mrs Green had found being hoisted uncomfortable and undignified. As Mr Green did not want to upset his wife, he continued to transfer her manually. Mrs Green has an indwelling urinary catheter and because of her multiple sclerosis suffers uncontrollable, intermittent muscle spasm. She has fragile skin and is assessed as being at 'high risk' of developing a pressure sore.

When the ward staff approach Mrs Green to transfer her from her bed to her wheelchair, she refuses to be hoisted and requests that staff lift her manually into her chair as her husband would at home.

Risk assessment

A risk assessment involves identifying hazards in the workplace and assessing the likelihood and severity of possible resultant harm. It allows for a proactive approach to the management of staff, patients and care. It systematically analyses actual and potential areas of risk and develops measures to address them. Manual handling can be identified as the hazard and injury to staff or the patient as the risk. The HSE (1999) places an obligation on the employer to actively carry out a risk assessment of the workplace and act accordingly. The assessment must be reviewed when necessary and recorded where there are five or more employees. It is intended to identify health, safety and fire risks. Manual handling risk assessment cannot be simplified to just completing a form, it requires a holistic approach that takes into account the task, individual capability, the load and environmental factors (TILE). It also needs to consider the interaction between these areas (Johnson, 2005). A full summary of TILE is available in Table 10.1.

Evidence suggests that nurses also acquire injuries from engaging in indirect patient care activities (Retsas and Pinikahana, 2000). When considering the task, the load may be

Table 10.1 Risk assessment: a full summary of TILE.

Task	**Individual capability**
How much can the patient do for themselves? Does the task involve poor posture: twisting, stooping, reaching upwards? Excessive lifting or lowering? Excessive carrying over distance? Repetition? Does the task involve pushing and/or pulling? Are there sufficient numbers of staff to assist with the task? Does it require frequent or prolonged physical effort? Insufficient rest or recovery times? Are there time constraints?	Adequate training? Level of experience? Attitude? Weight, height and shape? Familiarity with equipment? Existing injuries or pregnancy? Appropriate clothing and footwear? Age and general level of fitness?
Load	**Environment**
What are the patient's wishes? Weight, height and shape? Ability to bear weight? Physical ability? Medical condition? Pain, medication, drips, drains or catheters? Tissue viability? Infection control? Communication? Confusion? Challenging behaviour? Cultural issues? Sensory loss?	Space constraints? Uneven floor surfaces? Temperature, humidity and ventilation? Poor lighting? Slip and trip hazards? Noise? If using equipment is it readily available? Sufficient space to use equipment? Has equipment been maintained and does it comply with equipment regulations?

the patient or an object such as a piece of medical equipment or a bedside chair. Moving pieces of equipment is often seen as a day-to-day activity, and if it does not involve direct patient contact, the task is often not perceived as hazardous. However, nurses have been found to be engaged in indirect patient handling activities more frequently during an average shift than direct patient care activities, and evidence suggests that they are a significant cause of injury (Retsas and Pinikahana, 2000).

When the handling task involves a patient, common tasks include transfers, personal care and specialist procedures. Transfers that actively involve moving a patient are referred to as a dynamic load, whereas personal care and wound dressing require the handler to remain in the same position for a long period of time and are referred to as a static load. Unless working on a neonate unit, all patients will be above the HSE guidelines for safe lifting and in accordance with the HSE (1992), the risk must be reduced to the

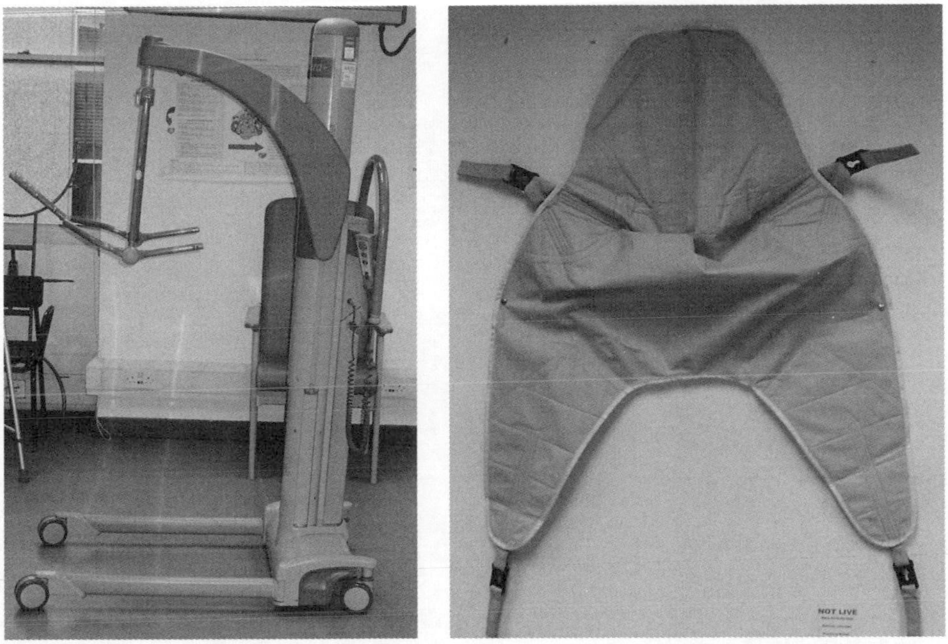

(a) (b)

Figure 10.3 A hoist and a sling.

lowest level possible. For patients unable to assist themselves, transfers are usually mechanised by the use of a hoist and sling (Figure 10.3).

For lateral transfers when the patient is lying flat, a PATSLIDE slide and low-friction sliding devices such as slide sheets may be used (Figure 10.4).

It is also possible to hoist a patient while they are lying flat. There are many makes and types of hoist and sling available including portable hoists, standing hoists (Figure 10.5), overhead ceiling mounted and gantry type hoists (Figure 10.6).

Gantry hoists are similar to overhead hoists but have their own frame instead of the track being fixed to the ceiling. The type of hoist and sling used will depend on the needs of the patient and availability of equipment. The person who performs the risk assessment is responsible for the final decision. If the patient is unable to assist with their personal/hygiene care in any way, this will normally be done on the bed or the patient hoisted into a specialist bath or shower trolley. It is important to ensure that this type of equipment is height adjustable to prevent nursing and care staff having to adopt awkward or stooping postures. An example of specialist care may be supporting a limb during a surgical procedure. This is a controversial handling procedure as one leg could weigh as much as 30% of the person's total body weight and an alternative method to support the limb should be found. Similarly, lifting patients' legs into bed forces the handler to adopt poor spinal posture with side flexing and rotating of the spine. Manual and powered leg lifters are widely available and the use of these devices, particularly in the community, can provide independence for patients allowing them to stay in their own home when they otherwise may have needed to go into residential care (Demain et al., 2000).

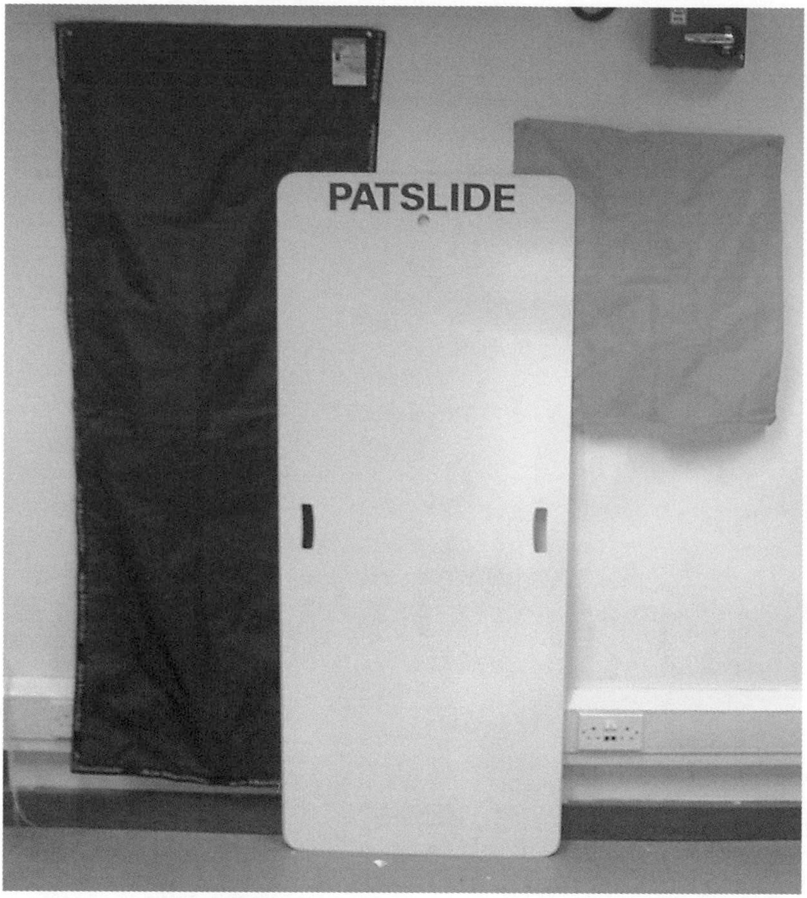

Figure 10.4 Slide sheets and PAT slide.

The individual capability section of TILE refers to the handler. Considerations for risk assessing the individuals' capability include the need to know if the individual has received appropriate training. If the individual has received training, are they capable and confident to perform the required handling task? It is also important to know if the task may be undertaken on an occasional basis by visiting staff, for example therapists. If this is likely they will need to be informed of the risks and included in the policy and action plan (Johnson, 2005). If handlers who may be required to perform the task have an existing injury or are pregnant, the potential risk to them will also need to be assessed and the risk reduced. The handler's clothing also needs to be considered, for instance does it restrict movement causing the handler to adopt poor posture? To prevent injury to the patient, it is important that handlers remove jewellery or any items that may scratch or otherwise injure a patient during the course of manual handling activities. Where protective safety equipment must be worn, the risk assessment should identify if this affects the task (Johnson, 2005).

Assessing the load when a patient can often be complicated as people unlike a static object can be unpredictable and depending on their health status their needs may vary

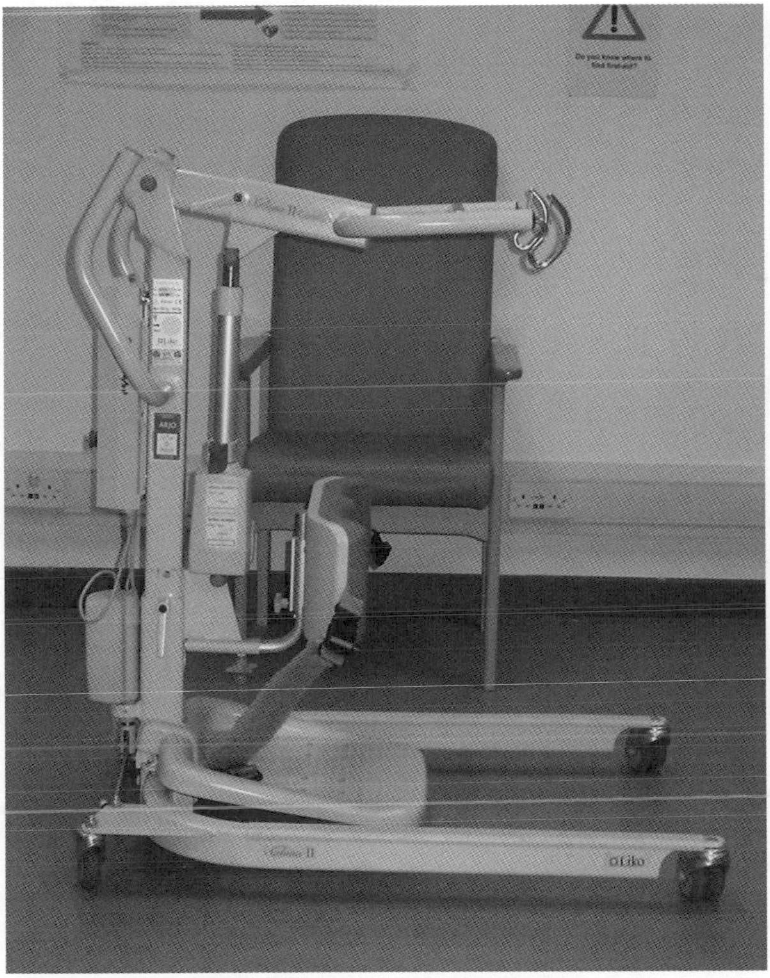

Figure 10.5 A standing hoist.

from day to day. There have also been some tensions, particularly in the community setting, between the needs of patients and the safety of staff. There is a legal requirement for local authorities to attain a balance between the safety and human rights of care staff with the care needs and human rights of patients; however, this balance is not always easy to attain (Mandelstam, 2005). It is important to remember that all manual handling activities are patient centred and must, at all times, take into account the patient's concerns and preferences (Nursing and Midwifery Council, 2008). The patients' manual handling care needs should always be discussed and agreed with the patient whenever possible and carefully documented. It may at times also be appropriate to involve relatives, particularly if the patient is elderly or a child. Whatever method of handling is chosen, it should aim to promote independence as far as possible and be comfortable for the patient. The first consideration of the risk assessment in relation to the load is how much the patients can do for themselves. As mentioned previously,

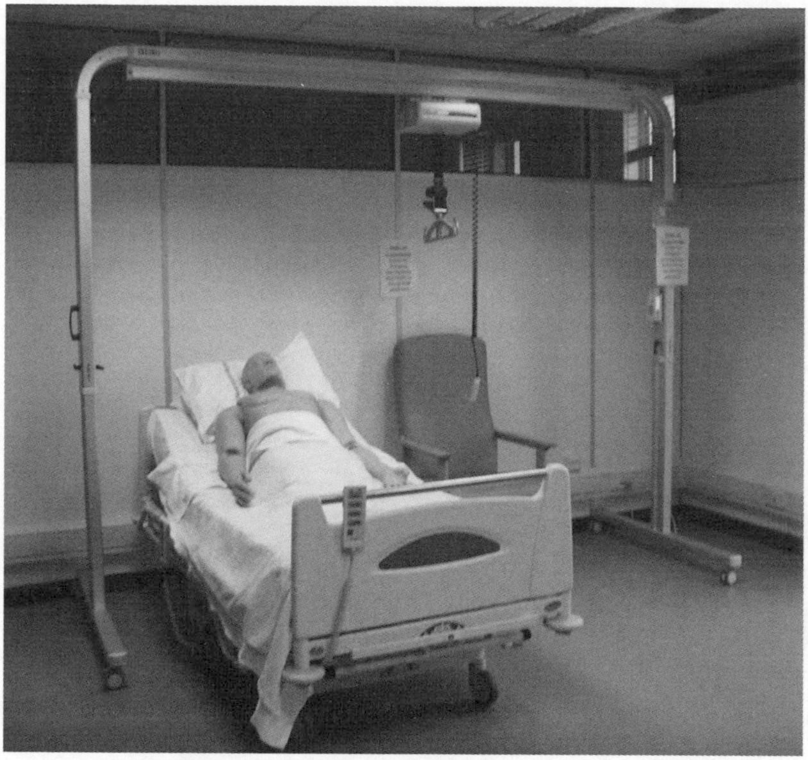

Figure 10.6 A gantry-type hoist.

a patient's health can vary from day to day and the risk assessment needs to reflect this. A patient may have sporadic muscle spasms, pain and epilepsy or have undergone surgery which may intermittently affect their ability to move and undertake activities of living. A patient susceptible to falls should have an assessment using an appropriate falls assessment tool (Johnson, 2005). Cultural considerations must also be kept in mind as these may affect acceptance of authority and expectations of gender in relation to personal care (Johnson, 2005).

Another important consideration for the risk assessment is the patients' ability to communicate. Communication can be impaired in a number of ways, for example as a result of stroke, sensory impairment, loss of consciousness, neurological disorders or dementia. Some patients also display challenging behaviour and may be uncooperative during manual handling. Issues related to tissue viability and infection control also need to be considered (Johnson, 2005). For example a patient with an infection may need disposable equipment, whereas a patient with a sacral pressure sore should not be moved up the bed with sliding sheets.

The height, weight and body shape of a patient also needs to be considered (Johnson, 2005). Patients may need specialist equipment if they have a body mass index (BMI) over 30 and custom-made hoist slings if they have an unconventional body shape and height.

The environment section of TILE examines the way the environment impacts on handling activities. The most obvious risk to handlers is space constraints and the resultant poor postures that need to be adopted because of this. Evidence suggests that an average bed space in a hospital is insufficient to use a mobile hoist safely (Hignett, 2005a). In the community, when working in a patient's home, there is often limited space with the additional hazard of the handler trying to push a mobile hoist with a patient in it on a carpeted surface. An obvious solution to this would be to provide an overhead or gantry hoist. However, cost and space constraints may make this to be a not viable option. As well as carpets, the levels of flooring need to be considered, for example are there steps, edges or uneven surfaces that need to be negotiated? When working in bathrooms, hot, humid and slippery conditions can present a hazard to the handler as can poor lighting when working at night. Reducing risk for individual patients is not always straightforward and each risk assessment will be unique to the patient and their environment.

See a case study given in Box 10.1 and Figure 10.7 provides the risk assessment and handling plan for the patient in the case study. The risk assessment demonstrates how the principles of safe handling are applied in the workplace. The following paragraph is a discussion of the issues raised by the scenario.

Although the risk assessment and manual handling care plan have been completed, indicating a high risk, the issue of Mrs Green refusing to be hoisted has still to be addressed. It would obviously be extremely hazardous for Mrs Green and her handlers to manually transfer her, but her wishes need to be taken into account. If they are not, it could be construed as a breach of the Human Rights Act (article 3) (HMSO, 1998), which is the right not to be subjected to inhuman or degrading treatment. A careful and thorough assessment is required to address exactly why Mrs Green does not want to be hoisted. Issues of comfort may be overcome by the provision of a specially adapted hoist sling, perhaps with added padding that does not cause Mrs Green discomfort. Mrs Green also needs to be made aware of the risks of being manually lifted to herself and her carers. Mr Green's health is also of importance as he is at high risk of injury from lifting Mrs Green when at home. He will need to be made aware of the risks to himself and be included in all discussion. Issues of dignity require reassurance and possibly a demonstration of hoisting technique with explanation. If, after all these measures have been put in place, Mrs Green continues to refuse to be hoisted then her right to refuse must be respected. However, as stated previously, the rights of the carers must be balanced with those of Mrs Green. To manually lift Mrs Green would breach the employer's duty under the MHOR (HSE, 1992) and put the carers at unacceptable risk. In this instance, there is little option other than nursing Mrs Green in bed during her hospital stay. All actions taken must be thoroughly documented and demonstrate that all safe options have been offered and refused. It must also be demonstrated that Mrs Green has been provided with appropriate safe care while being nursed in bed to avoid accusations of negligence.

Controversial techniques and hazardous tasks

Early methods of moving patients involved manually lifting them. Evidence now suggests that this puts the handler at high risk of musculoskeletal injury as well as causing patients

Patient Name: Mrs J Green Hospital Number:0086712

Patient Name: Mrs J Green Hospital Number:0086712
Patient's Weight: 70 Kgs Patient's Height (please state if estimated): Estimated 5'4
Date of assessment: 20.2.08
Staff Name (print): Jo Bloggs Job Title: Staff Nurse Signature: J Bloggs

This form must be countersigned by qualified staff if completed by any unqualified staff (i.e. HCA, Student Nurse)

A PATIENT'S PHYSICAL CAPABILITIES	B PATIENT'S COGNITIVE CAPABILITIES	CABILITY TO COMMUNICATE	D ENVIRONMENT	E TASK AND ADDITIONAL FACTORS	RISK STATUS
❑ Independent ❑ Independent with aids ❑ Other..................	❑ Co-operative ❑ Alert ❑ Fully conscious ❑ Other............	√ Fully understands and can respond appropriately ❑ Other	√ Room to manoeuvre with good posture √ Adjustable working height & levels √ Good lighting & ventilation √ Suitable equipment ❑ Other	❑ Access to relevant information regarding tasks and patients	**LOW** Score is low if all ticks are in this row
❑ Walks with carer and aid ❑ Walks with carer/s ❑ Needs some help with transfers ❑ Pain/Weakness ❑ Restricted movement in joints ❑ Other...............	❑ Poor short term Memory ❑ Disorientated ❑ Other............	❑ Needs precise Instruction ❑ Can copy if shown ❑ Hearing problems ❑ Language difficulty ❑ Other..................	❑ Temperature problem ❑ Variations in lighting ❑ Moveable clutter ❑ Limited handling aids ❑ Other............	❑ Plaster of Paris ❑ Drains ❑ Catheter ❑ Distance involved ❑ Other attachments e.g. lines and leads ❑ Other	**MEDIUM** If ticks are in the low **and** medium row, score as medium risk.
❑ Unsteady/History of falls √ Unable to assist at all with transfers √ Poor or no sitting balance √ Neurological Impairment (e.g. Spinal injury) ❑ Patient's abilities are Inconsistent ❑ Other............	❑ Unpredictable ❑ Behavioural problems ❑ Confused √ Very anxious ❑ Uncooperative ❑ Sedation ❑ Severe learning disability ❑ Other............	❑ No effective means of communication ❑ Other............	❑ Unsuitable or wet floor surface ❑ Fixed height bed or working surface ❑ Restricted space ❑ Immovable objects ❑ No appropriate Equipment ❑ Other..................	√ Repetitive ❑ Time constraints √ Poor postures involved √ Tissue viability Consideration ❑ Insufficient information about tasks and/or patient ❑ Lack of staff to assist ❑ Other..............	**HIGH** If **any** ticks are in the high row, the score is high risk

Overall Risk Level (please circle) **LOW** **MEDIUM** **HIGH**❑

Figure 10.7 Patient handling plan form (Continued).

PATIENT HANDLING CARE PLAN

TASK	EQUIPMENT REQUIRED	**Additional Information for Transfer** (e.g. No. of carers, type and size of equipment and method)
Bed Manoeuvres	**Please state type of equipment required:**	
Turning/rolling	☐ No equipment required ☐ ✓ Sliding sheet ☐ Other (please specify)...............	
Lying <> Sitting	☐ No equipment required ☐ Rope ladder ☐ Hoist ☐ ✓ Bed Mechanics ☐ Monkey pole ☐ Other (please specify)...............	
Moving up the bed in lying	☐ No equipment required ☐ Sling hoist ☐ Independent + sliding sheet ☐ Stretcher hoist ☐ ✓ Sliding Sheet	
Moving up the bed in sitting	☐ No equipment required ☐ Hoist ☐ ✓ 1-way glide ☐ Monkey Pole ☐ Independent + sliding sheet ☐ Hand Blocks	
Transfers		
Bed < > Chair / Wheelchair / Commode	☐ No equipment required ☐ ✓ Hoist ☐ Transfer board +/- sliding sheet ☐ Hand / feet blocks	
Bed < > trolley	☐ No equipment required ☐ Sliding sheet ☐ ✓ Sling Hoist ☐ Transfer board (e.g. Patslide) ☐ Stretcher hoist	
Wheelchair <> Car	☐ No equipment required ☐ Transfer board +/- sliding sheet ☐ Other (please specify)...............	

Figure 10.7 Patient handling plan form (Continued).

Standing / Mobilising			
Sit < > Stand (e.g. from edge of bed, wheelchair or toilet)	☐ No equipment required ☐ Standing hoist	☐ Handling belt	
Walking	☐ No equipment required ☐ Frame (Rollator) ☐ Frame (Zimmer)	☐ Crutches ☐ Stick/s ☐ Handling belt	
Bathing / Washing	☐ No equipment required ☐ Perching stool ☐ √ Shower trolley ☐ Wheel in shower chair	☐ Bath board ☐ Grab rails ☐ Bath hoist ☐ Bed bath	
Toileting	☐ √ No equipment required ☐ Bedpan ☐ √ Hoist onto commode ☐ Free standing toilet frame ☐ √ Pads / catheter insitu	☐ √ Padded toilet seat ☐ Grab rails ☐ Raised toilet seat ☐ Commode	

Figure 10.7 Patient handling plan form (Continued).

discomfort and possible injury (Ruszala, 2005). Pulling and/or grasping a patient's limb may cause pain and bruising. For patients with fragile skin, it may also lead to skin tears. Manually lifting a patient, for example up a bed, often means their buttocks and heels are not lifted clear of the bed subjecting these areas to high levels of friction and shear that may predispose them to pressure sores. Pulling on the patient's shoulder puts pressure on the soft tissue around the shoulder and glenohumeral dislocation and fractures of the humerus have been reported (Ruszala, 2005). With improved aids for manual handling that remove the need to manually lift patients, the acceptability of manually lifting is highly questionable (Ruszala, 2005).

In emergency situations, for example in the case of cardiac arrest, health care professionals may sometimes jeopardise their own safety as they are distracted by the stress and pressure of the situation and the need to maximise the outcome for the patient. It is important, however, that the health care professional who finds the collapsed patient carries out a rapid risk assessment that takes account of the risks to both the patient and themselves (Resuscitation Council (UK), 2001). In a hospital setting it is likely that help is readily available and cardiac or respiratory arrest is rarely unexpected as there would have been a previous deterioration in clinical signs. It is also argued that within a hospital setting, cardiac arrest is not an emergency but a foreseeable event (Resuscitation Council (UK), 2001). Patients can be safely resuscitated at floor level, if necessary sliding sheets can be used to pull a patient into a position that provides adequate space for resuscitation to be given. Once stable, the patient can be hoisted onto a more appropriate surface. The Resuscitation Council (UK) (2001) recommends that slide sheets should be readily available and, if space permits, kept on or near the emergency resuscitation trolley.

Falls amongst patients are a familiar occurrence and present a high risk of injury to both patient and handlers (Betts and Mowbray, 2005). The Royal College of Nursing and the National Back Pain Association (NBPA) (1997) suggested sometime ago that to catch or control a falling person is unsafe for the handler. The situation presents an ethical dilemma for health care professionals who feel allowing a person to fall breaches their duty of care to that person, but they are also aware that they have a duty to protect themselves. There are also significant risks to the falling person if no intervention is attempted, especially to the frail elderly who may suffer fracture and complications (Betts and Mowbray, 2005). Managing falls is best achieved by prevention wherever possible and this entails a careful risk assessment for the person susceptible to falling, including the potential injuries they may sustain, as this will help determine what strategies are put in place (Betts and Mowbray, 2005). Organisations must have a documented policy and procedure for managing the falling and fallen patient including guidelines for training requirements (Betts and Mowbray, 2005). However, practicing high-risk manual handling interventions for the falling patient may expose health care staff to unacceptable risk. Betts and Mowbray (2005) suggest that if these techniques are not demonstrated or practiced, they must be discussed. Falls may cause disability or mortality due to injury and the DH (2001) has published a National Service Framework for Older People that addresses the cause of falls and suggests interventions to prevent them. Patients may fall for various reasons that are intrinsic, including poor balance, sensory decline, medical condition, cognitive decline, for example dementia, and problems with gait. Extrinsically the falls may be caused by medication, unsuitable footwear, furniture, lighting and variations in floor level (Betts and Mowbray, 2005). It can be seen that a frail elderly person may also have a combination of both intrinsic and extrinsic factors contributing to their susceptibility to falls. A risk assessment that considers both intrinsic and extrinsic factors may require that a chair is positioned half way between the toilet and the person's normal day time seat or that the person is assessed for the suitability of a walking aid. At the same time a person's medication may be reviewed to identify if it is causing undue drowsiness or if there is an interaction between the various medicines being taken. In a community setting the environment may need to be assessed for slip and trip hazards such as rugs, steps and variations in floor levels.

It was previously suggested that a falling person could be guided to the floor by the handler with the handler using the front of their own body to support the falling patient and at the same time bending their knees and sinking to the ground with the patient. Inevitably, at some stage during the manoeuvre the handler will take all of the person's body weight. The rationale for using this technique was that the person would be less likely to be injured being supported in this way. The technique is dependent on the handler being slightly behind and to the side of the patient, the person falling backwards rather than forward, there is no significant height or weight difference between the person and the handler, the person cooperates and there are no obstructions in the immediate environment. In reality there is a very slim chance that this set of circumstances would occur and it may be all the handler can do to move obstacles out of the way or try to redirect the direction the person is falling in, to prevent them from striking objects that may further intensify their injuries. If the falling person's head can be protected without risk of injury to the handler, for instance if a person sinks to the ground from the knees, there may be a slim chance of protecting the head. If a person is falling some distance away, the handler may have no option other than to let the person fall. Attempting to guide a falling person to the ground requires a high level of skill and physical fitness on the part of the handler.

Managing the person when fallen involves ensuring that they have not sustained an injury or require resuscitation. If the person is able, they should be given verbal instructions to rise from the floor. A chair should be placed at the person's head and the person should be instructed to roll onto their side, draw up their knees and raise themselves on the lower elbow. They should then be instructed to press down with the lower elbow and upper hand to rise up on all fours. The person can then lean on the chair using both arms, place one foot flat on the floor and push up to straighten the legs and turn to sit on the chair (Betts and Mowbray, 2005). If the fallen person is unable to raise themselves from the floor due to poor muscle strength or joint mobility, they should be raised using a hoist. Manual lifting from the floor should only be undertaken with small children, in an emergency or in exceptional circumstances due to the high-risk nature of the manoeuvre (Betts and Mowbray, 2005).

The management of bariatric patients

We live quite literally in a growing society that is rapidly getting heavier. Almost two-thirds of adults and one-third of children are either overweight or obese (Department of Health [DH], 2008). Treatment of the overweight and the obese has been estimated to cost the NHS £48 million a year (DH, 2001), and this figure does not take into account the cost of lost working days and productivity to industry. The term *bariatric* originated from the Greek word for heavy, which is 'barros', and 'iatric', which means medical treatment (Rush, 2008). The BMI, which is calculated by dividing the individuals' weight in kilograms by the square of their height in metres, is the accepted body fat measurement (Rush, 2008). A healthy BMI is considered to be 18.6–24.9. A person with a BMI greater than 30 is considered obese and greater than 40 as morbidly obese (Hignett et al., 2007). A person with a BMI of over 40 would also be classed as bariatric (Rush, 2008).

Waist circumference has also been found to be significant. A waist circumference of more than 40 inches in a man and 35 inches in a woman indicates obesity (Rush, 2008). It has been suggested that waist circumference may be a more accurate measure of being overweight than the BMI (Campbell, 2004). The rise in the number of people with obesity has presented significant challenges for health and social care services in both the provision of suitable equipment and manual handling. It has also raised issues concerning the dignity and safety of these patients. For example, a morbidly obese patient may be too large to exit their home through its doorway or exceed the safe working load of an ambulance stretcher. Obesity is seen by society as under the control of the individual and obese people suffer discrimination and prejudice by society because of this (Rush, 2008).

Hignett et al. (2007) undertook a study considering risk assessment and process planning for bariatric patients. They found that a significant risk factor was the lack of policies relating specifically to manual handling of bariatric patients. They suggest that policies are important because they encourage staff to plan when admitting bariatric patients. Ideally, if the admission is planned, all equipment and environment adaptations can be made before the patient arrives. As previously discussed a manual handling risk assessment must be performed for all handling tasks. For bariatric patients the same process is used but with some additional risk factors that need to be considered.

Most hoists will lift up to 200 kg, so any patient over this weight will require a specialist hoist for taking heavier loads. Equipment such as beds, commodes, shower chairs or wheelchairs may not be strong or wide enough for bariatric patients and specialist equipment will be required. Whether these items are purchased or rented varies from organisation to organisation. A number of companies that specialise in manual handling equipment now also manufacture equipment for obese patients and the choice of equipment is increasing steadily. It is worth noting that with heavier equipment plus the weight of the patient, part of the assessment should be to consider the safe working load of the floor, particularly if equipment is being installed on first floors or above (Rush, 2008). Larger equipment also requires more space and it is important to ensure that care staff are left with enough room around the bed space to perform necessary tasks without compromising their posture. It is recommended that there should not be less than 1.5 m between the walls of the room and the equipment (Rush, 2008). If the patient is being cared for in their own home, doorways will often need to be widened to accommodate large pieces of equipment. Research suggests that although readily available for purchase or rent a significant number of trusts and ambulance services do not have specialist bariatric equipment and that some trusts have only limited equipment (Hignett et al., 2007). It was also reported that specialist equipment was not always used consistently and a possible explanation for this was limited space (Hignett et al., 2007).

The obese person's body shape like the rest of the population varies from individual to individual. Broadly speaking, bariatric body shape can be divided into four categories: anasarca, which is a severe generalised oedema; apple; pear and bulbous gluteal region, which is excessive buttock tissue (Rush, 2008). If the patient requires hoisting body shape will affect the type of sling used. For example, if an individual is pear shaped, there may be excessive weight around the thighs which will require the use of a sling with long leg pieces to ensure a comfortable and safe fit (Rush, 2008). Most bariatric patients experience breathing difficulties due to excessive weight on the chest and upper abdomen and are unable to lie down. Using a bed that can convert to a chair can benefit the patient and help therapists and care staff (Rush, 2008). Most bariatric patients are unable to use a bath so a shower chair is the preferred option. If a shower is not available, bed bathing may be the only option. This can be challenging for staff as skin folds can be heavy, particularly the abdomen. Ordinary bathrooms and toilets are usually unsuitable for bariatric patients as they tend to offer limited space. A commode by the patient's bed may be the only option unless the toileting area allows for a commode to be wheeled over the toilet with side access for hygiene purposes (Rush, 2008).

Caring for a bariatric patient requires a holistic approach ensuring that psychosocial needs are met as well as the more obvious physical needs. The aetiology of obesity is complex and care is also truly multidisciplinary involving nurses, carers, physiotherapists, occupational therapists, dieticians, doctors and sometimes the emergency services. A thorough assessment of an individual's needs and planning is crucial for a satisfactory outcome and could make the difference between enabling a patient to be supported in their own home or being admitted to hospital in some instances. At the centre of the assessment and planning process should be the patient with their wishes and preferences supported as far as possible.

Conclusions

Safe manual handling presents a significant challenge to health care staff. Injuries to staff remain unacceptably high despite HSE guidance and current legislation. This would appear to indicate that simply teaching staff safe manual handling techniques is an inadequate approach to the problem. There has been an increasing movement by organisations such as the National Back Exchange, National Back Pain Association and University Ergonomists to move towards evidence-based practice in manual handling. Because manual handling is multifaceted, it would be an impossible task to test or measure everything, so clinical experience will always be an important component in most situations. However, systematic reviews of current literature and the encouragement of new research increase assurance in the knowledge of manual handling guidance and interventions (Crumpton and Hignett, 2005).

The use of ergonomic principles to identify risk and study the safety of work environments allows for a proactive approach towards manual handling for both staff and patients by analysing actual and potential risks. This is particularly pertinent when we are faced with a situation where two-thirds of the population is being classified as either overweight or obese. With the emphasis on safety, it is worth reiterating that manual handling is also a patient-centred activity. With any manual handling intervention, if possible, the patient should be consulted at every step. As directed by the Nursing and Midwifery Council (2008), patients' concerns and preferences must be responded to.

Glossary

Bariatric	Originating from the Greek word 'barros', meaning heavy, and 'iatric', which means medical treatment. Patients with a body mass index above 40 are termed bariatric
Cardiac arrest	Cessation of the heart beat
Ergonomics	The science of work that is concerned with fitting the job to the person, rather than fitting the person to the job. It is concerned with the design of safe systems of work
Extrinsic	From outside
Facet joints	On the superior and inferior surfaces of the neural arch, there are two articular processes for articulation with the vertebra above and below. These are known as facet joints. The facet joints provide a locking mechanism between consecutive vertebra which limit twisting movements and stop forward sliding of the vertebrae
Hoist	A mechanical device for supporting the full weight of an individual. It is used to transfer an individual from one area to another, for example from bed to chair
Intrinsic	Inherent. From within
Ligaments	Flexible bands of fibrous tissue that bind joints together and connect various bones and cartilages
PAT slide	A flat, solid, low-friction board designed to bridge the gap between transfer surfaces which the patient is slid across
Risk assessment	A risk assessment involves identifying hazards in the workplace and assessing the likelihood and severity of possible resultant harm
Slide sheets	Soft, low-friction sheets used for sliding patients into position
TILE	The four areas of an ergonomic risk assessment – task, individual capability, load and environment

Post-chapter quiz

1. Describe the functions of the intervertebral discs
2. What do you understand by the term 'bariatric'?
3. What would be considered a healthy body mass index?
4. What does the HSE (1992) Regulation 4 state?
5. When carrying out a risk assessment, there are four areas that need to be considered. These can be thought of as TILE. What do these letters stand for?
6. What is the name of the central portion of the intervertebral disc?
7. Why is it important to raise the height of the bed when turning a patient?
8. What are the functions of the spine?
9. Why are the curves of the spinal column important?
10. Discuss the reasons why an individual's centre of gravity is important when performing manual handling tasks

References

Adams, M. and Dolan, P. (2005) Biomechanics of low back pain. In: Smith, J. (ed). *The Guide to the Handling of People*, 5th ed. Teddington, Middlesex: Back Care, pp. 45–55.

Adams, M.A., Bogduk, N., Burton, K. and Dolan, P. (2002) *The Biomechanics of Back Pain.* London: Churchill Livingstone.

Betts, M. and Mowbray, C. (2005) The falling and fallen person and emergency handling. In: Smith, J. (ed). *The Guide to the Handling of People*, 5th ed. Teddington, Middlesex: Back Care, pp. 241–272.

Campbell, I. (2004) Obesity and men's health. In: Kirby, R., Carson, C., Kirby, M. and Farah, R. (eds). *Men's Health*, 2nd ed. London: Taylor & Francis.

Carrivick, P.J., Lee, A.H. and Stevenson, M.R. (2001) Consultative team to assess manual handling and reduce the risk of occupational injury. *Occupational and Environmental Medicine* 58: 339–344.

Crumpton, E. and Hignett, S. (2005) Evidenced based practice. In: Smith, J. (ed). *The Guide to the Handling of People*, 5th ed. Teddington, Middlesex: Back Care, pp. 111–115.

Demain, S., Gore, S. and McLellan, D. (2000) The use of leg lifting equipment. *Nursing Standard* 14(39): 41–43.

Department of Health (2001) *Older People: National Service Framework for Older People.* London: The Stationery Office.

Department of Health (2001) *Tackling Obesity in England.* London: The StationeryOffice.

Department of Health (2008) Healthy *Weight, Healthy Lives: A Cross-Government Strategy for England.* London: The Stationery Office.

Griffith, R. and Stevens, M. (2004) Manual handling and the lawfulness of no-lift policies. *Nursing Standard* 18(21): 1–9.

Health and Safety Executive (1992) *Manual Handling Operations Regulations 1992 – Guidance on Regulations.* L23, London: HSE Books.

Health and Safety Executive (1999) Management of Health and Safety at Work Regulations. Available at www.legislation.hmso.gov.uk/si/si1999/19993242.htm. Accessed 12 June 2005.

Health and Safety Executive (2008) Musculoskeletal disorders – Why tackle them? Available at http://www.hse.gov.uk/healthservices/msd/whytackle.htm. Accessed 29 October 2008.

Hignett, S. (2005a) Determining the space needed to operate a mobile and an overhead patient hoist. *Professional Nurse* 20(7): 40–42.

Hignett, S. (2005b) Ergonomics in health and social care. In: Smith, J. (ed). *The Guide to the Handling of People*, 5th ed. Teddington, Middlesex: Back Care, pp. 37–44.

Hignett, S., Chipchase, S., Tetley, A. and Griffith, P. (2007) *Risk Assessment and Process Planning for Bariatric Patient Handling Pathways.* London: HSE.

Hignett, S. and McAtamney, L. (2000) Rapid entire body assessment (REBA). *Applied Ergonomics* 31: 201–205.

HMSO (1998) Human Rights Act. Available at www.legislation.hmso.gov.uk/acts/acts1998/19980042.htm. Accessed 29 October 2008.

Johnson, C. (2005) Manual handling risk assessment – theory and practice. In: Smith, J. (ed). *The Guide to the Handling of People*, 5th ed. Teddington, Middlesex: Back Care, pp. 89–110.

Mandelstam, M. (2005) Manual handling in social care: law, practice and balanced decision making. In: Smith, J. (ed). *The Guide to the Handling of People*, 5th ed. Teddington, Middlesex: Back Care, pp. 15–36.

National Back Pain Association/Royal College of Nursing (1997) *The Guide to the Handling of Persons: Introducing a Safer Handling Policy*, 4th ed. London: National Back Pain Association.

Nursing and Midwifery Council (2008) *The Code.* London: NMC.

Owen, B. and Staehler, K.S. (2003) Decreasing back stress in home care. *Home Healthcare Nurse* 21(3): 180–186.

Resuscitation Council (UK) (2001) *Guidance for Safer Handling During Resuscitation in Hospitals.* London: Resuscitation Council (UK).

Retsas, A. and Pinikahana, J. (2000) Manual handling activities and injuries among nurses: an Australian hospital study. *Journal of Advanced Nursing* 31(4): 875–883.

Royal College of Nursing (2002) *RCN Code of Practice for Patient Handling.* London: RCN.

Rush, A. (2008) Overview of bariatric management. Available at http://www.dlf.org.uk/pdf/professional/Overview%20of%20Bariatric%20Management.pdf. Accessed 9 October 2007.

Ruszala, S. (2005) Controversial techniques. In: Smith, J. (ed). *The Guide to the Handling of People*, 5th ed. Teddington, Middlesex: Back Care, pp. 273–289.

Sanders, M. and McCormick, E. (1992) *Human Factors in Engineering and Design*, 2nd ed. New York: McGraw-Hill.

Wilson, A. (2002) *Effective Management of Musculoskeletal Injury.* London: Churchill Livingstone.

Chapter 11
Maintaining Body Temperature

Guy Dean

Learning opportunities

This chapter will help you to:

1. Understand the maintenance of body temperature
2. Identify the factors influencing body temperature
3. Describe temperature regulation
4. Identify factors involved when measuring body temperature
5. Define nursing interventions related to extremes of body temperature
6. Understand why the nurse might need to measure and monitor a person's temperature

Pre-chapter quiz

1. Why should you take a patient's temperature?
2. How is temperature controlled?
3. What factors influence body temperature?
4. How does the body balance heat loss and gain?
5. List the methods that may be used to take the temperature of a patient
6. What is the most accurate method of taking a temperature?
7. Name the extremes of body temperature
8. What are the three basic phases of fever?
9. Describe the nursing interventions required to assist the patient in each phase of fever
10. What does the term 'pyrexial' mean?

Introduction: temperature and metabolism

Taking the temperature of a patient in both the hospital and the community setting is a common procedure performed by nurses. Assessment and monitoring of the rise and fall of a patient's body temperature can give a good indication to changes in the condition of the patient and assist in the diagnosis of illness and disease.

Temperature is taken for a number of reasons, for example to establish a baseline, to identify the possibility of infection or inflammatory condition, to establish whether a patient is suffering from hypothermia, in critically ill patients, during an operation and when a patient is receiving a blood transfusion (Mooney, 2007).

To ensure any clinical intervention is effective when dealing with a change in body temperature, the nurse should ensure that the measurement is accurate, record their findings and act upon it appropriately (Nursing and Midwifery Council (NMC), 2008a). According to Dougherty and Lister (2008), there are two reasons why the assessment of body temperature is carried out:

- To determine the patient's body temperature on admission in order to use this as a baseline for comparison with future measurements
- To monitor fluctuations in temperature

Control of temperature

In all forms of life, temperature is a fundamental concern, and we, as human beings, are no exception. The cellular processes that constitute metabolism are no more than chemical reactions. How quickly these chemical reactions can happen determine whether life is sustained or not and is of some concern. One of the most important by-products of the metabolism is heat. The higher the temperature, the faster the metabolic rate and the faster more heat will be produced. The lower the temperature, the slower the metabolic rate and heat will be produced more slowly.

However, the body temperature of an individual is not only dependent on the rate of heat production; it is the sum total of the balance between heat produced within the body and heat lost from the body to the environment. An extremely hot environment and anything above the normal body temperature range for humans are considered to be between 36 and 38°C (Berman et al., 2008).

The body is separated into two distinct thermal zones known as the core temperature and the shell (surface temperature). The core temperature can be up to 9°C higher than the shell temperature and normally remains within the range of 36.4 and 37.3°C with very little change (Dougherty and Lister, 2008).

The tissues that make up the core all have a fast metabolic rate to support their cellular activity and are adversely affected by low temperature. The core tissues are often described as:

- The brain and central nervous system
- The organs of the chest, the lungs and heart
- The organs of the abdomen and pelvis, the liver, spleen, pancreas, the gastrointestinal tract and the urinary system

Table 11.1 Comparison of temperature readings.

Route	Normal temperature
Oral	36.5–37.5°C
Axillary	36–37°C
Rectal	37–38°C
Tympanic	36.8–37.8°C

The shell tissues are described as:

- The skin
- The subcutaneous tissues
- The fat cells

The temperature of the large skeletal muscles found in the thigh and calf lies somewhere between the core and shell temperature. On a very cold day the thigh muscles could be as much as 4°C cooler than the core tissues and the calf muscles cooler by a further 2°C. Table 11.1 shows how temperature readings compare.

Factors influencing body temperature

It is important to recognise that there are many factors that can influence body temperature. It is imperative to note the patients' dependence–independence status as well as their age. Walker (2003) considers the following factors:

- Psychological
- Environmental
- Politico-economic
- Sociocultural
- Physical

The nurse must take into account the effect of a person's psychological state. If an individual's psychological state is impaired because of illness, i.e. depression, or affected as a result of medications such as sedatives, they may neglect to respond to changes in temperature.

Extremes of heat in severe winters and extremely warm summers can, as would be expected, have an impact on body temperature. These environmental issues cannot be thought of in isolation and the nurse needs to consider the patients and specifically the environment they may be living in.

Politico-economic factors must also be considered as an indirect factor that may have major implications for maintaining an ideal body temperature. The nurse needs to establish if the patient can afford to keep warm and recognise that keeping warm costs money. The recommended room temperature for an elderly person is 21°C compared to

18°C for others. Maintaining an environmental temperature as recommended may be a major concern depending on an individual's economic status (Peate, 2008).

It is important for the nurse to note that sociocultural factors have a role to play in maintaining body temperature. In some cultures there are particular customs concerning clothing, i.e. it may be that some women must, as a consequence of religious custom, be required to wear full covering of the body even in extreme heat. Being aware of the social and cultural needs of the patient can help to understand their requirements in a more meaningful manner. The multicultural context of health care is an important issue and should be considered by all involved in health care (Helman, 2007).

There is no such thing as a 'normal temperature'; however, consideration should always be given to the following factors when assessing an individual's temperature:

Time of day: The body temperature is lowest when the individual is asleep and their smetabolic rate is slowest. This is around 0400–0600 hours and at its highest between 2000 and 2400 hours for day workers. Individuals who work in nights may exhibit a different temperature pattern. The differences of temperature between these times of day are known as diurnal variation and the temperature of an individual may differ up to 1°C between these times. This is important when considering the social and employment history of the patient during an initial assessment of the patient.

Exercise or strenuous physical activity can elevate the body temperature significantly.

Hormonal activity can elevate body temperature.

Stress and anxiety create responses within the body which increase the metabolic rate and thus elevate the body temperature.

Ageing tends to lower the body temperature, as metabolic rate declines with age.

The environment that the individual is in or has recently been in and the length of time the individual has been exposed to those conditions.

Body heat considerations

Production and loss

To balance the heat production (thermogenesis) versus heat loss (or gain) equation, it should be recognised that a variety of events take place inside and outside the body. There are five factors that influence heat production within the body and a further five factors that influence heat loss from the body. For heat production these are:

Basal metabolic rate: This is described as the rate of energy consumption in the form of carbohydrates, fat and proteins for an individual just to exist and without any extra activity, such as when an individual is asleep. The higher the basal metabolic rate, the higher the rate of basic heat production, and as metabolic rates tend to decline as an individual gets older so does their resting body temperature (Berman et al., 2008). As heat production relies on increasing the metabolic rate of tissues, it is not surprising to find that the remaining four events change metabolic activity in specific tissues or the body as a whole. Where this is achieved by means of chemical agents the process is known as chemical thermogenesis (Marieb, 2008).

Raising cellular metabolic rate throughout the body is achieved by the secretion of the hormone thyroxine (known as T4) by the thyroid gland. Under the influence of this hormone the cells of the tissues produce more heat because of their elevated metabolic rate.

Raising cellular metabolic rate throughout the body is also achieved by the activity of the immune system and the chemical signalling agents released during the process of inflammation, such as prostaglandins.

The fight-or-flight response of the body increases the metabolic activity in the brain, heart, skeletal muscles and the liver. The chemicals involved are noradrenaline from the sympathetic division of the autonomic nervous system and adrenaline itself.

Involuntary muscle activity, such as shivering, and voluntary muscle activity, such as exercise, also produce a rise in temperature (Berman et al., 2008).

Heat loss from the body occurs in following five ways:

- Radiation
- Evaporation
- Conduction
- Convection
- Insensible loss

These processes occur across the surface area that the body presents to the environment, this includes the skin and the upper and lower respiratory tract. Heat transfer always proceeds in the direction from high temperature to low temperature, evaporation proceeds in the direction of high humidity (wet) to low humidity (dry).

Radiation is the transfer of heat from the surface of one body to another without touching by means of emission of energy from the infrared part of the electromagnetic spectrum, such as the heat felt from the sun or a fire. This is the fundamental method by which a person loses heat from the skin surface; the more skin that is exposed, the greater the heat loss.

Evaporation occurs when there is insufficient surface area for radiating the heat away, sweat begins to appear on the skin of an individual, the water of the sweat takes heat from the skin by conduction and is turned into vapour and the skin is cooled. Heat is also lost by evaporation in the respiratory tract, the heat being lost on breathing out. However evaporation can only contribute to the cooling process if the water can vaporise into the atmosphere and is dependent on the humidity of the air that is surrounding the individual. Under severe conditions, such as those found in the desert regions of the world, up to 4 L of water per hour can be lost from the body through sweating, although the usual daily loss is approximately 600 mL.

Conduction of heat takes place through direct molecular contact, such as the skin molecules to air or water molecules. Under normal circumstances, very little heat is lost from the body in this manner; however, heat can be lost very rapidly from the body by conduction in situations such as immersion in very cold water.

Convection is similar to conduction, the heat is transferred from the skin molecules to warm the air molecules, these warmed molecules then move away to be replaced by cold molecules and the process of heat loss from the body occurs at an increased rate. It is this replacement of the cold air molecules that prevents the body warming its surroundings until equilibrium of temperature is achieved, thus an individual can lose body heat very rapidly. This is the principle behind the use of fans and the wind chill effect.

Heat is also lost from the body with urine and faeces. These factors of heat production and loss provide the reasons that underpin nursing interventions related to body temperature.

Temperature regulation

The ability to regulate the internal temperature of the body is known as homeothermy. In the brain, there is a centre known as the hypothalamus that coordinates many of the responses required for homeostasis, homeothermy being just one of them.

The hypothalamus receives nerve impulses from specialised cells called thermoreceptors found in the core and shell tissues, processes these impulses and then sends signals via nerve impulses or hormones to the active tissues to alter the rate of heat production and adjust heat loss as required.

Once the temperature adjustment has been made, the thermoreceptor impulses change and the hypothalamus stops its signalling to the active tissues (Marieb, 2008) – this is an example of a negative feedback system. Activity in the hypothalamus also creates the feelings of cold and warmth. This allows us to decide if we need to take off or put on more clothes depending on the weather.

In response to the shell being sufficiently cooled, the shell thermoreceptors send impulses to the hypothalamus which coordinates activity with its own cold sensing receptors; the following responses may happen:

- The blood vessels of the skin constrict to decrease heat loss
- Cellular metabolic rate increases by noradrenaline and secretion of adrenaline
- The skeletal muscles begin to contract rhythmically to increase heat production
- Heat loss responses are inhibited

In response to stimulation of thermoreceptors in the shell and its own warmth sensing receptors, the hypothalamus may initiate the following:

- The blood vessels of the skin dilate to increase heat radiation
- Stimulation of sweat gland activity

Measuring body temperature

The body measures its own temperature by comparing the activity of core (body) and shell (environment) thermoreceptors, the difference of activity between the two generating the feeling of either warmth, comfort or cold (see Table 11.2)

It is therefore the temperature difference that gives the patient not only the sensation of relative warmth or coldness and behavioural response, but the physiological response of shivering or sweating as well. This can explain why a patient with a raised temperature complains of feeling cold in a warm room, and exhibits shivering which would not normally happen at this temperature.

Table 11.2 Body heat considerations.

Hypothalamus core thermoreceptors [internal temperature]	Shell thermoreceptors [external temperature]	Resultant sensation
Warmth [37°C]	Warmth [22°C]	Comfort
Warmth [37°C]	Hot [40°C]	Hot
Warmth [37°C]	Cold [10°C]	Cold

When measuring the temperature of a patient, it is the core temperature that is the most meaningful with regard to their metabolism (Berman et al., 2008); unfortunately, the core temperature is difficult to measure. The more convenient measurements of skin temperature are unreliable at best and inaccurate in cases of low body temperature. The type of thermometer that is available to measure the temperature also needs to be considered when deciding which site of the body to use for temperature measurement (Nichol et al., 2005). All probes that are inserted into body orifices should either have a disposable cover or be disposable themselves to prevent cross-infection between individuals.

There are four sites usually utilised to assess temperature: oral, axillary, rectal and tympanic. Each site has its own advantages and disadvantages depending on the type of thermometer used (Berman et al., 2008). It should be noted that for consistency and accuracy the same site should be used for each patient rather than varying from one site to another.

Rectal

This site has been considered the most accurate in assessing core temperature. Here the temperature of the rectum, supplied with blood from branches of the mesenteric arteries, is considered to be that of the core.

The difficulties in using this site for temperature measurement are inconvenience and loss of dignity for the patients having their temperature taken, especially those who have difficulty in turning to the side. There is also the potential hazard of perforation of the rectum with such an invasive procedure, which should not be ignored especially in children. The presence of a stool may also interfere with the thermometer placement (Berman et al., 2008).

Oral

Traditionally this is the commonest site for temperature measurement and is convenient with the best chance of some degree of accuracy. The desired site for placing of the thermometer is under the tongue into the crease made by the base of the tongue and the floor of the mouth, next to the frenulum. At this site the tissue is heated by blood coming from the sublingual artery and so should provide a reading very close to core temperature (Nichol et al., 2005). Traditionally, estimations have stated that temperatures measured at the sublingual site are between 0.5 and 1°C lower than the core temperature. The oral site does offer some consistency in the placement of the probe and thus some continuity in measurement. The oral site does, however, have a tendency to inaccuracy, the time taken for a measurement to be made can exceed the individual's willingness to tolerate any discomfort from the probe under the tongue, the mouth temperature of an individual can vary due to hot or cold drinks, tobacco smoke or mouth breathing. The individual may bite the probe causing damage to the probe or their mouth. The oral site may not be the most convenient to use for some individuals as there may be an oxygen mask or endotracheal tube in use.

Axillary

This is another convenient site with the least amount of accuracy specifically in children. The site for probe placement is in the armpit of the individual. This site is the least invasive and is not near the oropharynx (as is the case with the oral approach) so is not affected by drinking or smoking and does not interfere with the person's airway. However, individuals can have hollows in their armpits, particularly if the individual is very slender, so the probe will not contact the skin and registers the temperature of the air in the hollow of the armpit.

For the most accurate temperature measurement that this method can provide, the probe must be left in place for a long time, up to 6 minutes (Brooker and Waugh, 2007), when compared with the oral or rectal sites. The body temperature measured in the axilla is 1–1.5°C below the temperature of the core temperature. The length of time that a thermometer should be left in situ at a particular site for the most accurate reading depends on the thermometer type. Electronic probes have their time for optimal temperature measurement preset by their manufacturers relating to the rate of thermal change in the probe and the user has little choice other than to wait for the thermometer to announce its measurement is complete with an electronic sound.

Mercury bulb glass thermometers have been the subject of some research as to which length of time gave the most accurate temperature measurement for which site. These thermometers have ceased to be used routinely in the clinical situation.

Tympanic membrane (eardrum)

The tympanic membrane is supplied by arterial blood from the external carotid artery just as the oral site is; however, the tympanic membrane is not subject to the same factors that can cause inaccuracies of temperature measurement at the oral site.

The tympanic membrane thermometer measures the temperature of the tympanic membrane by its infrared radiation; to do this the infrared detector needs to 'see' the tympanic membrane. The infrared detector collects the infrared radiation from the tympanic membrane in a fraction of a second, so the temperature measurement is very rapid and generally accurate and reliable (Brooker and Waugh, 2007).

However, this method is not without its disadvantages. The accuracy of the measurement relies on the knowledge the user has of the outer ear as the tympanic membrane is difficult to see being at the end of a passage which is at a slight angle to the external ear. Poor positioning of the detector results in the measurement of the temperature of the wall of the external auditory passage. If the passage or tympanic membrane is obstructed by earwax (cerumen), blood, a foreign body, excessive hair, infection or ear or neurosurgery then the reading may be affected (Brooker and Waugh, 2007). It should be noted that hearing aids should always be removed before this procedure is undertaken.

Chemical thermometers usually rely on a chemical changing colour at a given temperature to produce a reading. There is a tendency to rely on interpretation of the colour change by the user to decide upon the value of temperature measured and so the accuracy of these thermometers is questionable. However, they are convenient in use; the strip is easily placed on the forehead of an individual, as an alternative to the liquid crystal thermometer which is placed under the tongue.

Taking the temperature

The nurse must explain to the patient what he/she is about to do in order to gain consent and cooperation from the patient (NMC, 2008a); explanations can allay any fears and anxiety they may have. The patient should be advised to refrain from eating or drinking as cold or hot liquids can interfere with circulation and body temperature and provide an inaccurate measurement which may have an adverse effect upon the nursing intervention required.

All equipment should be gathered together before participating in this procedure as this may prevent any interruptions. Privacy may need to be maintained, according to the site, and the nurse must wash his or her hands and, if appropriate, put on gloves prior to contact with the patient to reduce the transmission of microorganisms. Disposable sheaths should be used on any equipment and electronic equipment should be used as stated in the manufacturer's instructions. Disposable sheaths should be used for each patient and should be disposed of after use.

Once the procedure is over, gloves should be removed and the hands washed again. The reading should be recorded as per policy and in line with the NMC (2008b) guidelines for records and record keeping.

Body temperature

There are four basic body temperature states that an individual can be in; these are the normal range, pyrexia, hyperpyrexia and hypothermia. The characteristic temperature ranges are:

Hypothermia: The core body temperature ranges from 35 to 26°C, with the metabolic rate diminishing to standstill and death between 28 and 26°C.

Normal temperature range: The core body temperature ranges between 36 and 38°C. The individual is said to be apyrexial or afebrile.

Pyrexia: The core body temperature ranges between 37.7 and 40.9°C. The individual is said to have a fever or said to be febrile.

Hyperpyrexia: The core body temperature ranges between 41 and 43°C. At temperatures in excess of 41°C, nerve damage is known to occur and at 43°C death occurs. In this range, the individual is said to have a high fever.

Extremes of body temperature and the nursing interventions

There are three basic phases in fever: the onset (chill phase), the course and the crisis (flush or fevervescence phase) (Berman et al., 2008). The nursing interventions at all stages attempt to monitor and support the physiological changes within the individual's body, ease physical discomfort and help with complications.

Onset of fever

The onset of fever is characterised by complaints of (Berman et al., 2008):

- Increased heart rate
- Increased respiratory rate and depth
- Shivering and pallid cold skin with 'goose bumps'
- Feeling cold
- Cyanotic nail beds
- Cessation of sweating

The nursing interventions at this phase in the fever process would be to provide warmth, but not to excess, and to prevent heat loss while the individual is complaining of feeling cold. Attention to adequate fluid intake and nutrition is required to meet the increased metabolic demand of the individual's body. Measurement of the patient's intake and output of both fluid and nutrition must be required. Attention to the individual's personal hygiene is important at this stage to ensure the comfort of the individual throughout the three phases of fever. Oral hygiene is required to maintain the moisture of the mucous membranes of the mouth and is one procedure that may be neglected.

Prescribed antipyretic drugs such as paracetamol, ibuprofen or aspirin may be given to reset the individual's hypothalamus to a lower set point temperature; this reduces the feeling of being cold.

Course of fever (plateau phase)

This phase is characterised by (Berman et al., 2008):

- Absence of chills
- Warm skin
- Photosensitivity and 'glassy eyed appearance'
- Increased pulse and respiratory rates
- Increased thirst
- Dehydration
- Drowsiness, restlessness, delirium and/or convulsions
- Herpetic lesions of the mouth
- Loss of appetite
- Malaise, weakness and aching muscles

The nursing interventions during the course phase of the fever process would be to continue with attention to adequate fluid intake and nutrition to meet the continued increased metabolic demand of the individual's body. Measurement of intake and output becomes important due to increased insensible fluid losses through sweating.

Oral hygiene requires more attention to prevent the mucous membranes from drying out due to the elevated body temperature and increased rate of fluid loss. Antipyretic drugs continue to be administered, and active temperature lowering interventions need to be employed.

The use of tepid sponging can increase the rate of heat loss through conduction and evaporation; the careful use of fans can increase the rate of heat loss by convection. It should be noted that if the temperature-lowering activities are too aggressive, the individual's shell can be cooled too quickly to such an extent that the individual's temperature retaining reflexes are activated. Core body temperature rises contrary to the nursing intent to reduce the core body temperature. Provision of dry bedding and clothing are important for maintaining the comfort of the individual.

Crisis of fever/flush phase

This phase is characterised by (Berman et al., 2008):

- Skin that appears flushed and feels warm
- Sweating
- Decreased shivering
- Dehydration

The nursing interventions during the crisis phase of the fever process support the continued heat loss from the individual's body and reduce excess heat production. The removal of excess bed linen and use of light clothing help heat loss. Active temperature-lowering interventions of tepid sponging and/or use of fans may continue to be employed. In this phase, close attention to the individual's personal hygiene and provision of clean dry bed linen significantly contributes to the comfort of the patient.

Not every fever is resolved by a crisis phase, some fevers gradually subside as the stimulus that has caused the hypothalamus to raise the set point temperature diminishes steadily.

Hypothermia

At body temperatures in the range of −26 to 30°C, the site of measurement of the body temperature needs to be as close to the core temperature as possible. Traditionally, the rectal route is held to be the most accurate site for measuring core temperature in individuals suffering from hypothermia.

The signs of hypothermia that an individual exhibits become progressively more serious with the fall in the core body temperature. As the core body temperature falls from 35°C to approximately 30°C, the hypothalamus induces shivering of the skeletal muscles to generate heat, at core temperatures of 34°C and below, thought processing and coordination becomes impaired, progressive loss of heat leads to the hypothalamic reflexes of heat conservation failing and heat being lost from the core into the shell region of the body. As the body temperature falls lower than 30°C, the heart rate and respiratory effort of the individual diminishes, reducing the blood flow to the brain and the individual becomes very drowsy progressing to comatose. At these low temperatures, the heart muscle becomes unstable and is susceptible to ventricular fibrillation, pulmonary oedema can occur affecting the lungs and the kidneys producing scant urine output.

The intent of the nursing interventions for an individual is to remove the individual from the cold environment and warm the individual's body; however, these interventions must be applied in concert with the individual's heat retaining and generating reflexes, otherwise complications may result. An individual who has a very low body temperature will have constricted the blood vessels of the skin (which gives rise to the pallor associated with being cold); their skin temperature may be much lower than their core temperature. If heat is then rapidly applied to their skin over a wide surface area of their body in an attempt to warm them up, the resultant reflex is potentially quite harmful.

The thermoreceptors of the skin send impulses to the hypothalamus that the environmental temperature is no longer cold but very warm; this causes the heat loss reflexes to be initiated. The blood vessels of the skin dilate, warm blood from the core flows into the cooler skin and heat is lost to the environment. This causes a sudden heat loss from the core, and as the core cools, the hypothalamus still monitors a situation where the environment is warmer than the core. Thus the heat loss reflexes will still occur as long as the body tissues are at a sufficient temperature to respond. If the temperature continues to decline eventually, muscle tissue will no longer function and vasoconstriction of the skin blood vessels ceases which may lead to fatal heat loss.

Therefore the choices of interventions to re-warm an individual depend upon how cold that particular individual is, and how long that individual has been in the hypothermic state. In all events, re-warming should be a steady process seeking to raise the temperature of an individual by 0.5–1.0°C an hour.

The re-warming process of the body may be quite passive, but this would only be suitable for core body temperatures of 34–35°C. Here the individual may be re-warmed by ensuring that the skin is dry and covered with adequate layers of dry clothing or bed clothes; heat reflective blankets may also be used. Warm drinks may be given, blood warmed by the fluid in the gastrointestinal tract helps to raise the core temperature. In mountain and cave, rescue warmed air is also administered for breathing, so there is no further possible heat loss from the lungs and to counter any possible cold-induced pulmonary oedema. If the individual is capable then exercising the skeletal muscles can help to raise the core body temperature.

Active re-warming is required if the individual's core body temperature is below 34°C (Foss and Farine, 2000). A core body temperature of between 30 and 34°C is thought to be moderate hypothermia, whereas a core body temperature of lower than 30°C is considered to be severe hypothermia. Active re-warming can be divided into external and internal interventions.

External re-warming

External re-warming involves the application of heat over the skin surface area by the use of warmed blankets, heat reflective blankets, heating pads, radiant heat lamps (infrared) and warm baths. If applied too quickly or to excess then the complications of re-warming may occur.

Internal re-warming

Internal re-warming seeks to raise the core temperature in the face of severe hypothermia. Body compartments may be irrigated with warm fluid. The fluids are warmed to above normal core body temperature but below 42°C. This can include warmed intravenous fluids, peritoneal lavage, gastric lavage, oesophageal warming and inhalation of warmed respiratory gases (Foss and Farine, 2000).

Conclusions

The nursing interventions that are applied to an individual with temperature regulatory problems should be evaluated as to how they will work in concert with the individual's body to restore the core body temperature to its normal range. Each intervention also needs to be continuously evaluated as to its effectiveness and the degree of benefit the individual derives from that intervention, and finally each intervention needs to be carefully evaluated for any potential hazard that it might pose for the individual.

Glossary

Apyrexia	An absence of fever or febrile condition
Baseline observation	A set of observations normally taken on admission to hospital (temperature, pulse, respiration rate and blood pressure)
Core temperature	The operating temperature of a living being, specifically in the deep structures of the body in comparison to temperature of the surface
Shell (surface) temperature	The shell tissues are described as that of the skin, subcutaneous tissues and fat cells
Thermogenesis	The generation or production of heat, especially by physiological processes within the body
Hypothalamus	A portion of the brain whose main function is to maintain the body's status quo. Factors such as blood pressure, body temperature, fluid and electrolyte balance and body weight are held to a precise value called the set point
Frenulum	Frenula of the mouth include the frenulum linguae under the tongue, the frenulum labii superioris inside the upper lip, the frenulum labii inferioris inside the lower lip and the buccal frena which connect the cheeks to the gum
Tympanic membrane	The tympanic membrane is also called the eardrum. It separates the outer ear from the middle ear
Hypothermia	Abnormally low body temperature. The condition needs treatment at body temperatures of 35°C or below. Hypothermia becomes life-threatening below body temperatures of 32.2°C
Pyrexia	A fever or febrile condition. Can be said to be present if body temperature exceeds the normal range
Hyperpyrexia	An abnormally high fever or febrile condition

Post-chapter quiz

1. Explain the term fever
2. What mechanism is important in the control of temperature?
3. What areas of the body constitute the core tissues?
4. Name the shell tissues of the body

5. Give the normal temperature readings for the following sites
   a. Oral
   b. Axillary
   c. Rectal
   d. Tympanic
6. Describe the main factors influencing body temperature
7. What factors influence heat production and heat loss?
8. Describe how you would take a patient's temperature and what factors should be considered when undertaking this procedure
9. Identify the three phases of fever
10. What interventions can be taken to assist a patient with a raised temperature?

References

Berman, A., Snyder, S.J., Kozier, B. and Erb, G. (eds) (2008) *Fundamentals of Nursing: Concepts, Processes and Practice*, 8th ed. New Jersey: Pearson/Prentice Hall.

Brooker, C. and Waugh, A. (eds) (2007) *Foundations of Nursing Practice: Fundamentals of Holistic Care*. London: Mosby Elsevier.

Dougherty, L. and Lister, S. (2008) *The Royal Marsden Hospital Manual of Clinical Nursing Procedures*, 7th ed. Oxford: Wiley-Blackwell Publishing.

Foss, M. and Farine, T. (2000) *Science in Nursing and Health Care*. Harlow: Prentice Hall.

Helman, C.G. (2007) *Culture, Health and Illness*, 5th ed. London: Hodder Arnold.

Marieb, E. (2008) *Human Anatomy and Physiology*, 6th ed. California: Addison-Wesley.

Mooney, J.P. (2007) Temperature. Available at http://www.nursingtimes.net/nursing-practice-clinical-research/temperature/200193.article. Accessed 29 June 2009.

Nichol, M., Bavin, C., Bedford-Turner, S., Cronin, P. and Rawlings-Anderson, K. (2005) *Essential Nursing Skills*. Edinburgh: Mosby.

Nursing and Midwifery Council (2008a) *The Code: Standards of Conduct, Performance and Ethics for Nurses and Midwives*. London: NMC.

Nursing and Midwifery Council (2008b) *Guidelines for Records and Record Keeping*. London: NMC.

Peate, I. (2008) Keeping warm-health risks and vulnerable people. *Nursing and Residential Care* 10(12): 606–610.

Walker, S. (2003) Controlling body temperature. In: Holland, K., Jenkins, J., Solomon, J. and Whittam, S. (eds). *Applying the Roper, Logan and Tierney Model in Practice*. Edinburgh: Churchill Livingstone, pp. 257–282.

Chapter 12
Work and Leisure

Jackie Hulse

Learning opportunities

This chapter will help you to:

1. Raise your awareness of health issues related to work, unemployment and leisure
2. Consider why we discuss 'occupation', working patterns and leisure interests when assessing a patient
3. Explore how we define work and play
4. Examine how work and play can be affected by illness and accident
5. Discuss how the nurse can contribute to promoting health in the workplace and beyond
6. Outline the unique role and function of the nurse when helping or assisting others in relation to work and leisure

Pre-chapter quiz

1. What do you understand by 'work and play'?
2. What health problems do you think are associated with unemployment?
3. How do you think occupation might affect health?
4. Why do think nurses ask patients about occupation and leisure interests?
5. How do you think stress can affect health?
6. What is the official UK age for retirement?
7. What is the role and function of the Occupational Health Department?
8. What is the key purpose of the Health and Safety Act 1974? To whom does the Health and Safety Act 1974 apply?
9. What are the benefits of exercise?
10. How much is payable is respect of the current state pension?

Introduction

Work is traditionally seen as paid employment, and may occupy more of an individual's time than either sleeping or 'playing', that is leisure time. It may provide an income for the individual and dependants and may often be regarded as a necessity rather than a pleasure. However, work may also confer status, provide social opportunities and enhance an individual's feeling of worth and belonging (Bilton et al., 2002). How often is 'what do you do for a living?' one of the first questions that new acquaintances exchange? Talking informally to a new patient about their work or leisure interests may start to build the relationship that is at the centre of care.

It is worth remembering that work may not always bring a salary, for example when working as a volunteer, homemaker or family carer. It has been determined that in the UK some 6 million adults act as unpaid carers for family, friends or neighbours (Bullard, 2007). In 2006, some 14 million women (or 56% of the female population) were working outside the home, and the majority of these were full-time workers (www.statistics.gov.uk).

Thus, the nurse really needs to consider the impact of illness and accidents on adults of all ages and not just on the traditional 'breadwinner'.

Leisure time may be seen as that which remains after sleeping and working and is often jealously guarded. Nowadays, there is an astounding choice of entertainment, activities and travel opportunities available to us in our leisure time. As children may use play to learn and develop, an adult may use leisure time to acquire new skills, enjoy new experiences or simply as an antidote to the perceived stressors of modern life. Work and play may become inextricably linked to health status since an individual may need to work to generate the income to enjoy leisure activities and clearly needs to enjoy the positive health to do so. Similarly, as the range of sporting activities becomes more varied and some activities become extreme, the leisure pursuits themselves may cause injury or disability that affect an individual's working life.

Thus, this simple introduction has suggested that the nurse is asking questions about work and play with the purpose of interpreting any difficulties that may arise due to health problems and with the intent of offering appropriate and practical advice where possible. This chapter will proceed to consider the role and purpose of 'work' in more detail together with a consideration of the problems of unemployment.

As identified earlier, work may be paid or unpaid and is traditionally seen to occupy the years from adolescence and/or the end of compulsory education until retirement and consequent eligibility for retirement pension payments. It is worth noting that the retirement age is under constant review by government and a universal retirement age of 65 years will be phased in from 2010. This may be a reflection of increased absolute life expectancies and improved health in later years (Evandrou and Falkington, 2000), or it may be, as Clarke (2001) discusses, as a result of the perceived financial burden of pensions and health care created by an ageing population. Thus, the nurse needs an awareness of such changes in demography and related social policy in order to properly understand the situation and expectations of patients.

To 'work for a living' has long been customary in the UK. It developed from offering service or labour in feudal times through literally working for a living to feed and clothe the family to working outside the home in the industrialised society. The Victorians introduced poor relief and the now notorious workhouses for those unable to support themselves and this has developed into the systematic provision of state-funded benefits that operates today. Young people in schools and colleges are frequently offered 'work experience' as a taster of adult working life and as part of the important task of choosing a career. Thus, the idea of working to support oneself and one's dependants is central to our society.

Work provides adults with the means to be financially independent and so make choices about lifestyle. It may even provide a place to live and social activities, as in the armed forces. Paid work will finance leisure activities and hobbies, it may allow for travel and holidays and it may provide personal transport such as a car. However, work also becomes a much more significant part of the individual's profile and identity. Whilst the nurse will be mindful of the potential adverse consequences of stereotyping (Eysenck, 1996), it may hold true that individuals will choose a career that they feel reflects qualities or interests that are central to their sense of self. Nursing, for example, is consistently associated with a desire to care for people, whilst a hospital technician might focus on an interest in laboratory investigation and scientific measurement. Occupation is used by many governments including the UK as one measure of social class. This approach is considered a rather blunt tool, and often criticised, but Robinson and Elkan (1999) maintain that such scales are 'a rough guide to the way of life and living standards experienced by the groups and their families'. Certain occupations may be seen as higher status than others and may require a higher level or education and formal qualifications. Interestingly, these occupations may not offer greater financial rewards, although there are still correlations between education and income (Robinson and Elkan, 1999). Bilton et al. (2002) remind us that even if unemployed, we may still define ourselves through our jobs such as an unemployed coal miner or out-of-work actress to give just two examples.

Work and the workplace may also provide opportunities for socialising and making friends. Indeed, historically, many large employers perceived a duty to offer welfare and social activities as part of the employment package. Nowadays, opportunities may occur more informally but still remain an important part of being a worker. After all, an employee may spend more of the day with colleagues than with their family. Colleagues may find that the shared interests and aspirations that find them in the same employment are mirrored in common social interests. For those workers who live alone, work may provide invaluable and pleasurable social contact and support. The workplace may also offer support outside the usual circle of family and friends especially in times of illness or bereavement.

This all assumes that 'work' is a place where a person physically goes on a regular basis, but changes in working patterns mean that this model of work is by no means universal. With the advent of the internet and continuous developments in information technology, home working is increasingly popular, with 14% of men and 8% of women doing so (McOrmond, 2004), as it is perceived as a way of earning a living and pursuing a career without the complications of leaving one's home. It is seen by many as an ideal way forward for those with children or other domestic responsibilities who might otherwise find their options limited. It may also be seen as helping the 'green' agenda by reducing unnecessary commuter travel. It means that access to work may be widened for some people such as the physically disabled who might not have been able to work in some capacities before. However, some of these ways of flexible working are also seen as less secure than more traditional employment, which Naidoo and Wills (2001) suggest may bring other problems and they argue the need for more research into the psychosocial aspects of work in order to be aware of current and future risks. The government, however, suggests home working as a useful 'transition' to employment for those with mental health and other chronic health problems (Sainsbury, 2008). However, not all changes in work patterns are so obviously beneficial to the worker. McOrmond (2004) outlines that much work is now non-standard or flexible which includes greatly increased amounts of shift working to meet the needs of a fast-moving society, and an increase in temporary or casual labour in which the worker may have reduced employment rights.

Family life and gender

It is also worthwhile to consider how working patterns may be affected by gender, ethnicity and disability. Bilton et al. (2002) consider that women are still disproportionately represented in jobs such as teaching, catering and retail which may be regarded as an extension of home life. They also point out that these types of jobs tend to be less lucrative and women's careers tend to progress less rapidly than that of their male counterparts. This is usually attributed to women's role in child bearing and rearing, and whilst many mothers do engage in paid work, this itself may bring other dilemmas. The Joseph Rowntree Foundation supports a programme of social research into issues impacting on family life. The study by Joseph Rowntree Foundation (2003) reviewed the factors that working families identify as problematic. A key discussion point seems to be the conflicting feelings that working parents, and particularly mothers, experience. These include feeling that it is beneficial to be able to provide better in material terms, but feeling anxious about potential emotional and social disadvantages. The Foundation did publish a study (Ermisch and Francesconi, 2001) that suggested that pre-school children of mothers who work full-time may do less well at school in the long term than those of 'at home' mothers. The difficulties are clear to see for the working mother who needs to contribute to the family income, or as a lone parent, may be the only earner.

Employment and inequalities

Government statistics present an extremely varied picture of the employment patterns of members of ethnic groups. Parallels are drawn between ethnic minority members and women by Bilton et al. (2002), who say that 'prejudice and discrimination in the labour market lead to the racist equivalent of the glass ceiling experienced by women'. Whilst Davey Smith et al. (2000) state that 'minority ethnic groups are often concentrated in less favourable locations within a given occupational grade.' This chapter will consider *unemployment* and ill health later, but Davey Smith et al. (2000) do present a powerful review of some of the psychological distress and physical problems that may be caused by such inequalities whilst in employment.

There is a raft of government legislation (Disability Discrimination Act 1995 and Disability Discrimination Act 2005) to promote equality and opportunity for those with disabilities. Indeed, employers today appear proud to display the 'positive about disabled people' logo on corporate notepaper. However, just after the first Act in 1998, a large-scale study painted a bleak picture for the disabled in the workplace, including frequent reports of discrimination or unfair treatment and being more commonly employed in lower paid manual or low-skilled jobs (Institute of Employment Studies, 1998). More recent reports suggested heightened employer awareness of legislation but that employment practices still vary, with most positive attitudes occurring in the public sector (Simm et al., 2007).

Unemployment

Having discussed the purpose of work and emerging trends and patterns amongst the workforce, it is also worth considering the situation of those who cannot work or who work and then become unemployed. Haralambos and Holborn (2008) present an interesting review of the effects of unemployment on the individual and on society itself. They highlight studies which suggest that in times of high or rising unemployment 'divisions within society are likely to grow. The unemployed and those in unsatisfying work may blame weak groups in society for their problems .... Immigrants and ethnic minorities may be used as scapegoats with the result that racial tensions increase.' At the time of writing, the government is suggesting reforms to the benefits system, with the intention that all members of the community should contribute in some way to the economy.

The most immediate and most obvious consequence of unemployment is that of reduced income and potential reliance on state benefits. This reduction in income may affect the food eaten, clothes worn, places visited and so on. If unemployment continues, any savings are used up and real hardship may ensue. Since they are subject to change and individual variations, there is little purpose in quoting benefit payment rates here, but suffice it to say, as does Clarke, 'that there is no disputing that the unemployed and their dependents suffer considerable financial hardship and material deprivation.'

With regard to the effects on health, Wilson and Walker's (1993) early study suggested links between unemployment and stress and alcohol-related illnesses and mental illness. Since then a number of other studies have already identified strong links or associations between unemployment and an increase in psychological and psychiatric difficulties (McKee-Ryan, 2005; McLean, 2005). Prior and Hayes (2003) found that a quarter of unemployed men and women reported symptoms such as fatigue, sleep disturbance and feelings of irritability and worry. According to Peate and Greeno (2001), it appears that men still suffer the most dramatically from unemployment despite the changes in the labour market that have been discussed and they review studies that highlight the increased mortality rates amongst the unemployed as against comparable groups in employment. Amongst men, particularly, work may be seen as part of the masculine identity and its lack may cause feelings of uselessness and lack of purpose (Fagin and Little, 1984).

Thus, if not having work can make you ill, it seems ironic that work itself can also cause illness. We will now consider the health problems that may be caused by work.

Health and safety

Despite the application of well-established health and safety legislation in the UK, the Health and Safety Executive (2006) still reported that 36 million working days were lost through work-related ill health. This may be due to industrial and occupational accidents or incidents or may be work-related, such as stress. The six most commonly occurring work-related problems reported by the government (www.statistics.gov.uk) are:

- Musculoskeletal disorders
- Mental ill health
- Respiratory diseases
- Skin diseases
- Audiological problems
- Infections

The nurse may be surprised to read that the same government source reported 220 fatal work injuries in 2004–2005, which is actually a reduction on previous years. This was across all industries, although 72 of these deaths occurred in the construction industry alone. As Naidoo and Wills (2008) point out that 'the burden of occupational ill health is not shared evenly between all groups in society' and those who are already economically disadvantaged tend to work in hazardous conditions with less favourable working conditions. Naidoo and Wills (2001) also highlight the changes in patterns of occupational illness that may be expected as work itself changes. Some of these may be positive such as the decline in lung disease suffered by coal miners, but these will be replaced by newer problems. The musculoskeletal disorders best known in manufacturing and industry will be experienced increasingly by those whose work involves using the computer keyboard and mouse. Men are currently more likely to suffer a work-related accident, but as women form more and more of the workforce, their risk is obviously increased. It will be helpful for the nurse to ascertain that any patient presented with a work-related injury is aware of their rights and responsibilities under health and safety legislation.

Many nurses will become familiar with Holmes and Rahe's (1967) Social Readjustment Rating Scale and will see that events related to work such as change in role, working hours or difficulties with the boss score significantly in heightening stress. A recent report of Institute of Employment Studies aimed at encouraging awareness of good employment practices amongst employers and estimated that work-related stress still accounts for over one-third of all work-related ill health (Lucy, 2007). Nor must we forget that the nursing press carries regular features on stress in nursing itself. In a thorough literature review of stress, McVicar (2003) concluded that 'workplace stress is having a greater impact on today's workforce' and that 'sources of stress, that is workload, leadership/management issues, professional conflicts and the emotional demands of caring have been identified by nurses consistently for many years'. These issues will still resonate with many nurses, although a more recent *Nursing Times* report appeared to suggest that stress levels amongst nurses surveyed by it were reducing (Mooney, 2008).

Investigating the links between stress and ill health is a popular area for researchers in several disciplines. Ogden (2007) summarised the research that suggests a link between stress and illnesses such as gastric ulcers, heart disease, arthritis, kidney disease and reduced ability to fight infection. Clearly, it is more problematic to determine how much stress is needed over how long a period to cause these problems but both the causative and contributory role of stress seems beyond doubt. Literature on smoking and alcohol consumption offers an interesting insight into the links between stress and changes in behaviour, and Ogden (2007) reviews a range of studies that highlight how individuals' consumption of tobacco and alcohol increases in times of perceived stress. Thus, it is useful for the nurses to be aware of indications of stress in their patients, and indeed in themselves. Occupational health services may be a useful resource for nurses and patients alike. It is commonly possible to 'self-refer', that is go along without a general practitioner recommendation, and this service may be able to advise and support before problems become overwhelming. Indeed, in 2003, the Department of Health issued guidelines for occupational health professionals which urge them to take a more active role in public health and the prevention of coronary heart disease, cancer and mental health problems.

Informal carers

A relatively neglected group in the literature on work-related ill health are the informal, that is non-professional, carers. This is probably because problems are just beginning to emerge as the numbers of carers increase. Wilson (2004) reminds us that the government-driven move from acute to primary care has contributed to this increase with more people having to depend on family carers. However, as long ago as 1995, the British Medical Association tried to draw attention to the need to support carers. Acting as an informal, unpaid carer is clearly work, yet may bring few of the benefits that we have discussed as being associated with employment. Ironside (2004) states that 20% of these carers are also in full-time employment, which places enormous pressures on them. Those carers who are not in paid work may have given up a lucrative and interesting career in order to take on the care role for a family member. Sale (2004) discusses social isolation and lack of professional support as just two of the factors that lead carers to 'reach breaking point when their own needs . . . impact on their ability to care', whilst Northorne (2000) refers to the existence of the 'overlooked and overworked caregiver'. Sale points out several extreme and high-profile cases that have resulted in violence by carers, and whilst she acknowledges that such cases are rare, they have served to highlight the situation of those who are 'caring but not coping'. The nurse will certainly meet many elderly people who are acting as carers for partners of a similar age and needs to be aware of the difficulties that acute or chronic illness can cause to these families. Many carers may be embarrassed to discuss difficulties for fear of feeling that they are failing in the role (Sale, 2004) and so the nurse may need to explore these sensitive issues carefully in order to help. At a national level, the government has established carers' site 'Caring for Someone' at www.direct.gov.uk and a working knowledge of relevant local services and carers' support groups would be invaluable to the nurse. In England and Wales, the Carers (Equal Opportunities) Act of 2004 was intended to 'acknowledge that carers are entitled to the same life chances as others and should not be socially excluded because of their caring role' (Cass, 2005). Concerns remain, though, about its implementation, including even its definitions of 'carers'.

Illness and employment

For those who are in work, certain illnesses or accidents may have implications for their ability to continue with that work. Those who are self-employed are clearly vulnerable. A self-employed building worker with a tendon injury may not be able to earn for weeks or months and will obviously need urgent advice regarding his or her status and right to benefits. A bus driver who has a heart attack may worry that he will not be able to resume his work, and thus anxiety is added to the stress of heart disease and hospitalisation. In fact, after a full medical review, the bus driver may well return to work (www.dvla.gov.uk), but the nurse will need to reassure him and his family and he will need to be informed of the process. Some people may not be able to continue in work due to disabling illness or accident and some may need to be supported in changing work or roles. It is therefore vital that the nurse is aware of the multiple implications that this may have for the individual and family and that the patient and family are referred to the agencies that are available to offer support and advice. Nursing itself offers a perfect illustration of this potential problem. Nurses are still having to leave work entirely or leave the nursing work of their choice due to back injuries (http://www.rcn.org.uk/support/services/work_injured_nurses last; accessed 2 July 2009). In its most recent report, the National Audit Office (2003) indicated that there were still disappointing levels of accidents and back injuries amongst NHS staff with 285 of trusts actually reporting an increase in occurrences.

Retirement

Retirement has long been regarded as a significant and transitional event in the lifespan. After a full and rewarding working life, one might assume that people look forward to retirement. Many doubtless do, but this is by no means universal. Bilton et al. (2002) suggest that the pattern is changing and that retirement is not seen as being as bleak as in earlier decades. However, both Clarke (2001) and Bilton et al. (2002) acknowledge the difficulties which some retired people face. These are presented as financial due to reduced income, and lack of the social identity and activity offered by work. Many white-collar workers may continue to earn in some capacity once retired, but this may not be possible for manual workers. Thus, as Bilton et al. (2002) suggest 'for less advantaged social classes, retirement may well be accompanied by a sense of social retirement and exclusion'. Interestingly, it is the situation of women which is most likely to change for the better according to Evandrou and Falkington, who report that in this century far more women will be financially better off, having worked to secure their own pension rights. Clarke (2001) suggests that despite some evidence to the contrary, ill health is not commonly a consequence of retirement, but may be the reason for it. Indeed, it appears that many retired people even report feeling in better health after retirement.

As discussed earlier, the number of carers in the UK is rising consistently, and so the nurse must remember that although not in paid work, many retired people provide a vital contribution to family and society. A grandparent may care for his or her grandchild in order to enable his or her adult child to earn a living. Thus, any change in that grandparent's health may have an impact on the circumstances of the whole extended family.

Leisure

One of the problems that has been shown as being identified by carers and the retired is their own isolation and lack of social outlets and this links to the role of 'play' in maintaining health. 'Play' for adults may be sharing the company of friends or neighbours, learning new skills and so on. Most people might simply regard 'play' as enjoyable time away from work or other responsibilities, but it may also have more concrete links with health status. Indeed, 'social support' has been implicated in helping to improve the experience of those suffering from cancer (Naidoo and Wills, 2008) and to reduce work-related stress (Ogden, 2007), to give just two examples. Clarke (2001) also discusses well-documented links between social support and mental illness and considers that whilst a lack of a social network may be a cause of mental illness, having a strong social network may have a positive therapeutic effect on those with problems.

However, just as we have considered the ill health associated with work, it must also be recognised that 'play' may also cause illness and accidents. Ogden (2007) discusses the concept of the 'risky self': an individual whose health is at risk as a result of their own apparent choices and behaviour. This is a distinct change from early in the last century when the medical literature largely depicted risks as external ones such as those from a virus, bacteria or water and other environmental pollution. Very obvious examples of this might be involvement in a potentially dangerous yet relatively accessible sport such as skiing. Individuals may consume potentially damaging alcohol or tobacco as part of leisure activities. Whilst the effects of tobacco consumption may take time to become evident, the problems of alcohol misuse will be familiar to many nurses. This will not just be in the form of alcohol-related disorders such as liver damage but in alcohol-mediated problems such as falls, accidents and even violence and disorder that leads to police involvement. The Department of Health (2008a) estimates a cost of £2.7 billion annually to the NHS for alcohol-related illness and accident. Indeed, primary care trusts with the highest hospital admission rates due to alcohol are now to be offered funding from National Alcohol Support Teams under the DH plan 'Reducing Alcohol Harm'. Of equal concern is the consistently increasing use of illegal drugs as a seemingly integral part of leisure activities for many people. In 2008, the Department of Health reported a national survey which found that 10% of young people had taken drugs in the previous month and 20% had drunk alcohol in the previous 7 days (DH, 2008b). Whilst deaths of young people from drugs are often reported widely and often amidst sensational headlines, the nurse will also need to consider the effects of drug use amongst all ages, including the children of parents who may be using drugs, and across all socioeconomic groups. Concern is also rising about the link between drug use and road traffic accidents (DH, 2008c), which clearly mirrors the 'drink-drive' dilemmas of previous decades. Illegal drugs are costly and there is incontrovertible evidence that links drug use to theft and other criminal activities; 'between a third and half of all acquisitive crime is estimated to be drug related' (DH, 2008c). Whilst it is obvious that the nurse may not have the specialist skills needed in this area of care, it is also clear that it is the role of the nurse to offer non-judgemental support and referral to any patients with problems relating to drug or alcohol consumption. Roper et al. (1996) point out the irony that means that something which often begins as a leisure activity may result in loss of employment due to absenteeism and poor performance, and they describe that the 'deterioration of the self that spills over to affect many other activities of daily living'.

Conclusions

This chapter has provided the nurse with a great deal of interesting background material when considering 'working and playing' for adults. It is clear that in asking apparently simple questions about employment patterns or leisure interests, the nurse is actually looking at aspects that define the whole person and much about their lives. It is to be hoped that the nurse will be aware of the need to make no assumptions about who is a family breadwinner, or about the vital role of a grandparent in maintaining family life. The nurse will need to express understanding of the difficulties and even despair faced by those without work or of those who seem pressured to return to work despite poor health. Nursing care will be most successful if offered in partnership with the patient and family, and this partnership will only result from a thorough understanding and acceptance of the patient and his or her situation in life.

Glossary

Acute illness	Illness over a limited period and may occur suddenly
Attendance allowance	State benefit payable to a person who looks after or 'attends' another person at home
Carer	Person in a care-giving capacity, may be a paid professional or family member or friend
Chronic illness	Illness that continues beyond the acute phase and/or occurs on several occasions
Discrimination	Distinction that disadvantages people for being different, for example through age or gender
Disability	Restriction or impairment of normal ability to perform an activity
Inequality	Unequal treatment or unfairness
Incapacity benefit	State benefit payable to those whose health restricts their ability to work
Risk	Exposure to chance, hazard or danger
Stress	Feelings, usually unpleasant, of pressure, anxiety or tension which may lead to distress
State pension	State benefit for older people who reach retirement age
Well-being	A positive state of health

Post-chapter quiz

1. What do you understand by the term 'risky self'?
2. When was the latest Disability Discrimination Act enacted?
3. What are the most common causes of work-related illness/absence?
4. Which piece of legislation is intended to support informal carers?
5. Do you know how many people in the UK act as informal carers?
6. What do you understand by 'COSHH'?
7. What state benefits may be payable to an unemployed person?
8. What is the role and function of the Department for Work and Pensions?
9. What detrimental effects can loneliness create?
10. How can the detrimental effects of loneliness be reduced?

References

Bilton, T., Bonnet, K., Jones, P., Lawson, T., Skinner, D., Stanworth, M. and Webster, A. (2002) *Introductory Sociology*, 4th ed. Basingstoke: Palgrave.

British Medical Association (1995) *Taking Care of the Carers*. London: BMA.

Bullard, R. (2007) *A Little Oasis*. London: Community Care, pp. 17-18.

Cass, E. (2005) *Guidance to Help Health Professionals Implement the Carers' Act (2004)*. London: Community Care, pp. 38-41.

Clarke, A. (2001) *The Sociology of Healthcare*. Harlow: Pearson Education.

Davey Smith, G., Charsley, K., Lambert, L., Paul, S., Fenton, P. and Ahmad, W. (2000) Ethnicity, health and the meaning of socio-economic position. In: Graham, H. (ed). *Understanding Health Inequalities*. Buckingham: Open University Press.

Department of Health (2003) *Taking a Public Health Approach in the Workplace*. London: DH.

Department of Health (2008a) *Reducing Alcohol Harm*. London: DH.

Department of Health (2008b) *Drug Use and Smoking Amongst Young People in England and Wales in 2007*. London: DH.

Department of Health (2008c) *Drugs: Protecting Families and Communities*. London: DH.

Ermisch, J. and Francesconi, M. (2001) *The Effect of Parents' Employment on Children's Lives*. London: Jospeh Rowntree Foundation.

Evandrou, M. and Falkington, J. (2000) Looking back to look forward: lessons from four birth cohorts in the twenty first century. *Population Trends* 99: 21-30.

Eysenck, M. (1996) *Simply Psychology*. West Sussex: Psychology Press Hove.

Fagin, L. and Little, M. (1984) *The Forsaken Families*. Harmondsworth: Penguin.

Haralambos, M. and Holborn, M. (2008) *Sociology Themes and Perspectives*, 7th ed. London: Unwin Hyman.

Health and Safety Executive (2006) *Statistics of Fatal Injuries at Work*. London: HSE.

Holmes, T. and Rahe, R. (1967) The social readjustment rating scale. *Journal of Psychosomatic Research* 11: 213-218.

Institute of Employment Studies (1998) *Employment of Disabled People: Assessing the Extent of Participation*. London: IES.

Ironside, V. (2004) *Just give me a break. The Times*, April 3, p. 6.

Joseph Rowntree Foundation (2003) *Families and Work in the Twenty First Century*. London: Joseph Rowntree. Available at http://www.jrf.org.uk. Accessed 2 July 2009.

Lucy, D. (2007) *Stress and Psychological Trauma*. London: Institute for Employment studies.

McKee-Ryan, F. (2005) Psychological and physical well being during unemployment: a meta analytic study. *Journal of Applied Psychology* 90(1): 53-76.

McLean, C. (2005) *Worklessness and Health - What Do We Know About the Causal Relationship?* London: Health development Agency.

McOrmond, T. (2004) Changes in working trends over the last decade. *Labour Market Trends* Jan 2004: 25-34.

McVicar, A. (2003) Workplace stress: a literature review. *Journal of Advanced Nursing* 44(6): 633-642.

Mooney, H. (2008) How happy and healthy are nurses? *Nursing Times* 104(42): 8-9.

Naidoo, J. and Wills, J. (2001) *Health Studies: An Introduction.* Basingstoke: Palgrave.

Naidoo, J. and Wills, J. (2008) *Health Studies: An Introduction*, 2nd ed. Basingstoke: Palgrave.

National Audit Office (2003) *A Safer Place to Work.* London: HMSO.

Northorne, L. (2000) The overlooked and overworked caregiver. *Social Science and Medicine* 50: 271-284.

Ogden, J. (2007) *Health Psychology: A Textbook*, 4th ed. Buckingham: Open University Press.

Peate, I. and Greeno, M. (2001) The consequences of male unemployment. *Practice Nursing* 12(11): 460-462.

Prior, P. and Hayes, B. (2003) *Gender and Health Care in the UK.* Basingstoke: Palgrave Macmillan.

Robinson, J. and Elkan, R. (1999) *Health Needs Assessment: Theory and Practice.* London: Churchill Livingstone.

Roper, N., Logan, W. and Tierney, A. (1996) *The Elements of Nursing*, 4th ed. Edinburgh: Churchill Livingstone.

Sainsbury, L. (2008) *Mental Health and Employment.* London: Department for Work and Pensions.

Sale, A. (2004) *Caring But Not Coping.* London: Community Care 29 April to 5 May, pp. 32-33.

Simm, C., Aston, J. Williams, C., Hill, D. and Bellis, A. (2007) *Organisations' Response to the Disability Discrimination Act.* London: Department for Work and Pensions.

Wilson, S. and Walker, G. (1993) Unemployment and health: a review. *Public Health* 107: 153-162.

Wilson, V. (2004) Supporting family carers in the community setting. *Nursing Standard* 18(9): 47-55.

Chapter 13
The Sexual Being

Ian Peate

Learning opportunities

This chapter will help you to:

1. Understand the difference between sex and sexuality
2. Define a number of key terms associated with sex and sexuality
3. Begin to understand how sexuality is expressed
4. Discuss ways in which the nurse can help people fulfil their needs with regards to their sexuality
5. Describe some of the key issues related to sexual health assessment
6. Outline the way the nurse can help to enhance a person's sexual health

Pre-chapter quiz

1. Sexuality is best described by which of the following definitions?
   a. Sexual function
   b. A composite of feelings and behaviours specific to gender
   c. Sexual activity and the love and caring that accompany it
   d. Body image, gender roles, patterns of affection, family and social roles, and genital sex
2. What do you understand by the term 'holistic care'?
3. List all of the issues that you can think of that could enhance a person's sexual health
4. Describe some of the barriers that may impinge on a person's ability to enjoy good sexual health
5. Think about some of the effects illness may have on an individual's sexuality
6. Discuss what is meant by body image
7. Describe the normal changes that can occur as the body ages and the effects this may have on a person's sexual health
8. List five commonly used medications and the effects these may have on an individual's sexual health

9. Why do you think some nurses and people find discussing sexual health and issues associated with sexuality difficult?
10. How do you think you might react to a person who expresses their sexuality differently to the way you express your sexuality?

Introduction

The National Strategy for Sexual Health (Department of Health [DH], 2001a) provides insight into the government's aims and objectives in relation to the sexual health of people, setting out an ambitious 10-year programme to tackle sexual ill health as well as modernising service provision. The key aim is to ensure that the population is in good sexual health and well educated in how to protect themselves against sexually transmitted infections (STIs) and unplanned pregnancies (Independent Advisory Group on Sexual Health and HIV, 2008). This chapter introduces the reader to the various complex concepts associated with sexuality and sexual health, reinforcing the notion that people are sexual beings.

In order to offer care that is safe and effective, the nurse must also ensure that the important issue of sexuality is addressed when providing a holistic approach to care provision; this must be undertaken in a supportive and non-judgmental way. To fully address the holistic needs of people (and this will incorporate their sexual health needs), it is vital that important concepts impinging on sexuality are understood.

Sex is a common strand of all of our lives, not only at our conception but hopefully considered amongst some of our most positive experiences. Sex should be something we rejoice in not fear; it should be seen as a positive influence in our overall health and well-being. Katz (2007) points out that sexuality is a natural part of life and as such should be given attention by nurses and other health care professionals. Sexual health is an important issue for all of us, young and old. Adler (2003) notes that young people are becoming sexually active at an earlier age. Young people - those aged between 16 and 24 years - are the age group that is most at risk of being diagnosed with an STI; this age group accounted for 65% of all chlamydial infection, 50% of genital warts and 50% of gonorrhoea infections diagnosed in genitourinary clinics in the UK in 2007 (Health Protection Agency, 2008); however, Bauer et al. (2007) observe that there is a growing concern about the transmission of STIs amongst the older population.

The issue of sexuality has often been ignored by the nursing profession despite the benefits it brings to the psychosocial well-being of people (Anderson and Kitchen, 2000; McCann, 2000). Chapters 1 and 2 of this text consider the important role and function of the nurse and promotes the notion of holistic nursing care; Earle (2001) notes that despite this claim to caring for the whole person, a framework for care that should include the biopsychosocial needs of people is often excluded from nursing practice. There may be many reasons why nurses fail to address the complex issues of sexuality; barriers to some of these are addressed later in this chapter.

The Nursing and Midwifery Council (NMC, 2008) makes it clear in their Code of Conduct that the nurse must make the care of people his or her first concern, treating them as individuals and respecting their dignity. The nurse must not discriminate in any way against those in their care, people must be cared for kindly and considerately.

Policy and key drivers

The government has put in place a number of policies, guidance and national initiatives that focus on improving sexual health. A number of government policies can be seen as key drivers in ensuring that the nation enjoys positive sexual health and avoids negative sexual health. In the government White Paper, 'Choosing Health' (DH, 2004), sexual health is identified as one of the key national priorities for action. Commitments are made in this document to improve sexual health services.

The first ever strategy for sexual health and HIV was published by the DH in 2001 (DH, 2001a); in Wales, the Welsh Assembly has published its approach to sexual health (Welsh Assembly, 2000) and the Scottish Executive (2005) also has a strategy and action plan for improving sexual health of the people of Scotland.

The Medical Foundation for AIDS and Sexual Health (2005) recommends standards for sexual health services. These standards are for use in a number of health care settings, for example general practice, hospital and community-based clinics, pharmacies, voluntary and independent organisations. This document recognises that there may be some challenges to helping people attain optimum sexual health.

The World Health Organization (WHO, 2000) notes that the protection of health is a basic human right; therefore, sexual health encompasses sexual rights and as a result of this they also deserve protection. Eleven sexual rights have been declared as universal (see Box 13.1).

Box 13.1 WHO declaration of sexual rights.

- The right to sexual freedom
- The right to sexual autonomy, sexual integrity and safety
- The right to sexual privacy
- The right to sexual equality and fairness
- The right to sexual enjoyment
- The right to emotional sexual expression
- The right to sexually associate freely
- The right to make free and responsible reproductive preferences
- The right to sexual information based on a sound evidence base
- The right to an inclusive sexuality education
- The right to sexual health care

Source: Reproduced from WHO (2000).

The National Institute for Health and Clinical Excellence (NICE) has produced guidance for health care professionals and the members of the public (NICE, 2007) that focuses on the prevention of STIs and reduction in the rate of conceptions in those under 18 years of age, with specific reference to those in vulnerable and at-risk groups. SIGN (Scottish Intercollegiate Guidelines Network) also produces guidance in relation to sexual health (www.sign.ac.uk).

Sexual ill health costs the National Health Service (NHS) over £700 million per year (Health Protection Agency, 2004). For individuals who experience sexual ill health, this may range from a brief period of discomfort to infertility and in some cases death as the result of HIV/AIDS.

Defining key terms

It is important to have some commonly agreed definitions of the terminology used in the discipline of human sexuality and sexual health. Definitions of key terms are needed in an attempt to communicate effectively, to disseminate information and to develop activities that can be used to promote sexual health. Challenges do occur, however, when attempting to agree about the chosen definition.

Human sexuality is a concept that can prove difficult to define (Bauer et al., 2007). Often definitions are influenced by the particular sociocultural and historical context and process in which the definition is constructed. It must be remembered that some definitions that are used do not receive a wide consensus from the various communities who use them, different communities use the terms in different ways. The definitions provided here are only intended to be used as practical tools.

Sexuality

There is no agreed definition of what sexuality is, but there are several to choose from. Sexuality is an all-encompassing term that considers sexual character in its widest sense and is made known in the way a person expresses their preferences as a sexual being. Humans are sexual beings and how a person communicates their sexuality is determined by a number of factors. Regardless of whether a person is healthy, ill or disabled, they are sexual beings all of the time according to McCann (2000).

Sexuality is an important characteristic of daily life, it brings pleasure and enjoyment and it also has the potential to bring about anxiety, uncertainty, unhappiness and danger. Expressing sexuality is an important feature of self-esteem, self-acceptance and general well-being; it allows a person to define themselves to others and failure to experience sexual intimacy can result in depression (Hajjar and Kamel, 2003).

Sexuality refers to a core definition of what it is to be a human being and encompasses sex, gender, sexual and gender identity, sexual orientation, eroticism, emotional attachment/love and reproduction. It is, therefore, a multidimensional, fluid, dynamic construct that is much more than the penetrative sexual act, meaning different things to different people; it changes across time and place. People can express their sexuality in a number of ways, for example in thoughts, fantasies, desires, beliefs, attitudes, values, activities, practices, roles and relationships. There is the interaction of biological, psychological, socioeconomic, cultural, ethical and religious/spiritual factors (see Figure 13.1).

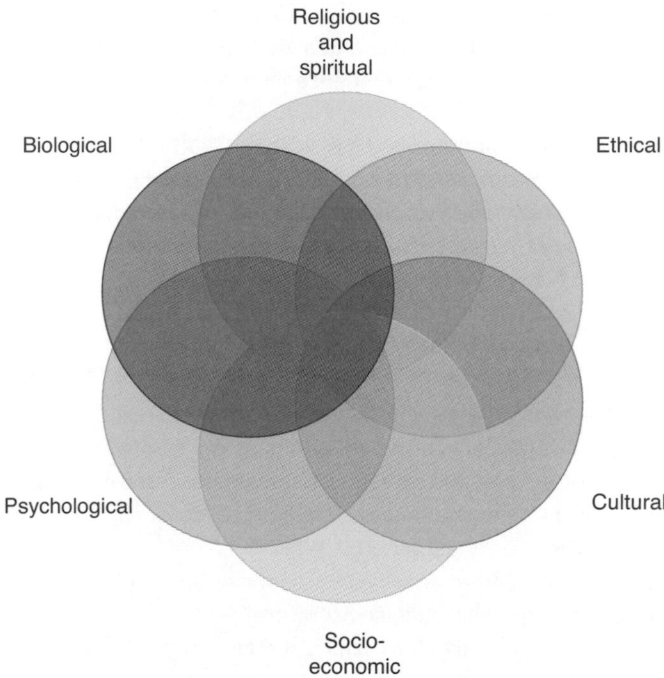

Figure 13.1 The interaction of key issues associated with sexuality.

Sexual health

Sexual health is one aspect of an individual's sexuality (Cherry, 2008). There are a number of definitions available to help understand this complex, fluid and dynamic activity. A broad definition of sexual health is provided in *Choosing Health* (DH, 2004):

> Sexual health is an important part of physical and mental health. It is a key part of our identity as human beings together with the fundamental human rights to privacy, a family life, and living free from discrimination. Essential elements of good sexual health are equitable relationships and sexual fulfilment with access to information and services to avoid the risk of unintended pregnancy, illness or disease.

In this definition, sexual health is seen as central to physical and mental health; the definition acknowledges a person's rights to live their life free from discrimination as well as to enjoy privacy and family life. Other topics can be addressed when using this definition as a starting point, for example teenage conceptions, STIs and their impact on a person's health and well-being, sexual assault, sexual knowledge, attitudes and behaviours. The definition also allows for consideration of inequalities that are prevalent in sexual health amongst some women, teenagers and young adults, gay men, black and ethnic minority groups and socially deprived groups. In England there are higher numbers of people diagnosed with HIV from deprived and socially excluded populations (Health Services Commission, 2007).

The WHO (2002) defines sexual health as:

> A state of physical, emotional, mental and social well-being related to sexuality; it is not merely the absence of disease, dysfunction or infirmity. Sexual health requires a positive and respectful approach to sexuality and sexual relationships, as well as the possibility of having pleasurable and safe sex experiences, free of coercion, discrimination and violence. For sexual health to be attained and maintained, the sexual rights of all persons must be respected, protected and fulfilled.

This definition again, an all-encompassing one, values respect for self and others as well as supporting mutuality, trust and love in relationships. An acceptance of diversity of beliefs is also inherent in this statement along with freedom from inequity, violence or intimidation.

A final definition of sexual health is offered by the Royal College of Nursing (RCN, 2000) which define it as:

> ...the physical, emotional, psychological, social and cultural well-being associated with a person's sexual identity and capacity to enjoy and express sexuality, freely and without physical or emotional harm, exploitation and oppression.

Sexuality is defined as a person's self-concept that is shaped by their personality and expressed as sexual feelings, attitudes, beliefs and behaviour expressed through heterosexual, bisexual, homosexual or transsexual orientation.

Sexual health promotion

This can be defined as those activities which proactively and positively support the sexual and emotional health and well-being of individuals, groups, communities and the wider public (DH, 2003). By including emotional health in this definition, one acknowledges the strong link between an individual's emotional well-being and his or her ability to take control over decisions and choices that will impact on their sexual health.

The aims of sexual health promotion are to:

- Improve the positive sexual health of the general population and to reduce inequalities in sexual health
- Reduce rates of new and undiagnosed HIV infection
- Reduce rates of STIs
- Reduce unintended pregnancies
- Reduce psychosexual problems
- Facilitate more satisfying, fulfilling and pleasurable relationships

Gender

A person's gender refers to the social and cultural attributes and opportunities associated with being male or female in a particular point in time. Children, during developmental phases of their lives, usually acquire a fixed sense of themselves as male or

Table 13.1 Socially constructed descriptions of masculinity and femininity.

Masculinity	Femininity
• Strong • Powerful • Rational • Self-reliant • Breadwinner	• Soft, gentle • Weak • Emotional • Dependent • Child raiser

Source: Reproduced from Laws (2006).

female. They acquire what some developmental psychologist's term gender identity (Smith et al., 2003).

Gender, according to Gray et al. (2000), does not live within the person; it is the product of social interactions and transactions and is better understood as a verb than as a noun; in this way, gender can be viewed as a dynamic, gendered, social structure (Crawford, 1995). Gender stereotypes are used by people when they try to construct gender; gender is a living system of social interactions. The stereotypes put together represent the characteristics that are usually supposed to be typical of men or women. Society has strong and well-established beliefs of what men and women should and should not do, and what is masculine or feminine. Table 13.1 identifies some common socially constructed features (generalisations) of masculinity and femininity.

Sex

It is important to note that there is a distinction between sex and sexuality. The term sex refers to the biological characteristics that define people as either female or male. Sex is not only decided on by the appearance of the external genitalia, but advances in technology have also allowed for the determination of sex by examination of chromosomes; most men usually have external genitalia and one Y and one X chromosome, whereas women usually have internal genitalia with X chromosomes.

Some people do not have discernable external genitalia and some have combinations of chromosomes that do not follow the normal description of man or woman - in this case, their sex may be described as atypical. In approximately 1% of live births, some element of sexual ambiguity may exist (Blackless et al., 2000).

When some people talk about sex, they are often referring to sexual activity and not to sex as a biological entity where there are differences between anatomical and physiological aspects.

Assessing sexual health

Assessment, as Sibson explains in her chapter in this text (Chapter 3), is a complex skilled activity that is often undertaken using a tool or a model. Nurses have a role to play in assessing sexual health, developing plans of care, providing that care and evaluating it when helping people with their sexual health.

Most patients do not automatically offer information about sexual problems; because of this the nurse should incorporate at least a brief sexual assessment into routine health assessments. It is acknowledged that not every nurse can be a sexual counsellor, listening to the concerns of patient and family, offering factual information in a non-threatening manner, caring for people with non-complex disease and treatment-related symptoms as well as providing appropriate referrals can be easily incorporated into routine care.

According to Shell (2007), assessing the sexual health care needs of people effectively means that this should be an in-depth, fact-finding activity that puts into context the person's life, for example:

- Age
- Relationship status
- Living arrangements
- Career status
- Parental status

Despite this, Carpenito-Moyet (2006) suggests that most nurses do not carry out this important activity nor do they have the time to do so.

The sexual health assessment should be conducted in private, if possible, with an explanation of its purpose. Doors should be closed or the curtains drawn around the bed with the nurse speaking in a low tone. If this is problematic then the nurse should consider moving to another area where privacy may be guaranteed, for example an office.

It is vital that the patient (and, if appropriate, partner) is reassured with regard to confidentiality. The nurse should meet privately with the patient first unless otherwise requested and then include the partner (Shell, 2007). At all times the nurse must bear in mind the tenets of the NMC's *Code of Conduct* (NMC, 2008) with regard to confidentiality. The nurse must respect the person's right to confidentiality, informing them about how and why information is shared by those who will be providing their care.

As early as possible during the assessment, the nurse should initiate discussion about sexuality and any sexual concerns. This approach implies that sexuality is an important aspect of good health. The nurse should use sexual terms before expecting the patient to. It is imperative that the nurse uses the language the patient chooses to use so as to ensure that communication between both parties is effective; it is unacceptable to use threatening language, for example, by using technical terms or jargon. The use of open-ended questions is vital and this has been alluded to many times in this book, as Briggs does in Chapter 5.

When the nurse and patient are communicating effectively on this very intimate activity then patient-centred goals can begin to emerge. It may be that there are no issues, as sexuality may not be seen by the patient to feature as a part of, or impinge on his or her quality of life. Every person is an individual and not all people have partners or want one and not all people experience sexual satisfaction in the same manner.

During the period of assessment, a positive, relaxed and professional attitude is needed. If the person chooses to reveal personal and intimate details, the nurse should not appear shocked or surprised, but should remember that the shock and surprise can be revealed both verbally and non-verbally. The key aim for the nurse is to demonstrate to the person that they are truly interested in them, which can communicate acceptance.

There may be occasions when referral to other health or social care agencies is needed. Referral must be appropriate and with the person's consent. The nurse can only do this effectively if he or she is aware of and knows who to refer to.

Wilmoth (2006) notes that often when talking to patients about sexuality and issues associated with sexuality this can occur by chance, usually in an informal and unexpected way. The nurse must be alert and sensitive to these hidden cues when talking to patients and then follow them up with open-ended questions to elicit more details, with the intention of helping.

Approaches to assessment

There are a number of approaches to assess sexual health. Two models - the PLISSIT model (P, permission; LI, limited information; SS, specific suggestions; IT, intensive therapy) (Anon, 1974) and BETTER model (B, bring up the topic; E, explaining sexuality as part of quality of life; T, tell patient about appropriate resources; T, timing; E, educate about side effects; R, record in patient chart) (Mick et al., 2003) - may be helpful and provide sexuality information for patients and partners. A brief outline of the BETTER model is present and a more in-depth look at the PLISSIT model in practice is provided.

BETTER model

Bring up the topic

People who have, for example, long-term conditions may have questions about how their condition and treatment may affect their sexuality. The nurse can ask 'Do you have any questions?'

Explain

The nurse should explain to the person that he or she is concerned with quality of life issues. The nurse may explain that 'I am concerned with issues related to quality of life, for example, your body image and sexuality is also one of those issues.' 'I will do my best to answer your questions as far as I can.'

Tell

'I am aware that you are concerned with the affects of the radiotherapy associated with your treatment for your prostate cancer and what effects this will have on your ability to achieve and maintain an erection.' The nurse should tell the person that he or she will endeavour to provide appropriate resources to address their concerns. The nurse can provide information for the person and also give them written information (or direct the person to other resources); this will reinforce what has been said.

Timing

If the timing does not seem right during the first encounter with the person then the nurse can acknowledge this and tell them that they can ask for information at any time.

Educate

Providing the person with oral and written information or other resources using a variety of formats can help them understand treatment and any potential side effects.

Record

All interactions with the person should be documented according to policy and procedure and in line with guidance produced by the NMC (2007).

PLISSIT model

This model was developed in 1974 by an American psychologist and was intended for use in sex therapy. The model can also be helpful to nurses as it provides a framework that can help the nurse to assess and plan care interventions, working with patients to address their sexual health concerns. The model provides a number of suggestions for initiating and maintaining the discussion of sexuality, particularly with older adults. The approach used includes the use of open-ended questions about sexuality.

The aim of the assessment is to collect information that permits the patient to communicate his or her sexuality safely as well as being able to feel uninhibited by normal or pathological problems. It is usual for nurses to feel uncomfortable when assessing a patient's sexual desires and functions. Nevertheless, a sexual assessment should be undertaken as a routine part of the nursing assessment. Knowledge, skill, and a sense of one's own feelings and sexuality will make available the comfort that is needed for the nurse to assess the sexuality of adults effectively.

Permission

This is the first step in the model and is used to ask permission to begin the sexual assessment; this could also be interpreted as giving the patient permission to discuss issues associated with sexual health. The nurse introduces the subject of sex and encourages the patient to discuss sexual concerns and ask questions. The nurse may say 'I always ask whether patients are having any relationship or sexual problems. Your sexual health is an important part of your life. There are times when an illness or the medicines you are taking can affect your sexuality. Tell me how your relationships have been lately?' This strategy uses an open-ended approach. Other examples could be 'What questions can I answer for you about how the proposed treatment might impinge on your sexuality?'

Limited information

At this stage the nurse can provide the person with limited information about normal and pathological changes that can impact on sexuality as well as the side effects of treatment. This is an opportunity for the nurse to dispel any myths or misconceptions.

Specific suggestions

Specific suggestion aspect of the model and how it is enacted will depend on the responses the patient has given the nurse to the open-ended questions that have been asked. This is why it is important that the nurse actively listens to the patient (see Chapter 5). These specific suggestions might include providing the patient with written materials about sexuality and their illness. The nurse might suggest, for example, that prior to intercourse the patient takes analgesia or adopts a different position during the sex act.

Intensive therapy

This final element of the model requires further in-depth education and the nurse may have to refer the patient to another expert health care professional, for example a sex therapist, psychologist or counsellor.

Older people's sexuality and health

Sexuality for older people is an important component of their lives, just as it might be for anyone else. Nay (2004) points out that sexuality for older people can be as much about intimate kissing, cuddling, masturbation or intercourse as it can be about companionship, looking and feeling good, talking dirty and enjoying explicit magazines and movies.

According to Reed (2007), sexuality and the older person has been underdiscussed; the sexual needs and concerns of older people have not been addressed as fully as they could have been in the past. Those studies that have been undertaken point out that most individuals in later life retain sexual interest and ability. Regular sex has the potential to improve cardiovascular function and can help to sustain well-being, for example relationships. The biggest single factor that mitigates against older people enjoying sexual health is the attitude of society, and nurses are a part of society.

A satisfying sexual relationship throughout life is an important aspect of that life; it is not always easy to achieve this as a person ages. The ageing process impinges on the whole body and because of this it is certain that it will have a bearing on sex.

When discussing sexuality it is wrong to homogenise older people as each person is a unique being. It is important to respect, however, whatever the older person defines as sex and what it means to them. Not all older people may want to engage in sexual intercourse or even to express their sexuality and that is their privilege. Just like some younger people, there are some older people who prefer to abstain from sex.

Policy often focuses on younger people and the importance of education, for example, related to unintended pregnancy, and sometimes this is to the disadvantage of the emotional and well-being elements associated with sex and sexuality for older people. Sex education often highlights how to cope with coming into adulthood and can fail to deal with the sexual changes that occur to an individual as they age. Much has been written about the transition between a child and an adolescent and the challenges that the person may face with respect to sex, but there is very little concerning the complex transitions that occur as people become older. The National Service Framework (NSF) for Older People (DH, 2001b) specifically concerns older people, yet this document fails to address sexual health for the older person and as such this portion of the population has been done a disservice.

The older person (and the nurse) may feel unprepared when faced with the normal changes associated with the ageing process; they could feel just as uncomfortable about sex at the age of 75 years as they did when they were engaging in their first sexual experiences when they were an adolescent. As people live longer and the population ages, there could be an expectation that they will remain sexually active for the greater part of their years.

Often the media assumes that sex is only for the young and beautiful. This is an incorrect assumption as intimacy is ageless and sexual activity can be an essential aspect of any relationship; it offers enjoyment, fun, excitement, personal fulfilment and intimacy.

There are several negative stereotypes that are linked with older people, for example often they are depicted as decrepit, frail, and these negative stereotypes have the ability to strengthen feelings that if an older person expresses an interest in sex they are somehow dirty or perverted. Negative stereotypes can affect how older people feel about themselves.

It must be acknowledged that the older person might not experience the same enjoyment of sex that they enjoyed when they were in their 20s, nevertheless this does not mean that it cannot be just as fulfilling and enjoyable as it was then. People can, regardless of age, experience fluctuations in sex drive; this is normal. There are aspects of sex that will change or alter as a person ages, but there are ways in which the older person can adjust to these changes and these changes can impact on the whole sexual experience and not just the physical act. If sexual problems continue they can cause anxiety and distress, further exacerbating problems and inhibiting sexual enjoyment or fulfilment.

Sexual problems

There are a number of male and female sexual psychological and physiological changes that arise as the result of ageing; these changes can be related only to the psychological or only to the physical or they may be a combination of both. Sexual problems may begin as the result of an underlying physical cause that may have an effect on sexual performance and this may exacerbate issues for the person and his or her partner.

Physical changes

For a number of older women (and maybe their partner) a common physical change as a result of the ageing process is vaginal dryness. This is usually a result of oestrogen deficiency - a common feature of the ageing process. There are many ways in which the effects of vaginal dryness can be reduced, leading to better sexual activity for the woman and her partner. The use of prescribed oestrogen cream (if the woman is not already receiving hormone replacement therapy) applied topically, KY jelly or Senselle and some aroma-based oils may help with lubrication. There are some topically applied lubricants which may cause breakage or weakening of condoms and this should not be forgotten. If appropriate, referral to a gynaecologist or urologist may be required in order to seek specialist advice.

Erectile dysfunction is defined by the National Institutes of Health Consensus Development Conference (1992) as the persistent inability to obtain or maintain sufficient rigidity of the penis to allow satisfactory sexual performance; however, there are a number of other definitions available. In 30–50% of men aged between 40 and 70 years worldwide, some degree of erectile dysfunction is experienced, age is the variable mostly associated with erectile dysfunction (McKinley, 2000). Other reasons exist as to why a man may not be able to initiate and maintain an erection for satisfactory sexual performance, for example loss of libido.

There are several therapeutic options that are available for erectile dysfunction, with varying degrees of patient satisfaction. Options include pharmacologic agents, for example sildenafil (Viagra), intracavernosal alprostadil (Caverject) and transurethral alprostadil (MUSE). Non-pharmacologic treatments include vacuum erection devices, penile prostheses and penile revascularisation.

Pharmacological considerations

There are many drugs (prescribed and recreational) that have the potential to compromise sexual health. It is not easy to decide if any particular drug is responsible for bringing about sexual dysfunction, as a number of disease processes can also affect and impinge on sexual function. Many patients do not report sexual dysfunction as they may be embarrassed to do so.

Medications that have the ability to affect the sexual hormone system will also have the capacity to have some bearing on sexual function, for example depressing libido. When the patient does report sexual dysfunction as the potential result of the side effects of medications, a decision has to be made whether to carry on with the drug, alter the dose or think about changing the medication altogether; the decision can depend on the benefits of the medication outweighing the unwanted side effects.

Mechanisms concerning sexual function are multifaceted and not fully understood; what is known reveals that sexual function comprises a set of complex coordinated activities involving hormones, chemical messengers in the brain, such as dopamine and serotonin, as well as the sexual organs. Medications can therefore affect sexual function in a variety of ways. Table 13.2 provides a list of some medications that may affect sexual function.

Not all people will be subjected to side effects with the medicines that they are taking; sexual dysfunction may be entirely unconnected to the medications being taken. The person prescribing the medication must always reflect on the possible impact it may have on the whole person as well as their sexual function.

Long-term conditions

Long-term conditions, for example disability (Earle, 2001), cancer (Wilmoth, 2006), diabetes mellitus (Grandjean and Moran, 2007), the impact of surgery, the effects of restricted mobility and the side effects of some prescribed and recreational drugs, can have a bearing on how a person enjoys sex. Only by understanding what they are can the nurse help people who are experiencing sexual ill health.

Barriers to sexual discussion

Sexuality is a topic of great interest for many people. Given the exposure it receives in the media - electronic and print - it could be expected that nurses and other health care professionals will feel comfortable when communicating with people about sexual health

Table 13.2 A selection of medications that can affect sexual function

Medication	Key use/indication	Potential effect on sexual functioning
Antidepressants		
MOAIs (monoamine oxidase inhibitors) i.e. phenlazine SSRIs (selective serotonin re uptake inhibitors) i.e. fluoxetine Tricyclics i.e. amitryptiline	Depression	Decreased sex drive ED Delayed orgasm Absent orgasm Ejaculatory disturbances
Antiepileptics		
Carbamazepine	Epilepsy	ED
Antihypertensives		
ACE (angiotensin-converting enzyme) inhibitors i.e. enalapril Alpha-blockers i.e. prazosin Beta-blockers i.e. atenolol Calcium channel blockers i.e. verapamil Methyldopa Thiazide diuretics i.e. bendroflumethiazide	Hypertension Heart failure Glaucoma Angina	ED Ejaculatory disturbance Decreased sex drive Delayed or failure of ejaculation
Cholesterol-reducing medicines		
Statins i.e. simvastatin	High cholesterol	ED
Other		
Benzodiazepine	Anxiety and insomnia	Decreased sex drive
Cimetidine	Peptic ulcers	Decreased sex drive and ED
Cyproterone acetate	Prostate cancer	Decreased sex drive and ED and reduced volume of ejaculate
Disulfiram	Alcohol withdrawal	Decreased sex drive
Finasteride	Enlarged prostate	Decreased sex drive and ED and reduced volume of ejaculate
Metoclopramide	Nausea and vomiting	Decreased sex drive and ED
Omeprazole	Peptic ulcers	ED
Opioids i.e. morphine	Severe pain	Decreased sex drive and ED
Prochloperazine	Nausea and vomiting	ED
Spironolactone	Heart failure and fluid retention	Decreased sex drive and ED

(ED = erectile dysfunction)

issues. Katz (2005) notes that some clinicians (nurses included) express discomfort when discussing sexuality, or they avoid discussing issues concerning a patient's sexual worries or anxieties. When sexuality is discussed, because of the power of the media, this is often reserved for the young and healthy.

For people with chronic illnesses, for example those with cancer, if sexuality is considered then this is usually centred on those whose sexual function may be directly impacted by the cancer, for example cancer of the cervix, cancer of the prostate. Those whose cancer is not seen as being directly related to their sexual function, for example those with cancer of the lung or the stomach, may not, according to Katz (2005), receive help and support concerning sexuality and self-image. Shell (2007) identifies others who may be left out of discussions relating to sexuality:

- Older people
- Gay and lesbian
- Bisexual and transgendered
- Those of a different culture

This omission can provoke anxiety and discomfort; nurses who care for those people with a chronic condition are ideally placed to help encourage a more positive self-esteem for the patient by offering opportunities to talk about feelings and worries about treatment and how this can impact on sexuality.

Social and cultural forces have the ability to influence what is seen as normal or appropriate in relation to sexual behaviour, for example gender roles, sexual identity or the expression of sexual desire. Preconceived ideas, attitudes and values can mean that nurses may have their own cultural biases coupled with a discomfort when talking to patients about their sexuality and their sexual health needs.

Nurses need to develop strategies that will enable them to feel more comfortable with people when discussing sexuality; this means that they must first be comfortable with their own sexuality; Wilmoth (2006) calls this a process of self-exploration. Self-exploration can take place in a number of ways with the aim of becoming more at ease when talking about sexuality (see Box 13.2).

Box 13.2 Some examples of self-exploration.

Reading articles and books
Accessing the internet
Consulting or speaking with other nurses who are comfortable with sexuality, for example a clinical nurse specialist
Observing those who incorporate sexual assessment into their practice, for example a nurse working in the genitourinary medicine setting
Taking part in role play/simulation
Attending conferences, seminars, workshops
Undertaking self-assessment that considers your attitudes, values and beliefs about sexuality

Good communication skills can be developed and one effective way of doing this is through role-play. Working with others, you can start asking questions, experimenting, moving from less sensitive questions to more sensitive ones, noting how you and the other person is feeling. After you have been practising for a number of times, you are likely to become more comfortable, feel less embarrassed and act in a more confident manner.

Increasing your knowledge base in relation to sexual health can help you to help others. Revising the anatomy and physiology of the male and female reproductive tracts, delving deeper into important areas such as psychosexual development, the sexual response cycle, the implications for an individual's health and well-being from a cultural, religious and ethical perspective are issues that can be considered (Hyde et al., 2001; Rathaus et al., 2008).

Conclusions

Zanni et al. (2003) note that a central element concerning quality of life is sexuality and this can lead to the continuation of healthy interpersonal relationships, self-concept and a sense of integrity. Self-worth is aligned to one's sense of self-esteem and if this is deprived, the result, according to Hajjar and Kamel (2003), can have damaging effects on the person's sexuality, self-image, social relationships and mental health.

When sexual intercourse is no longer possible or desirable, the issue that becomes central to emotional connectedness and well-being is intimacy (Gott and Hinchliffe, 2003). There are other activities available for people to express their sexuality when the act of penetration, because of disability or choice, does not occur; these can consist of close body contact, kissing, taking time over appearance and holding hands.

The nurse in accordance with the NMC's Code of Conduct (NMC, 2008) has a duty to ensure that each person is treated with respect; failure to do this is tantamount to professional misconduct. With respect to the older population, the nurse should reconsider his or her approach to them and their sexual health needs; if nurses are unaware and uninformed about the older people's needs, it is highly doubtful that they will be offering services that fully address these needs.

Values, beliefs and attitudes have the ability to impact considerably on the health and well-being of all people and in particular the health and well-being of those with problems associated with their sexuality. Prior to attempting to address the needs of people and their sexual health, the nurse must focus on his or her own prejudices and the stereotypes they may have. Holding prejudice can dehumanise and as such this can diminish the quality of an individual's life.

Glossary

Chlamydia	A common STI caused by the bacterium *Chlamydia trachomatis*
Chromosome	An organised structure of DNA
Gonorrhoea	An STI caused by the bacteria *Neisseria gonorrhoeae*
Intimacy	A feeling of being emotionally close to another person

Intracavernosal	Within the chambers of the penis
Libido	Sexual desire
Prophylaxis	To guard or prevent against
Prostheses	An artificial extension (singular prosthesis)
Transgender	An umbrella term used to include many people whose lifestyles appear to conflict with the gender norms of society
Transsexual	A person who has achieved transsexualism by having a sex-change operation
Transurethral	An approach via the urethra
Transvestite	A person who masquerades and dresses in the clothes of the opposite sex (also known as cross-dressing)

Post-chapter quiz

1. Define the following terms:
   a. Chromosome
   b. Impotence
   c. Transvestite
   d. Gender dysphoria
2. List three of the most common male sexually transmitted infections
3. List three of the most common female sexually transmitted infections
4. When is world AIDS day?
5. Describe the issues that you would need to take into account when providing information to a person who has been diagnosed with an STI
6. What do you understand by the term 'sexual dysfunction'?
7. Briefly, describe the nurse's role and function when offering advice to a person concerning safer sex activities
8. What do you understand by post-exposure prophylaxis?
9. How is rape defined in the Sexual Offences Act 2003?
10. How should the nurse maintain sexual boundaries at work?

References

Adler, M. (2003) Report finds sexual health services to be a shambles. *British Medical Journal* 327: 62–63.

Anderson, P. and Kitchen, R. (2000) Disability, space and sexuality: access to family planning services. *Social Science and Medicine* 51: 1163–1174.

Anon, J. (1974) *The Behavioural Treatment of Sexual Problems*. Honolulu: Enabling Systems.

Bauer, M., McAuliffe, L. and Nay, R. (2007) Sexuality, health care and the older person: an overview of the literature. *International Journal of Older People Nursing* 2: 63–68.

Blackless, M., Charuvastra, A., Derryck, A., Fausto-Sterling, A., Lauzanne, K. and Lee, E. (2000) How sexually dimorphic are we? Review and synthesis. *American Journal of Human Biology* 12: 151–160.

Carpenito-Moyet, L.J. (2006) *Nursing Diagnosis: Application to Clinical Practice*, 11th ed. Philadelphia: Lippincott.

Cherry, A. (2008) Young people and sexual health: assessing risk. *British Journal of School Nursing* 3(1): 6–10.

Crawford, M. (1995) *Talking Difference: On Gender and Language*. Thousand Oaks: Sage Publications.

Department of Health (2001a) *National Strategy for Sexual Health*. London: DH.

Department of Health (2001b) *The National Service Framework for Older People*. London: DH.

Department of Health (2003) *A Toolkit for Primary Care Trust and Others Working in the Field of Promoting Good Sexual Health and HIV Prevention*. London: DH.

Department of Health (2004) *Choosing Health: Making Healthy Choices Easier*. London: DH.

Earle, S. (2001) Disability, facilitated sex and the role of the nurse. *Journal of Advanced Nursing* 36(3): 433–440.

Gott, M. and Hinchliffe, S. (2003) How important is sex in later life? The views of older people. *Social Science and Medicine* 56: 1617–1628.

Grandjean, C. and Moran, B. (2007) The impact of diabetes mellitus on female sexual well-being. *Nursing Clinics of North America* 42: 581–592.

Gray, R.E., Fitch, M.I., Philips, C., Labrecque, M. and Fergus, K.D. (2000) Managing the impact of illness: the experiences of men with prostate cancer and their spouses. *Journal of Health Psychology* 5: 531–548.

Hajjar, R. and Kamel, H. (2003) Sexuality in the nursing home part 1: attitudes and barriers to sexual expression. *Journal of the American Medical Directors Association* 4: 152–156.

Health Protection Agency (2004) *Annual Report, HIV and other Sexually Transmitted Infections in the United Kingdom*. London: HPA.

Health Protection Agency (2008) *Sexually Transmitted Infections and Young People in the United Kingdom: 2008 Report*. London: HPA.

Health Services Commission (2007) *Performing Better? A Focus on Sexual Health in England*. London: HSC.

Hyde, J., DeLamater, J. and Byers, E. (2001) *Understanding Human Sexuality*. Toronto, Ontario, Canada: McGraw Hill.

Independent Advisory Group on Sexual Health and HIV (2008) *Progress and Priorities – Working Together for High Quality Sexual Health*. London: Independent Advisory Group on Sexual Health and HIV.

Katz, A. (2005) The sounds of silence: sexuality information for cancer patients. *Journal of Clinical Oncology* 23(1): 238–241.

Katz, A. (2007) *Breaking the Silence on Cancer and Sexuality: A Handbook for Healthcare Provider*. Pittsburgh: Oncology Nursing Society Publishing.

Laws, T. (2006) *A Handbook of Men's Health*. Edinburgh: Elsevier.

McCann, E. (2000) The expression of sexuality in people with psychosis: breaking the taboos. *Journal of Advanced Nursing* 32(1): 132–138.

McKinley, J.B. (2000) The worldwide prevalence and epidemiology of erectile dysfunction. *International Journal of Impotence Research* 12: S6–S11.

Medical Foundation for AIDS and Sexual Health (2005) *Recommended Standards for Sexual Health Services*. London: MEDFASH.

Mick, J., Hughes, M. and Cohen, M. (2003) Sexuality and cancer: how oncology nurses can address it BETTER [Abstract]. *Oncology Nursing Forum* 30(supp 2): 152–153.

National Institute of Health and Clinical Excellence (2007) *One to One Interventions to Reduce the Transmission of Sexually Transmitted Infections (STIs) Including HIV, and to Reduce the Rate of Under 18 Conceptions, Especially Among Vulnerable and at Risk Groups*. London: NICE.

National Institutes of Health Consensus Development Conference (1992).

Nay, R. (2004) Sexuality and older people. In: Nay, R. and Garratt, S. (eds). *Nursing Older People: Issues and Innovations*, 2nd ed. Sydney: Churchill Livingstone, pp. 276–288.

Nursing and Midwifery Council (2007) Record Keeping. Available at http://www.nmc-uk.org/aFrameDisplay.aspx?DocumentID=4008. Accessed 19 October 2007.

Nursing and Midwifery Council (2008) *The Code of Conduct*. London: NMC.

Rathaus, L. (2008) *Human Sexuality in a World of Diversity*, 7th ed. Ontario: Pearson.

Rathaus, S., Nevid, J. and Ficher-Rathaus, L. (2000) *Human Sexuality in a World of Diversity*, 4th ed. Toronto, Ontario, Canada: Allyn and Bacon.

Reed, J. (2007) Sexuality. *International Journal of Older People Nursing* 2(1): 62.

Royal College of Nursing (2000) *Sexuality and Sexual Health in Nursing Practice*. London: RCN.

Scottish Executive (2005) *Respect and Responsibility: Strategy and Action Plan for Improving Sexual Health*. Edinburgh: Scottish Executive.

Shell, J.A. (2007) Including sexuality in your nursing practice. *Nursing Clinics of North America* 42: 685–696.

Smith, E.E., Nolen-Hoeksema, S., Fredrickson, B. and Loftus, G.R. (2003) *Atkinson and Hilgard's Introduction to Psychology*, 14th ed. New York: Thompson.

Welsh Assembly (2000) *A Strategic Framework for Promoting Sexual Health in Wales*. Cardiff: Welsh Assembly.

Wilmoth, M.C. (2006) Life after cancer: what does sexuality have to do with it? *Oncology Nursing Forum* 33(5): 905–910.

WHO (2000) *Promotion of Sexual Health: Recommendations for Action*. Antigua, Guatemala: WHO.

WHO (2002) *International WHO Technical Consultation on Sexual Health*, 28–31 January 2002. Geneva: WHO.

Zanni, G.R., Wick, J.Y. and Walker, B.L. (2003) Sexual health and the elderly. *The Consultant Pharmacist* 18: 310–322.

Chapter 14
Sleep and Rest

Debbie Davies

Learning opportunities

This chapter will help you to:

1. Understand the complexities associated with sleep
2. Define a number of key terms associated with sleep
3. Begin to understand the factors that may adversely affect the sleep and rest a person gets
4. Discuss ways in which the nurse can help promote sleep and rest
5. Describe some of the key issues related to sleep assessment
6. Outline the way the nurse can help to enhance the environment in which a person sleeps and rests

Pre-chapter quiz

1. Why is sleep important?
2. What do you understand by the term 'rapid eye movement'?
3. What are circadian rhythms?
4. What are some of the possible causes of insomnia?
5. What is an electroencephalogram?
6. How does the nurse prepare the patient safely for an electroencephalogram?
7. What are the environmental factors that may have a positive effect on sleep?
8. What are the environmental factors that may have a negative effect on sleep?
9. How might you notice sleep depravation in a patient?
10. How might you carry out a sleep assessment?

Introduction

The capacity to rest and sleep is the right of every individual (Fox, 1999). Quality sleep means that it is continuous and uninterrupted. As we get older, sleep may be disrupted due to pain or discomfort, the need to go to the toilet, medical problems, medications, poorly organised work or social schedules and sleep disorders. Myths about sleep abound. Thus, to nurse effectively, an awareness of the nature of sleep, the factors that influence sleep and sleep problems are essential in order to promote optimal sleep for the individual in a variety of care settings.

What is sleep?

Sleep is a universal process common to all people. It is, according to Marieb (2009), a state of natural unconsciousness from which a person can be aroused. During this time, the processing of sensory input is minimal, coordinated behaviour is eradicated and cognitive activity such as thinking, planning and reflection is suspended; it is that part of the day when people are unconscious and unaware of their surroundings (Scanlan, 2008).

Sleep is a complicated physiological phenomenon that intrigues scientists. It takes up a significant component of the lifespan; about one third of an individual's existence is spent in sleep. No human or animal has ever been shown to be able to go without sleep, although the amount needed varies.

Up until the 1950s sleep was considered to be a passive, dormant part of life associated with the simple withdrawal of wakefulness (National Institute of Neurological Disorders and Strokes (NINDS), 2003). More recently great strides have been made to clarify some of the mysteries of normal and abnormal sleep (Spangler, 1997).

The use of the electroencephalogram (EEG) to measure brain activity revolutionised thinking about sleep, with the discovery of distinct sleep states where sleep is found to be a dynamic process during which the brain is very active (McPherson, 1994). Thus, there are recognised stages of sleep, each of which is characterised by a different type of brain activity.

As knowledge and information about physiological processes has developed, current views (Thompson et al., 2001) are that these distinct sleep states, actively generated by different brain regions, are now considered to exert significant and specific influence to affect most, if not all, fundamental homeostatic mechanisms.

Sleep, then, is not just a way of taking a respite from everyday busy routines; it is an essential component for good health, mental and emotional well-being and personal safety (Jenson and Herr, 1993). Indeed it has been clearly demonstrated that sleep loss or a sleep disorder can lead rapidly to impaired physiological function, deteriorating health and even death (Rechtschaffen et al., 1983). Those people with chronic sleep disorders are more likely than others to develop several types of psychiatric problems and are likely to have higher blood pressure and suffer from excessive daytime sleepiness. Sleep loss influences the ability to undertake tasks that involve memory, learning and logical reasoning, leading to lost productivity, accidents, unsafe actions, strained relationships and unfulfilled potential.

Physiology of sleep

Sleep is controlled and regulated by two brain processes that respond to both internal and external stimuli (McPherson, 1994). The first is the restorative process when sleep occurs naturally in response to how long an individual is awake; the longer awake, the stronger the desire to sleep. The second process controls the timing of sleep and wakefulness during the day-night cycle and is known as the circadian rhythm or circadian biological clock.

Circadian rhythm

Circadian rhythms are regular changes in mental and physical characteristics that occur in the course of a day. Most circadian rhythms are controlled by the body's biological 'clock', a special centre in the hypothalamus of the brain known as the suprachiasmatic nucleus (SCN).

Scientists have found that there is an association between staying awake during the day when it is light and sleeping at night when it is dark (Fox, 1999). Light that reaches photoreceptors in the retina of the eye creates signals that travel along the optic nerve to the SCN, which, by sending signals to several brain regions in particular the pineal gland, works like a clock that sets off a set of activities affecting the whole body.

When exposed to the first light of day, the SCN initiates signals to these other parts of the brain associated with the sleep-wake cycle - hormone control, body temperature, urine production and blood pressure modification. Body temperature is raised, stimulating hormones such as cortisol. Blood levels of the hormone melatonin, which induces drowsiness and is associated with sleep onset, are much higher at night than in the day as production is suspended during daylight hours.

This 'clock' within the brain runs on a 24-hour cycle resulting in the feelings of sleepiness at its strongest around 0200-0400 h and in the afternoon between 1300 and 1500 hours, thus influencing the timing and duration of sleep.

Circadian regularity begins by the third week of life. From the early months of wakefulness during the early hours of the morning and late afternoon, by the time an infant is about 6 months old, it would have developed a circadian rhythm that corresponds with the adult cycle.

When travellers pass from one time zone to another, they experience a disruption in the biological circadian rhythm that is known as 'jet lag' whereby the sufferer 'loses' time even though he or she may have slept. People who work in shift patterns or nights will encounter similar symptoms.

The states and stages of sleep

Neurotransmitters and nerve-signalling chemicals control the sleep-wake cycle by acting on different groups of nerve cells, or neurons in the brain. These will keep some parts of the brain active when the individual is awake. Others begin signalling as sleep begins by 'switching off' those very signals.

As an individual sleeps, the sleep cycle passes through a range of differing, but predictable, states and stages throughout a typical 8-hour period. With continuous sleep, each of these states alternates every 90 minutes.

Orthodox and paradoxical sleep

Orthodox sleep is described as sleep with non-rapid eye movement (NREM), which can be identified through four distinct progressive stages (Patel et al., 2008).

Paradoxical sleep is depicted as sleep with rapid eye movement (REM) and constitutes the fifth stage of the sleep cycle. Although the time spent in these states and stages will

Table 14.1 Orthodox and paradoxical sleep.

NREM sleep	As sleep commences, the stages of NREM or orthodox sleep progress. NREM sleep is considered to be essential as restorative to the body.
Stage I	The eyes begin to close and the body relaxes. The eyes move very slowly and muscle activity is reduced. Sleep is light; drifting in and out, easily wakened. Mental activity is dreamlike and if wakened many individuals remember fragmented visual images. There may also be the experience of sudden muscle contractions known as hypnic myoclonia whereby there is often a sensation of falling before 'jumping' awake.
Stage II	Eye movements stop, with a slowing of brain activity. Breathing and heart rate become regular. Body temperature goes down. A person can still be easily roused.
Stage III	Delta sleep now occurs whereby very slow brain waves begin to appear, intermingled with bursts of rapid waves known as sleep spindles. It is more difficult to wake someone up in this stage.
Stage IV	The deepest and most restorative sleep. Blood pressure drops, breathing slows and there is no eye movement or muscle activity. Energy is regained and hormones for growth and development are released. It is difficult to wake someone during this stage of sleep. If they are awakened, the individual may spend some minutes feeling dazed and disorientated.
REM sleep	The first REM sleep period takes place approximately 90 minutes after sleep has been initiated as the sleep pattern ascends to a lower stage. During this time, vivid dreams occur, breathing and heart rate become more rapid and irregular and there is transient limb immobility. The eyes periodically move rapidly from side to side. Males may develop penile erections. This stage of sleep is considered to be essential for effective daytime performance and may be associated with memory consolidation. Excessive lack of REM sleep is known to lead to hallucinations, paranoia and short-term personality changes.

vary with age, it is generally agreed that 75% of the sleep cycle is NREM sleep and 25% REM sleep (see Table 14.1).

For a restful and restorative sleep, the balance and mix of both REM and NREM are essential components of the sleep cycle, which takes up to 90–110 minutes to complete and occurs four to five times a night. As the night progresses, REM sleep periods increase in length while deep sleep decreases (see Figure 14.1).

Theories of the need for sleep

The focus of the literature to date has acknowledged that the functions of sleep have yet to be proven (Redeker, 2002) but generally concurs the promotion of sleep as vital to the psychological and physiological restoration and repair of the body (Njawe, 2003). As more information and data is gathered by scientists in their quest to understand sleep, a number of theories are emerging to explain the function of sleep.

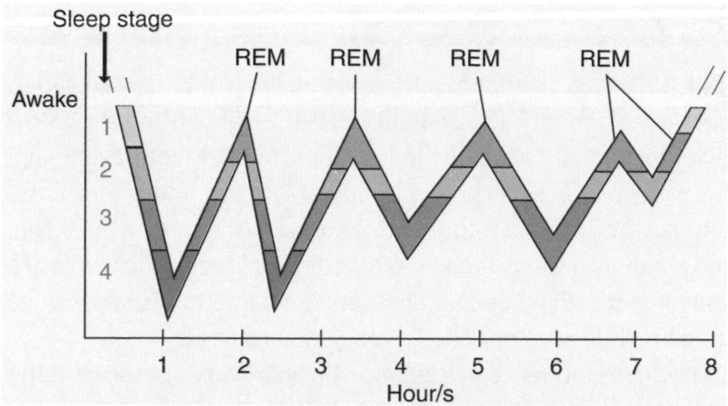

Figure 14.1 Periods of rapid eye movement (REM).

- *Developmental theory*: Sleep plays a role in the development of the brain. REM sleep is a major component of sleep for babies in utero and infants. It has been suggested that by activating visual, motor and sensory areas in the brain, sleep plays a role in preparing the individual for the outside world.
- *Conservation theory*: Sleep is physiologically vital to help the body recover from the work it does. By slowing down metabolism, sleep enables the body to conserve and restore energy and may have some association with effective immune system function. The physiological changes during NREM sleep include:
  - Arterial blood pressure falls
  - Pulse rate decreases
  - Peripheral blood vessels dilate
  - Skeletal muscle relaxes
  - Basal metabolic rate reduces
- *Restorative theory*: Sleep to enable physiological and biochemical repairs to take place. According to this theory, sleep is necessary for protein synthesis essential for cell growth and repair. This enables the central nervous system, more specifically neurons, to shut down and repair themselves. The secretion of growth hormone in children and young adults also occurs. Activity in parts of the brain associated with the control of emotions, decision-making processes and social interactions are also greatly reduced during deep sleep that corresponds to optimal emotional and social functioning during waking hours.
- *Adaptive theory*: Sleeping at night when vision is poor as a useful adaptive behaviour to protect individuals against predators.
- *Learning theories*: During sleep, it is suggested that REM sleep plays a role in memory retention and consolidation. It also enables the brain to reorganise and store information. The evidence suggests that when deprived of REM sleep during a single night, retention of complex materials such as stories is greatly reduced. There are a number of proposed theories associated with the purpose of dreams and dreaming (Hobson, 1998). These include resolving emotional preoccupations, altering mood, in adaptation, in creativity and for amusement. One of the most long-standing notions, however, has been the link between dreaming and learning.

Dreaming and sleep

Scientific studies of the brain have led to a range of theories of sleep and its association with dreaming coming under discussion (Crick and Mitchison, 1983; Hobson and McCarley, 1977). It is estimated that an individual spends at least 2 hours each night dreaming. Dreaming takes place in a variety of ways, occurring at any stage during the four basic elements of the sleep cycle but occurs most commonly during periods of REM sleep, usually starting an hour and a half into sleep. It has been demonstrated that dreams are not always composed of only images. Blind people and people unable to visualise while awake also dream, made up of mostly auditory and sensory experiences.

Originally, Sigmund Freud with his influence in the field of psychology put forward the notion of dreaming as a 'safety valve' for unconscious worries and desires.

Some scientists consider dreams to be attempts by the cortex of the brain to find meaning in the random signals that it receives during REM sleep. By trying to interpret these signals, a 'story' is created out of the fragmented brain activity (NINDS, 2003). Indeed, Crick and Mitchison (1983) propose dreams to be the process of discarding unwanted memories whereby information that is not required is wiped out by signals sent to the cortex. Dreaming enables the brain to process daily experiences and process them through dreams into an ongoing strategy for behaviour, whilst others argue that dreaming gives the brain the opportunity to scan the environment in case of danger, incorporating the external stimuli into the dream.

There is general agreement, however, that for the most part dreaming is caused by internal biological processes. Which processes are responsible, however, is open to debate. Of people who are wakened during REM sleep, as many as 70–95% report dreams, in contrast to 5–10% of awakenings during NREM sleep. REM sleep is produced by the excretion of the chemical acetylcholine in the part of the brainstem known as the pons. Other neurotransmitters produced by the pons are able to switch off REM sleep. Conversely, there is evidence in some neurological literature that in cases where there is loss of REM sleep, dreaming is still reported to occur, whereas if there is damage to the frontal lobe of the brain, the REM cycle may be unaffected but dreaming is impossible (Apsa, 1999). REM sleep is considered by some scientists as only one of a number of dream triggers.

The study of lucid dreaming, the ability of the dreaming individual to become aware of the dream and be able to control it, is in its infancy and is one of the many challenges scientists face when exploring the mysteries of sleep and dreaming.

Sleep needs over the life cycle

Sleep needs vary. Sleep patterns are individual and may change but the need for sleep remains the same, a drive that must be met. Getting enough continuous uninterrupted quality sleep will contribute to short-term performance and feelings; it also impacts on the overall quality of our lives (see Table 14.2).

Although an average of 7–9 hours sleep per night is generally recommended, the optimal amount will vary for each individual and over the life cycle. As can be seen in Table 14.2, newborns and infants require a lot of sleep and have several periods throughout a

Table 14.2 Sleep requirements and age.

Sleep requirements over the life cycle	
Infants/babies (includes naps)	0-2 months: 10.5-18.5 hours 2-12 months: 14-15 hours
Toddlers/children (includes naps)	12-18 months: 13-15 hours 18 months to 3 years: 12-14 hours 3-5 years: 11-13 hours 5-12 years: 9-11 hours
Adolescents	8.5-9.5 hours
Adults/older persons	On average: 7-9 hours

24-hour time cycle; this will include naps, which are important to children up to the age of 5 years. As adolescence is reached, the sleep pattern shifts to a later sleep-wake cycle, with around 9 hours' sleep considered the optimum. Throughout adulthood and old age, patterns of sleep may change but 7-9 hours a night will ensure effective functioning.

Factors influencing sleep

According to Sorenson (1996), sleep disorders are common, serious, treatable and generally under-diagnosed. They cost the nation financially, have health and safety consequences and cause decreased quality of life for many people. Sleep disorders can be categorised into primary sleep disorders whereon the individual's sleep problem is the main disorder and secondary sleep disorders. In the latter situation, the sleep problem is the result of a distinct clinical disorder. All sleep and arousal disorders can be grouped into one of the following categories:

- Disorders of initiating and maintaining sleep
- Disorders of excessive somnolence
- Disorders of the sleep-wake schedule
- Dysfunctions associated with sleep, sleep stages or partial arousals

An individual's ability to acquire appropriate quality and quantity of sleep and to wake effectively is thus affected by a number of factors (see Figure 14.2).

Psychological factors

Problems associated with sleep are considered to be closely related with mental health issues such as depression and schizophrenia. Anxiety and depression are often synonymous with sleep disturbance of which early morning wakening is a significant feature (Scanlan, 2008). An individual with personal problems may be unable to relax sufficiently to get to sleep. Anxiety and excitement increase the production of norepinephrine blood levels, a chemical change that results in less Stage IV NREM sleep, and in REM sleep there are more stage modifications and awakenings. In depressive conditions such as

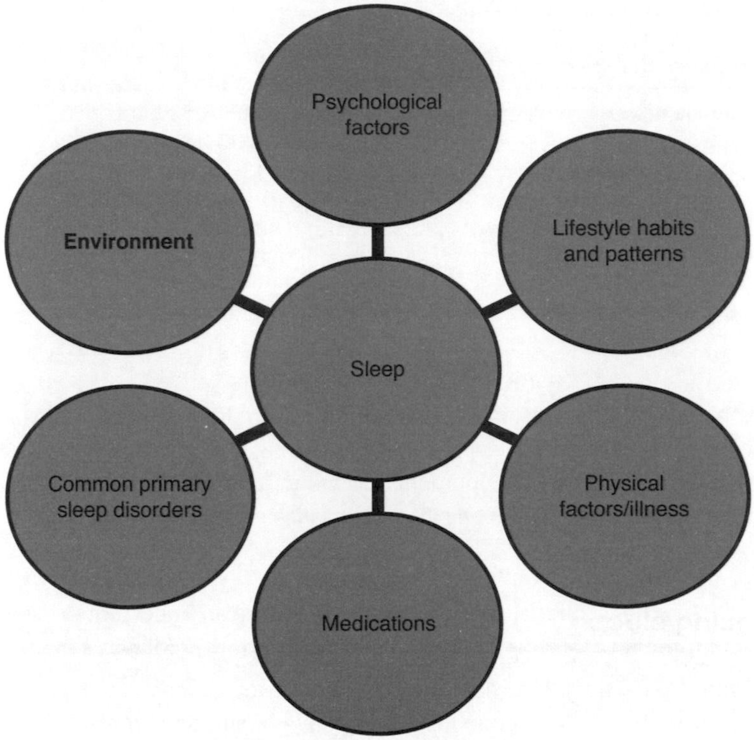

Figure 14.2 Some factors affecting sleep.

seasonal affective disorder (SAD), there may even be an increased quantity of sleep but of poor quality, which in turn increases fatigue. Post-traumatic stress disorder may lead to wakening by nightmares and an inability to return to sleep.

Sleep deprivation in itself can cause depression, even states of paranoia and hallucinations. It may also influence the symptoms of mental disorder, for example episodes of agitation in people with manic depression.

Motivation, the desire to stay awake, may often overcome a person's fatigue and even if tired the individual will stay awake if something interesting is going on. By contrast, without the motivation to stay awake, a person who is bored is more likely to fall asleep.

Lifestyle habits and patterns

Situations that disrupt circadian rhythms will influence the quality and quantity of sleep an individual achieves. A person who does shift work and changes shifts frequently may experience sleep disturbances (Samaha et al., 2007; Winwood, 2006).

Many blind people have sleep disorders because they cannot detect light and so their biological clock does not follow the usual 24-hour light-induced clock; jet lag is also a common cause of sleep disruption. Moderate exercise is considered to be conducive to sleep but excessive exercise may stimulate the sympathetic nervous system resulting in difficulty getting to sleep.

The use of chemicals/substances will influence sleep and the sleep cycle. Beverages that contain caffeine, such as coffee, tea and fizzy drinks, act as stimulants of the nervous system and thus disrupt sleep. Although initially hastening the onset of sleep, excessive alcohol intake actually disrupts REM sleep creating a rebound effect when the individual either wakes when the effects of alcohol wear off or has vivid dreams or nightmares.

Nicotine also has a stimulant effect on the nervous system. Many smokers describe themselves as light sleepers.

Bedtime rituals and routines influence an individual's ability to sleep effectively - good sleep hygiene routines assist the individual to have a good night's sleep - by creating a period of calmness and relaxation this may include the time of going to bed, a warm bath before bedtime, reducing stimulating situations will also encourage a good sleep routine.Going to bed when moderately tired is likely to lead to a restful sleep rather than being overtired.

A warm milky drink, which contains dietary L-tryptophan, an amino acid thought to induce sleep, is often used to promote sleepiness, as do peanut butter, cheese or nuts.

Environmental factors

The environment in which the individual seeks to sleep and rest is an important consideration. A familiar bedroom, beds, pillows, type of bedclothes, degree of light/dark, for example, will influence how well an individual sleeps.

Changes to the environment such as excessive, sharp or intermittent strange sounds and noise, extremes of heat and cold, a poorly ventilated room, unfamiliar surroundings and the issues associated with hospitalisation are examples of factors that may disrupt sleep (Dogan et al., 2005; Patel et al., 2008). Continuous care, treatment schedules and hospital routines lend credence to the old adage about patients being roused from sleep by the nurse in order to take a sleeping tablet. Sleeping with or without someone may influence sleep patterns - many people who have slept together in the same bed for a number of years with others may find a clinical environment where there may be a group of strangers to be stressful.Indeed, the relevance of the environment to sleep within the clinical context was explored in depth by Florence Nightingale in the 1860s.

Physical factors and the lifespan

As has been demonstrated, there are developmental sleep requirements associated with age. Although the amount of sleep required will vary between individuals, there are some general considerations that can be applied; life cycle changes are likely to influence sleep. Pregnant women are likely to need more sleep, particularly during the first 3 months of pregnancy. Having a new baby or small children will affect the ability to attain an undisturbed night's rest.

Getting too little sleep over a period of time creates a 'sleep debt' - even if an individual gets used to a sleep depriving way of life, judgement and reaction time continue to be disrupted.

Changes in the life cycle such as menopause exhibit symptoms such as insomnia. There is a tendency for people who are older to sleep more lightly and for a shorter time span, although it is generally agreed that they need the same amount of sleep as when they were in early adulthood. There is evidence that about half of all people over the age of 65 have sleeping problems such as insomnia, and the deep sleep stages essential to sleep often become reduced or stop completely (Mauk, 2008). This change may be considered to be a normal part of ageing or a result from medical problems associated with age, bladder problems and lack of mobility or environmental changes such as hospitalisation (Cole and Richards, 2007; Lee et al., 2007).

Illness and disease

Illness and disease can have an effect on sleep and sleep-related disorders. The converse also occurs when the process of sleep may itself influence the disease/illness process. In these situations, sleep onset may be prevented and wakefulness may occur; there may be difficulties with positioning or the need to eliminate.

During illness the individual often requires more sleep. Neurons that control sleep interact with the immune system. Potent sleep-inducing chemicals known as cytokines are produced by the immune system at the onset of infections such as influenza. These may enable the body to conserve energy and utilise its resources to fight the illness.

The pain, discomfort and fatigue caused by illness or medical intervention such as surgery may adversely affect sleep either by preventing sleep or by wakening the sleeper. The impact of illness on an individual can create fear and anxiety, disrupt day/night routines and in its wider context impact adversely on caregivers too.

The scope of medical problems that influence sleep and sleep patterns is wide ranging (Dirksen and Epstein, 2008; Kozachik and Bandeen-Roche, 2008). The exacerbation of asthma, for example, or the onset of an acute cerebrovascular accident has a propensity to occur more frequently at night, possibly due to the physiological changes associated with sleep that have previously been identified.

Some types of epilepsy are also affected by sleep. Sleep deprivation may trigger a seizure on the one hand, but another form of epileptic seizure may be exacerbated by deep sleep. REM sleep appears to help contain the spread of a seizure that originates in a confined region of the brain. Patients with neurological conditions such as Alzheimer's disease and head injury, for example, are also likely to experience problems with sleeping. This may be due to changes in regions of the brain and neurotransmitters that control sleep or from drugs used to control symptoms of the disorder.

Breathing difficulties such as shortness of breath, nasal congestion, cough associated with acute and/or chronic respiratory conditions, and cardiac disorders such as congestive cardiac failure are likely to lead to sleep disturbance (Closs, 1989). This in turn leads to an increase in fatigue that perpetuates the cycle of distress. Up to 45% of cancer patients have serious sleep disturbances (Katz and McHarney, 1998). Gastrointestinal problems such as reflux or peptic ulcers cause pain and discomfort often as the result of an increase in gastric secretions associated with REM sleep.

Medications

There are a number of groups of medications that influence the sleep-wake cycle. Examples of these include hypnotics that can interfere with the latter stages of sleep and REM sleep affect the quality of sleep. Some drugs used in cardiology, for example beta-blockers, are known to cause vivid dreams, nightmares and insomnia. Many drugs interfere with or suppress REM sleep. Morphine, a narcotic, is one of these drugs causing frequent wakenings and drowsiness. Tranquillisers, amphetamines and antidepressant drugs may also exhibit these properties.

Medications given to help patients sleep, act either by inducing sleep or by reducing anxiety. One of the side effects of these drugs is an increased tolerance and over-reliance. This may lead people to increase the drug dose or supplement them with alcohol. Other side effects are often exacerbated in elderly clients due to their altered rates of metabolism, absorption and body fat (Kozier et al., 2008). As a result, there has been a shift towards alternative ways of promoting sleep without the use, or only limited use of medication.

Common primary sleep disorders

Among the more common sleep disorders are insomnia, sleep apnoea, narcolepsy, restless leg syndrome and the parasomnias.

Insomnia

The most common sleep disorder is insomnia whereby people complain of inadequate or poor-quality sleep because of one or more of the following (Doghrami, 1999):

- Falling asleep with difficulty
- Waking frequently during the night with difficulty returning to sleep
- Premature waking
- Not feeling refreshed on waking

Insomnia can be classified as transient if it only lasts for up to a couple of weeks, and intermittent if transient insomnia occurs from time to time (Holcomb, 2007; Katz and McHarney, 1998). In these situations the sleep disorder is often associated with the influencing factors outlined previously. Insomnia is chronic if it occurs on most nights and lasts a month or more when the actual cause of the sleep changes may have been resolved long ago.

The condition affects both men and women but is the most common sleep-related complaint for women and often disrupts the individual's daily life (Doghrami, 1999; Holcomb, 2007). When it occurs, tiredness is a key issue and there is a tendency to worry about not getting enough sleep.

The use of sleep medication is deemed questionable when seeking to resolve insomnia, particularly in the long term when it is argued the situation can be made worse (Long et al., 1993).

Treatment for insomnia therefore has its focus on the development of new behavioural patterns to reduce sleep disturbance. It may take several months to reset the sleep-wake cycle using a plan that may have a range of interchangeable elements related to daytime activities, preparation for sleep and interpretation of the sleep experience. However, as Holcomb (2007) points out, if lifestyle and behaviour modification strategies are not completely effective, medications may be necessary, preferably for only short-term use.

The range of pharmacologic treatment is extensive but should always be approached with caution.

Sleep apnoea

Sleep apnoea, from the Greek word 4 'want of breath', is a disorder of interrupted breathing during sleep where airflow at the nose and mouth is absent for 10 seconds to a minute whilst the sleeping individual struggles to breathe.

The condition can be classified as obstructive, central or mixed depending on the presence or absence of respiratory muscle effort. People with apnoea are deprived of oxygen during sleep, although the severity of decrease in oxygen saturation will vary (Khawaja and Phillips, 1998).

In obstructive apnoea, airflow is physically blocked but abdominal and ribcage effort continues. It usually occurs in conjunction with fat build-up or loss of muscle tone associated with ageing and is common in men. There may also be airway problems such as enlarged tonsils or jaw abnormalities. In central apnoea, thought to be neurological rather than physical in origin, both types of movement are absent and are more common in women.

During an episode of obstructive apnoea, efforts to inhale air create a suction that creates a collapse of the windpipe. These involuntary cycles may be as high as 20–30 per hour throughout the night and are usually associated with loud snoring in between apnoeic episodes as the blood oxygen levels fall and the brain responds by waking the individual up enough to respond by tightening the upper airway muscles and opening the trachea. The person may snort or gasp and then continue to snore, although not everyone who snores has sleep apnoea.

As a consequence, many people with sleep apnoea describe it as a choking sensation that with the frequent wakenings leads to complaints of morning headaches, daytime sleepiness, irritability or depression and loss of libido (Brostrom et al., 2007; Khawaja and Phillips, 1998; Ye et al., 2008). At its most serious, sleep apnoea is linked to high blood pressure, irregular heartbeats, increased risk of cardiovascular catastrophe and even respiratory arrest.

Self-care treatments vary following diagnosis and range from weight loss, encouraging the individual to sleep on their side, and advice not to use alcohol, tobacco or sleep medication (Brostrom et al., 2007). More complex treatments may involve the use of devices such as nasal continuous positive airway pressure (CPAP), dental appliance or surgery to correct the obstruction.

Narcolepsy

Narcolepsy is a chronic sleep disorder that may be genetic in origin, the main characteristic of which is excessive and overwhelming irresistible daytime sleepiness; even with a normal amount of night-time sleep. Symptoms usually appear during adolescence (www.ninds.nih.gov).

A less common symptom of narcolepsy is cataplexy, an abrupt reversible loss of muscle function brought on by strong emotions such as fright, laughter or anger. The individual remains conscious throughout.

Sleep paralysis, also associated with narcolepsy, is a terrifying experience that occurs just before waking up or falling asleep, where there is a temporary inability to talk or move. Often accompanied by vivid frightening hypnagogic hallucinations, sleep paralysis terminates spontaneously after a few minutes.

The most effective treatment is with drug therapy such as central nervous system stimulants or tricyclic antidepressants. Daytime naps may help with daytime alertness.

Restless legs syndrome

A common, familial disorder found particularly amongst the elderly, pregnant and premenopausal women, that involves unpleasant sensations in the legs and feet, variously described by sufferers as creeping, crawling, tingling or pulling. Although not described as painful, the urge to move the limb is overwhelming. Restless legs syndrome can be experienced when awake or asleep and not necessarily in bed, but is associated with insomnia. Many of those with this disorder also experience a related sleep disorder called periodic limb movements in sleep in which involuntary jerking of the limbs at frequent intervals leads to difficulties with falling asleep and with maintaining sleep leading to daytime sleepiness.

Parasomnias

Parasomnias refer to the group of arousal behaviours that may interfere with sleep. Examples of a range of these dysfunctions are illustrated in Box 14.1.

Box 14.1 Some of the parasomnias.

- Nocturnal enuresis (bedwetting during sleep) is often associated with children over 3 years old, occurring 1–2 hours after falling asleep when moving from Stage III to IV NREM. More common in males.
- Somnambulism (sleepwalking) occurs during Stages III and IV of NREM sleep 1–2 hours after falling asleep. Episodic sleepwalkers require protection from danger.
- Sleep talking occurs during NREM sleep just prior to REM sleep.
- Nocturnal erections and emissions occur during REM sleep, starting in adolescence.
- Bruxism – clenching and grinding of teeth usually occurs during Stage II NREM sleep.

Promoting sleep

With the concept of individualised patient care as the cornerstone of modern professional nursing in society, the relationship between sleep, health and the patient experience should be of great relevance when undertaking holistic care. As Jenson and Herr (1993) point out, the role of the nurse is essential in the thorough assessment of sleep patterns, the identification of requirements and implementation of effective activities to enhance healthy sleep.

There is a plethora of research outlining specific and effective strategies to promote sleep for individuals with a variety of conditions and in a range of settings (Holcomb, 2007; Mauk, 2005; Njawe, 2003; Patel et al., 2008; Smyth, 2008).

Common themes amongst these strategies include good communication skills, the use of formal assessment tools to identify needs and problems and an individualised care programme that, when implemented and evaluated, ensures optimal sleep as an essential component of health and well-being.

Nursing assessment

The initial nursing assessment may take the form of obtaining a complete sleep history from the client. Initially, the history may be part of the general information gathered in order to plan care to specific needs and preferences. A more detailed history would be required if there is an indication that there is a sleep problem. This would establish the exact nature of the problem, its effect on the client and the success or otherwise of strategies in use to overcome it.

General information elicited will include the following:

- Usual sleeping pattern
- Bedtime rituals
- Use of sleep medication
- Effective sleep environment
- Recent changes in sleep pattern

If there has been a change in pattern or difficulty with sleeping, a more detailed history that explores the nature of the problem should be ascertained. This may include questions that:

- Clarify what happens at sleep onset
- Determine the extent of excessive daytime sleepiness
- Characterise the extent and content of awakenings
- Delineate sleep habits
- Review intake of chemical substances such as alcohol
- Establish the possibility of obstructive sleep apnoea

Other nursing assessment tools may be brought into play, for example the keeping of a sleep diary to obtain more detailed and precise information about a particular problem.

There are a range of scales that can be used to gain objective data for assessment, for example Epworth Sleepiness Scale (1991) and Stansford Sleepiness Scale (cited in Hoddes et al., 1973). More recent tools include the Pittsburgh Sleep Quality Index, a self-administered questionnaire which provides a subjective measure of sleep quality and patterns (Smyth, 2008). For children the Tayside sleep questionnaire has proved to be a reliable and effective assessment tool (McGreavey et al., 2005).

A physical examination by the nurse will elicit information to determine the extent of the problem. Whether the client looks fatigued, lacks energy, has darkened rings or puffiness around the eyes, is exhibiting irritable behaviours or confusion, or has a deviated nasal septum are all examples.

Planning care

The major outcome for the client will be the maintenance or re-establishment of a sleep pattern that enables the client to wake refreshed and able to have enough energy to complete day-to-day activities. The range of nursing strategies and interventions identified will reflect an understanding of the client's individual situation or problem.

Implementing care

Assisting the client to sleep, particularly in the formal hospital setting, requires the nurse to be creative with their knowledge and understanding about the nature of sleep and its relevance to the individual (Dines-Kalinowski, 2002). Key interventions to explore are:

- The creation of a restful environment by reducing environmental distractions
- Ensuring that the client feels physically and psychologically safe within the environment
- Supporting accustomed bedtime rituals
- Promoting comfort and relaxation
- Administering appropriate sleep medication
- Client teaching - new strategies to aid sleep, for example relaxation techniques

Evaluation

Success of client outcomes should be established through observation, monitoring and questioning. Observing the duration of sleep, signs of NREM and REM sleep and eliciting client's feelings about how they feel and the success or failure of specific strategies are key to evaluation.

Conclusions

Although the notion of sleep and rest is often one of the last activities of living to be considered, it is certainly not inconsequential. It has clearly been established that sleep is a complex phenomenon, the functions of which are essential to health, well-being and even to survival. A knowledge and understanding about the nature of sleep and the factors associated with sleep and sleep problems should be part of every nurse's repertoire. This will enable the nurse to consider objectively and creatively successful strategies to promote optimal sleep for each individual.

Glossary

Acetylcholine	A neurotransmitter found in the nervous system
Apnoea	The cessation of airflow, sleep apnoea refers to the cessation of airflow during sleep
Cortisol	A steroid
Cytokines	A type of hormone, a protein
Dilate	To widen
Electroencephalogram	A graphical record of the electrical activity of the brain
Hypnagogic	Sleep inducing
Hypothalamus	Situated in the centre of the base of the brain and regulates a number of key body functions
Insomnia	Difficulty in getting to sleep or staying asleep
Metabolism	The set of chemical reactions that occur in living organisms in order to maintain life
Narcolepsy	Sleep disorder characterized by sudden and uncontrollable episodes of deep sleep
Pineal gland	Very small gland located in the brain that secretes melatonin
Photoreceptors	Specialised types of cells that are photosensitive, that is sensitive to light
Somnolence	A near state of sleep
Suprachiasmatic nucleus	A tiny region on the brain that controls circadian rhythms
Transient	Short-lived

Post-chapter quiz

1. Describe the differences between orthodox and paradoxical sleep
2. Why might changes in the life cycle impact on sleep?
3. What do you understand by 'sleep debt'?
4. Why might an individual require more sleep when they are ill?
5. List some of the groups of medications that might influence the sleep-wake cycle
6. What is sleep apnoea?
7. List four parasomnias
8. What general information should be elicited when assessing a person's experiences of sleep?
9. Consider the different sleep and rest needs across the lifespan
10. What is the biological clock?

References

Brostrom, A., Johansson, P., Stromberg, A., Albers, J., Martensson, J. and Svanborg, E. (2007) Obstructive sleep apnoea syndrome - patients perceptions of their sleep and its effects on their life situation. *Journal of Advanced Nursing* 57(3): 318-327.

Closs, J. (1989) Patients sleep-wake rhythms in hospital parts 1 and 2. *Nursing Times* 84(2) 48–50 and 54–55.
Cole, C. and Richards, K. (2007) Sleep disruption in older adults. *American Journal of Nursing* 107(5): 40–49 May 2007.
Crick, F. and Mitchison, G. (1983) The function of dream sleep. *Nature* 304: 111–114.
Dines-Kalinowski, C. (2002) Nature's nurse: promoting sleep in the ICU. *Dimensions of Critical Care Nursing* 21(1): 32–34.
Dirksen, S. and Epstein, D. (2008) Efficacy of an insomnia intervention on fatigue, mood and quality of life in breast cancer survivors. *Journal of Advanced Nursing* 61(6): 664–675.
Dogan, O., Ertekin, S. and Dogan, S. (2005) Sleep quality in hospitalised patients. *Journal of Clinical Nursing* 14(1): 107–113.
Doghrami, K. (1999) Clinical frontiers in the sleep/psychiatry interface. Psychiatry treatment updates, *Medscape Inc. Satellite Symposium in American Psychiatric Association Meeting*, 22 June, 1–13.
Epworth Sleepiness Scale (1991) Measurement of sleep deprivation. *Sleep* 0161–8105 14(6): 540–545.
Fox, M. (1999) The importance of sleep. *Nursing Standard* 13(24): 44–47.
Hobson, J. (1998) *The Dreaming Brain*. New York: Basic Books.
Hobson, J. and McCarley, R.W. (1977) The brain as a dream state generator. *American Journal of Psychiatry* 134: 1335–1368.
Hoddes, E., Zarcone, V., Smith, H., Phillips, R. and Dement, W.C. (1973) Quantification of sleepiness: a new approach. *Psychophysiology* 10: 431–436.
Holcomb, S. (2007) Putting insomnia to rest. *The Nurse Practitioner: The American Journal of Primary Health Care* 32(4): 28–34.
Jenson, D.P. and Herr, K.A. (1993) Sleeplessness: advances in clinical nursing research. *Nursing Clinics of North America* 26(2): 385–405.
Katz, D. and McHarney, C. (1998) Clinical correlates of insomnia in patients with chronic illness. *Archives of Internal Medicine* 158(10): 1099–1107.
Khawaja, I. and Phillips, B. (1998) Obstructive sleep apnoea: diagnosis and treatment. *Hospital Medicine* 34(3): 33–36 and 39–41.
Kozachik, S. and Bandeen-Roche, K. (2008) Predictors of patterns of pain, fatigue and insomnia during the first year after cancer diagnosis in the elderly. *Cancer Nursing* 31(5): 334-344.
Kozier, B., Erb, G. and Berman, A. (2008) *Fundamentals of Nursing – Concepts Process and Practice*, 8th ed. New Jersey: Pearson.
Lee, C., Low, L. and Twinn, S. (2007) Older men's experiences of sleep in the hospital. *Journal of Clinical Nursing* 16(2): 336–343.
Long, B., Phipps, W. and Cassmeyer, V. (1993) *Medical Surgical Nursing: A Nursing Process Approach*. London: Mosby.
Marieb, E. (2009) *Essentials of Human Anatomy and Physiology*, 9th ed. New Jersey: Pearson.
Mauk, K. (2008) Promoting sound sleep habits in older adults. *Nursing 2007* 35(2): 22–25.
McGreavey, J., Donnan, P., Pagliari, H. and Sullivan, F. (2005) The Tayside children's sleep questionnaire: a tool to evaluate sleep problems in young children. *Child: Care, Health and Development* 31(5): 539–544.
McPherson, G. (ed.) (1994) *Blacks Medical Dictionary*, 37th ed. London: AC Blacks.
Njawe, P. (2003) Sleep and rest in patients undergoing cardiac surgery. *Nursing Standard* 18(12): 33–37.
Patel, M., Chipman, J., Carlin, B. and Shade, D. (2008) Sleep in the intensive care unit setting. *Critical Care Nursing Quarterly* 31(4): 309–318.
Rechtschaffen, A., Gilliland, M., Bergmann, B. and Winter, J. (1983) Physiological correlates of prolonged sleep deprivation in rats. *Science* 221: 182–184.

Redeker, N.S. (2008) Sleep disturbances in people with heart failure: implications for self care. *Journal of Cardiovascular Nursing* 23(3): 231–238.

Samaha, E., Lal, S., Samaha, N. and Wyndham, J. (2007) Psychological, lifestyle and coping contributors to chronic fatigue in shift workers. *Journal of Advanced Nursing* 59(3): 221–232.

Scanlan, M. (2008) Sleep disturbance in the patient experiencing depression. *Primary Health Care* 18(5): 19–21.

Smyth, C. (2008) Catching those Zs in hospital. *American Journal of Nursing* 108(5). Available at http://www.nursingcenter.com/pdf.asp?AID=788879. Accessed 7 July 2009.

Sorenson, D.S. (1996) Sleep module. Available at http://learn.sdstate.edu/sorensond/nurs760 Fall02.

Thompson, S., Ackerman, U. and Horner, R. (2001) Sleep as a teaching tool for integrating respiratory physiology and motor control. *Advances in Physiology Education* 25: 29–44.

Winwood, P. (2006) Disentangling the effects of psychological and physical work demands on sleep recovery and maladaptive chronic stress outcomes within a large sample of Australian nurses. *Journal of Advanced Nursing* 56(6): 679–689.

Ye, L., Liang, Z. and Weaver, T. (2008) Predictors of health related quality of life in patients with obstructive sleep apnoea. *Journal of Advanced Nursing* 63(1): 54–63.

Chapter 15
Death and Dying

Mary Greeno

Learning opportunities

This chapter will help you to:

1. Identify the signs for when a person is dying
2. Care for the needs of the dying patient
3. Care for the patient's diverse religious needs
4. Facilitate the family/next of kin
5. Carry out the last offices
6. Identify when a post-mortem may be required

Pre-chapter quiz

1. What signs do you expect to see when a patient is dying?
2. What are the needs of the dying patient?
3. What are the needs of the family?
4. What do you understand by the term 'last offices'?
5. When was the Liverpool Care Pathway introduced?
6. What do you understand by the term 'patient dignity'?
7. List the reasons why a patient may be referred for post-mortem
8. Identify the specific needs of the dying patient within the six main religions
9. What is the role of the hospice?
10. How is the dead patient's property disposed of?

Introduction

This chapter considers the care of a person facing death and loss. The psychological, physical, spiritual and religious needs and social support that may be required are addressed. The cause of death differs; there are different types of death. There is the expected death that may be caused by a terminal illness or old age, or a sudden or unexpected death that may result from a car accident or a sudden acute illness, such as a heart attack or stroke.

Although we may become familiar with death and caring for the dying patient, the nurse must remember that for the patient and his or her family it is a singularly unique experience. This experience may be painful, unfamiliar and frightening. The nurse is ideally placed to offer help and support to those who may be affected by the complex issues associated with death and dying. It must also be acknowledged that the nurse may also need help and support when caring for those who are dying or have died.

Death and dignity

When a patient is dying it is important that their self-esteem be preserved and their personal dignity not violated. The person must feel in control of their own destiny. Some of the nursing care that is provided may undermine a person's modesty and personal privacy; however, this can be minimised by explaining the procedure to be undertaken, so that there is understanding and cooperation through obtaining informed consent. For example, if the patient needs an enema to relieve constipation, this procedure, similar to catheterisation, can be very embarrassing for the patient. To minimise embarrassment, the nurse should expose the minimum amount of the patient's body and make sure that the curtain or door is closed in order to ensure patient privacy.

The Royal College of Nursing's (RCN, 2008) campaign *Dignity at the Heart of Everything We Do* has three principal aims:

- To give nurses the skills and confidence to deliver the kind of dignified care they would like and the confidence to challenge where standards fall short of what patients deserve
- To work with the government and employers on a range of dignity issues including the removal of obstacles to dignified care and the abolition of mixed sex wards and facilities. The investment in specialist equipment and the provision of adequate staffing levels
- Demonstrate to the public that patient's dignity matters to nurses and to the RCN

Ensuring the environment is prepared in such a way as to promote dignity and ensuring the nurse acts in a humane and sensitive way will demonstrate care and concern. Dignity should always be an integral part of nursing care and has special relevance when caring for the dying patient.

Caring for a dying patient can take place at home, in a hospital or in a hospice. Wherever it occurs, there should be adequate support systems in place for patients, relatives and staff. Where possible, this can be achieved through a multidisciplinary approach. It must be remembered that the relationships staff form in order to care for patients will cause some form of sadness or grief for them when death finally occurs.

By using examples of how people avoid talking about death, Freud (1918) claimed that no person really believed in his or her own mortality, clarifying that 'the aim of all life is death'. Jung (1959) stressed the value of beliefs about death and their importance for daily life. He claimed that the first half of one's life is concerned with the preparation for the life ahead and the second half with the preparation for death. Nursing is at the forefront of matters concerned with dying and death, and nurses are expected to become competent when caring.

Palliative care

The World Health Organization (2007) defined palliative care as an approach that improves the quality of life of patients and their families approaching life-limiting illness. Care can be achieved through prevention of suffering through early assessment and treatment of pain and other symptoms, which includes a person's physical, psychological and spiritual care. The terminal care of a patient is part of the palliative care and is frequently referred to the management of patients during the phase when their health is rapidly deteriorating.

During the 1960s, there was a move to improve the quality of care for patients who were dying and this occurred with the founding of the first hospice. This movement has inspired others to ensure patient dignity throughout end-of-life care (Clark, 2002).

Ellershaw and Wilkinson (2003) identified that patients who are terminally ill have complex needs and those needs are met to a high standard when patients are cared for in a hospice. However, not all patients receive this excellent hospice care and it has been identified that only 15% of terminally ill patients die in a hospice with approximately 50% dying in hospital. Taylor (2004) claimed that palliative care delivered in an acute hospital did not meet the patient's needs and the families were dissatisfied as they felt helpless and isolated.

The National Health Service (NHS) Cancer Plan (DH, 2000) recognised that patients experienced poor nursing care, distressing symptoms, inadequate social, psychological and communication interaction during the final stage of illness. It advises that the care of all dying patients must improve to the level of the best, and that excellence in palliative care is poorly understood and practised outside the hospice.

The National Institute for Health and Clinical Excellence (NICE, 2004) issued guidance acknowledging that the care of the dying patient received in hospitals was inadequate. They recommend that the Liverpool Care Pathway (LCP) be used in all care environments to provide managed systems to make certain of best practice in caring for dying patients. The LCP, according to Ellershaw and Wilkinson (2003), was developed by the Royal Liverpool University Hospital Trust and the Marie Curie Centre. The LCP allows end-of-life care to be provided for patients using the hospice model of care.

The LCP provides an evidence-based framework for end-of-life care. It contains the following sections:

- Initial assessment and care
- Ongoing care
- Care after death

The LCP ensures that all health care professionals caring for the patient record their notes in the same document. All health care professionals have a responsibility to ensure their practice is based on up-to-date, sound clinical evidence and that research evidence is incorporated into clinical practice (Nursing and Midwifery Council, 2008).

Fowell et al. (2002) claimed that the length of time a patient could be on the LCP could range from less than 1 day to 23 days, but can be taken off if his or her condition improves; however, others suggest that the average length of time on the LPC is 2 days. Two of the following must apply before a patient is put on the LCP (Ellershaw and Wilkinson, 2003):

- The patient is bed bound
- Semi-comatose
- Only able to take sips of fluids
- No longer able to swallow tablets

The NHS Cancer Plan (DH, 2000) acknowledges that patients with cancer should be able to live and, when possible, die in the place they choose.

Caring for the patient who has died should incorporate the patient's and family's wishes, respecting their religious, cultural and social beliefs. It is a privilege to be involved in the final stage of the patient's journey. This final stage of care which is referred to as 'last offices' must be constantly updated to ensure best practice. Health and safety guidelines must be followed to ensure the safety of families, hospital staff, mortuary staff and undertakers (Health and Safety Executive, 2007). Respect for the patient should continue after death. Neuberger (2004) suggests that care practices should encompass not only the patient but the family also, and their wishes should be accommodated as far as possible.

The legal requirements relating to death must be adhered to, such as washing and grooming, removal of unnecessary equipment and following the prescribed procedure regarding the correct identification of the patient (Costello, 2004). However, if the patient's death is referred to the coroner, this occurs in cases where:

1. There is reasonable cause to suspect a person has died a violent or unnatural death
2. There is reasonable cause to suspect a person's sudden death of which the cause is unknown
3. The person has died in prison or in such place or under such circumstances as to require an inquest

Those causes of death which should be reported to the coroner include accidents and injuries, abortions, alcoholism, anaesthetics and operations, drugs, crime or suspected crime, ill treatment, diseases, infant deaths if in any way obscure, pensioners whose death may be connected with a pensionable disability, people in legal custody, poisoning, septicaemia if caused by injury and stillbirths if there is a possibility that the child may have been born alive (Dimond, 2005).

Dimond (2005) also states that if it is likely to be a coroner's case then no official post-mortem should be undertaken without the coroner's approval. The coroner can order a post-mortem examination to be carried out before deciding to hold an inquest.

A post-mortem is the examination of a body after death. It may also be referred to as an autopsy. Post-mortems are carried out by a pathologist. Pathologists are medical doctors who specialise in the diagnosis of disease and the identification of the cause of death.

Post-mortems are carried out for two reasons:

1. If the death has been referred to the coroner and the coroner feels that a post-mortem is necessary to determine the cause of death. A coroner is a judicial officer who is responsible for investigating deaths, particularly those that happen under unusual circumstances, and for determining the cause of death
2. At the request of the hospital in order to provide information about an illness or cause of death, and to further medical research

If a post-mortem is ordered by a coroner, it must take place by law, whether the next of kin gives permission or not.

If, on the other hand, the post-mortem is requested by the hospital, written consent must be obtained from the deceased's next of kin. However the Secretary of State for Health can override the wishes of the next of kin and order a post-mortem to go ahead. This power is reserved for only the most exceptional circumstances, such as a public health emergency.

Relatives of the deceased can also request the hospital to carry out a post-mortem in order to learn more about the reasons why their relative died. However, if the hospital pathologist wishes to take samples of tissue or remove organs for further study or research then the next of kin must give consent (NHS, 2007)

The way this patient's body is prepared may differ depending on the circumstances in which they died. A legal post-mortem is a coroner post-mortem and may require specific preparation. NHS Trusts should provide up-to-date information on the legal requirements.

All deaths must be treated with equal respect (Green and Green, 2006). It is necessary that the patient's spiritual and cultural needs are met when preparing the person who has died. A patient's family should always be consulted; however, a patient's previous wishes should take precedence.

Where to die

Most people wish to die at home if there is appropriate help available. If people live alone then home care may include:

- Family support
- District/community nurses
- Night sitters
- Specialist nurses such as Macmillan nurses
- General practitioners
- Respite care

The district/community nurse's success at arranging maximum home support from all agencies is vital. Expertise in symptom control is vital if hospital admissions are to be avoided.

A hospital may be a secure place for some people who have had recurrent treatments. Hospice-attached day centres offer special treatments and social support for those living alone and for all patients and their families. However, the ability to return home nightly helps the patient to maintain independence for as long as possible. Hospice care is a philosophy of care that should spread throughout every hospital and primary care team. Admissions to a hospice are frequently for symptom control or family respite.

Some of the losses a dying patient or the family may experience

Patients may experience loss of health, weight, mobility, independence, financial income, youth, dignity and a role within the family and community. The family may experience the loss of a family member, home, financial income, security and company.

The death of a loved one brings with it the greatest experience of loss. Grief is frequently described as a feeling of deep sorrow associated with this loss and grieving can be described as the state of feeling grief, and bereavement is described as the time span during which this occurs.

It is commonly recognised that the person left behind is the one experiencing grief, but it must be recognised that when patients are facing their own death, they may experience many losses: the loss of their own life, leaving their loved ones behind, the hopes, dreams and expectations that may be unfulfilled.

If the relatives know in advance that their loved one is going to die, they may start their grieving before the death occurs in anticipation of the event. It is good if both the patient and the family can support each other by exploring the grieving path together, this can be achieved through openness, and not secrecy. The nurse's role at this time is to support both the patient and the family through their pain and grief. Importantly, people may show their pain in many ways.

Family involvement

Some families do not want anyone else involved in the care of the dying person but themselves, because they may fear that the nurse will not be gentle enough with their loved one and may try to take over the caring role. Many families may want to do the nursing and only want to be shown how to move the patient and carry out pressure care.

Nurses must respect the families' commitment and never take over. Their role is to teach, encourage and support the family, carry out nursing care, reassuring them that they are doing the right thing; in this way nurses can lessen regrets rather than increase them. A peaceful death can be a lasting comfort to the family.

There are many theoretical approaches relating to the dying process. Kubler-Ross (1969) classified the 'stages model', she identified five stages that dying people were understood to go through. The stages of dying are a pattern of thinking and behaving that most people go through after learning they are dying. It is noted that not all patients react the same or move through the stages in the same way or at the same time.

Denial

This is the first stage, when the patient is first diagnosed and told that the illness will lead to death, and which he or she may refuse to believe. It is a temporary defence against the overwhelming news. There may be a 'grasping at straws'. Sometimes reality can be faced but often not for long and not too frequently. Acceptance has to be in the heart as well as in the head.

Anger

In the second stage, the patient feels angry and resentful. It is marked by the phrase: 'It's not fair, why me?' This anger can be directed at anyone: God, hospitals, nurses or doctors. This can be a difficult stage for the family, friends and carers. There can be periods of fear and agitation, and support should be given to the patient during these times.

Bargaining

This has been identified as the third stage; the patient is calmer but attempts to bargain with God or a supreme being, making promises if death will be postponed.

Depression or anticipatory grief

This is the fourth phase. Kubler-Ross (1969) claims that the patient begins to accept dying and feels sadness and grief, and may start mourning for the imminent loss of life.

Acceptance

During this stage (the final stage) the patient has accepted the inevitability of death and may feel peaceful about it or may become withdrawn. The acceptance of death by both patient and family can be a painful pathway that can be trodden only a little at a time. Some people pass silently along the pathway, coming to terms with death inside themselves, voicing little of their thoughts, whereas others voice their feelings and reactions. However, for some it is not a happy state, but an end to the struggle.

It is important to remember that the dying person need not go through all the phases and not necessarily in the order outlined above.

The needs of the dying patient

Dying patients appear to share some common fears:

- Pain and suffering
- Loneliness and dying alone
- Fear for their relatives and how they will cope
- Fear about what happens after death

When nursing terminally ill patients, the nurse must remember that the emphasis moves from curative to palliative care.

As previously emphasised, palliative care must include up-to-date knowledge of the therapy required to achieve good symptom control. It is unacceptable that anyone should suffer severe pain or distress during a final illness. The nurse's role is to ensure that he or she has the skills and knowledge required to achieve this goal, otherwise the symptom control team in a hospital or the hospice team in the community can be requested to advise.

A dying patient may experience feelings of isolation for various reasons. Fears are expressed about dying by suffocating or choking and some patients are afraid to sleep for fear of failing to wake up. Patients may feel unable to share their thoughts about dying and are left alone with their emotions and fears. Buckman (2000) says that once patients have begun to speak their thoughts, feelings and fears, it is important to let them do so at their own pace. Reflecting back on their statements, ensuring correct interpretation of what they are conveying, shows that the nurse is actually listening. The use of non-verbal cues, e.g. nodding, encourages them to continue. At this time it is important that the patient and family talk to each other (if this is what they wish), so that their affairs may be put in order, because unfinished business may cause distress for both patients and their families.

Beauchamp and Childress (2001) identified four ethical principles that must be adhered to by all nurses; these are (1) autonomy, (2) beneficence, (3) non-maleficence and (4) justice. When considering patient autonomy, it is the patient's right to make decisions about their care. Patients should always be involved in planning their care and it is their right to accept or refuse any nursing or medical intervention. Beneficence is to do good or provide benefits to others, whereas non-maleficence dictates that we do no harm to others. Justice means that everyone receives a fair share of the available resources, namely they should receive care according to their needs.

Bradbury (2000) claims that Western society sees a good death as one where the patient does not suffer. This should be the aim of every nurse, to ensure that the patient is pain free and comfortable. The nurse should ensure that patients' physical, psychological, cultural and religious beliefs are respected and their individual needs met. It is important that patients are given time to discuss any fears about their imminent death. All questions should be answered truthfully with sensitivity and maintenance of patient confidentiality at all times to ensure trust.

Caring for patients who are dying and their relatives can be an alarming prospect, but for some nurses it is one of the most rewarding and fulfilling aspects of nursing practice. Often, it is envisaged that the people the nurses care for will get better; however, Henderson (1996) says that the nurse's unique position is to assist individuals, sick or well, in the performance of their activities, contributing to health or recovery or to a peaceful death. It must be remembered that every person is a unique individual, with his or her own personality, social, cultural and spiritual background and life experiences. The nurse must address the needs of the whole person through providing holistic care – body, mind and soul in unison.

Family members should be supported if they wish to participate in caring for their loved ones. They may wish to assist in bathing the patient, administering mouth care, giving sips of water or feeding the patient; however, control of the patient's symptoms becomes the main issue whether the patient is cared for at home, in a hospice or in hospital. Accurate assessment of the patient's needs is essential for good symptom control, which does not refer just to pain control; as Dickinson et al. (2000) point out, there may also be emotional pain and other symptoms such as nausea, constipation and breathlessness.

Wilson (2004) states that terminally ill patients would prefer to die at home or to spend as much time there as possible. For the dying person and the family, this can be a rewarding experience; however, it can also be both physically and emotionally draining. The community nursing services, the Macmillan nurse or the Marie Curie nurse can be accessed for support and respite so that the family can get some rest.

Some dying patients may fear being isolated both physically and psychologically. Some do not like being in a room alone; they prefer to be surrounded by people and the general activity of the ward. However, psychological isolation can be very painful, if the patient is afraid to discuss impending death with his or her family or carers for fear of breaking down. The patient should be encouraged by the nurse to talk, the nurse should be relaxed and unhurried when carrying out any procedure; good communication skills are essential in every aspect of nursing, but more so when caring for the dying patient and his or her family.

Good practice in caring for patients and relatives/friends before death

- Always welcome the relatives, irrespective of the time of day or night
- Respect and value their participation in caring for their loved one
- Respect patients' needs, having regard for their spiritual beliefs and culture
- All nursing care must be based on patients' individual needs

In a hospital setting, if the family is with the patient 24 hours a day, a single room may be appropriate to ensure privacy. However, if the patient does not have anyone sitting with him or her, then the main ward may be appropriate so that the patient is never alone and someone sits with him or her during the last hours of his or her life.

The aim of the care of the dying patient is complex and multifaceted; one of these aims may be to provide care that relieves the patient of pain, so that death comes in a gentle way and with dignity. This can be achieved only if the needs of the body, mind and soul are met together. The nurse must always remember that patients' attitudes towards death vary a great deal and cultural and religious beliefs may influence this and the spiritual needs of the patient should be respected and addressed. The nurse must remember that practices vary within each religion and culture; the nurse should always consult the patient or family about religious observances to ensure that no offence is inadvertently caused. Death may come quickly or slowly depending on the patient's condition. The nurse must continue to provide care up to and after death.

Buckman (2000) identified some of the fears experienced by staff when caring for terminally ill patients and their relatives:

- Fear of causing pain
- Fear of being blamed

- Fear of not knowing the answers
- Fear of unleashing and having to respond to strong reactions
- Fear of expressing personal feelings
- Fear of having to confront own fears of illness and mortality
- Fear of reaction from peers (who may not always be supportive)

Signs of approaching death

The following are some of the signs that may suggest that death is approaching:

- The person may feel cold regardless of the room temperature and the number of blankets covering them.
- The person may seem to become peaceful, not showing any signs of discomfort.
- Consciousness may give way to semi-consciousness/unconsciousness, with the patient drifting in and out of consciousness until eventually drifting into a coma. However, some patients may remain conscious until death.
- The nurse must always remember that the sense of hearing is the last sense to be lost, so the room where the patient is being cared for, or the area of the ward, should be quiet.
- The person's circulation may slow down, making the skin appear pale and possibly cold to touch.
- The pulse may become weak and irregular and you may be unable to feel it before the individual dies.
- The person's breathing may become irregular and laboured and the patient may develop Cheyne-Stokes breathing, where big gaps between breaths occur until the patient stops breathing altogether. Mucus in the throat and airways may make a sound that is often called 'a death rattle'.

In some patients the muscles may relax and the patient's body becomes 'limp', there is no pulse, respiration or blood pressure. The pupils become fixed and dilated.

Procedures after death

The following procedures may be undertaken after the death of the patient. These procedures are only guidelines and local policy and procedure must prevail.

- Medical staff must be informed and confirmation of death must be recorded in both the medical and the nursing notes. This is usually done by a doctor; however, if an expected death occurs during the night, a senior nurse on duty may confirm a death if an agreed policy is in place.
- Inform the appropriate senior nurse.
- Inform and offer support to relatives. Offer support of the hospital Chaplin if appropriate.
- Put on gloves and apron.

- Depending on the ward's protocol, the nurse may proceed gently to lay the patient flat on the bed with one pillow.
- Dentures must be inserted into the mouth immediately because it may be difficult to do this later when rigor mortis sets in.
- The person's eyes must be closed.
- Exudating wounds should be covered with a clean absorbent dressing and secured with an occlusive dressing.
- Inform other patients.
- A pillow or a rolled-up towel must be placed on the patient's chest under the chin to support the jaw.
- The arms and legs must be straightened.
- Remove any mechanical aids such as syringe drivers unless otherwise stated, for example in the case of an unexpected death that will be referred to the coroner.

The body is covered with a clean sheet and left for an hour, or whatever the ward's protocol is, before the last offices are performed. The last offices are when the body is prepared prior to removal to the mortuary.

If the relatives are not present at the time of death, the nurse must have ascertained previously if they wished to be called any time of the day or night when the event happens. Thayre and Peate (2003) claim that when contacting and notifying relatives of the death of their loved one, this is the first step in breaking bad news and is very important. They claim that it may present a dilemma as to whether you tell them over the telephone in order to avoid a distressed dash to the hospital, or by saying that the condition of their loved one had deteriorated and could they come to the hospital where the news of the death can be broken in a more gentle way. Thayre and Peate (2003) provide suggestions for a nurse's first contact with relatives:

- The nurse should identify himself or herself, the ward and the hospital clearly and slowly, confirm to whom he or she is speaking and the relationship with the patient.
- The nurse must explain clearly that the person has been admitted to either the accident and emergency department or a ward, or that the person's condition has unexpectedly deteriorated.
- The nurse must reassure the family that everything possible is being done; this may give relatives an insight into the seriousness of the patient's condition. If the nurse asks the family to come to the hospital, he or she could suggest that they should be driven by someone if possible, thus suggesting that the situation is serious.

The nurse must be aware that the family may be angry if they arrive too late and they must always be truthful and say whether the patient was already dead when the phone call was made. If the family is not told the truth, then feelings of guilt of not being with the patient may ensue. If there is anger, the nurse must acknowledge it and be aware of their grief. Gently explain the reasons why you felt that this was the best way to break the sad news and apologise if the family feels that it was the wrong approach.

When people are distressed the nurse may find it difficult to know what to say, especially if they do not know the family. It is important to be gentle, warm and honest in approach. Any offer of help may be rejected, especially if relatives are unhappy about the care given to their loved one. If appropriate, touch may be appreciated by the grieving relative; however, the nurse must be aware of when to withdraw, but never be afraid to show that he or she cares because relatives gain comfort when nurses show emotion on the death of their loved one.

The hospital should accommodate any wishes that the relatives may have as this may help the grieving process. The relatives should be given refreshments in private. If they were not present at the death, they may wish to discuss the death with a nurse.

Last offices

An opportunity to view the body should be offered to the family either before laying the body flat or after the last offices have been performed. 'Last offices' is the last act that nurses are privileged to carry out for a patient for whom they have cared. The family must always be offered the opportunity to participate in this procedure, but must never be forced to do so; the nurse must be aware of both cultural and religious requirements. The nurse must have confirmed with the family what they want done at the time of the patient's death. In some cultures, it is the members of the family or their religious group who perform the last offices. It must also be remembered that the way the body is handled forms an important part of how the bereaved view the hospital care and also helps them in their grieving process. Neuberger (2004) claims that it is essential that the correct procedures be followed during last offices, so that the wishes of the patient and the relatives are met, thus also ensuring holistic care. (However, if they are disregarded, we disregard both the patient's and the family's dignity.)

Most people have a spiritual aspect to their psyche. Some people call it their soul, others the inner energy that makes them whom they are. Spirituality is frequently linked to religious beliefs. Firth (2001) claims that the lack of research into the spiritual and religious needs of ethnic minorities may be the result of the belief that religious and spiritual care are provided by the faith communities.

Equipment for performing the last offices

The following is a list of equipment that may be used when performing the last offices. The equipment needed must be tailored to meet the individual needs of the person who has died:

- A bowl, soap, two towels, two face cloths
- A razor, comb, nail scissors
- Equipment for cleaning dentures and oral toilet
- Notification of death labels and two identification bracelets
- A shroud or patient's nightdress or pyjamas or clothes requested by the patient or family, or those needed for religious or cultural observance
- A body bag may be required if there is the possibility of leakage of body fluids or an infectious disease
- Dressing pack with tape or bandages if there are any wounds
- Sellotape

- Valuables envelope, valuables book and property book
- Skip for dirty linen and plastic bag for waste
- Mortuary sheet

All equipment must be taken to the bedside. The nurse should wear an apron and gloves. Patients in the beds nearby should be informed. All drainage tubes should be removed, unless otherwise stated, and covered with an occlusive dressing.

Wash the patient gently if permitted to do so by the family. A male patient may need to be shaved. The family may wish to assist in this procedure as a mark of respect for the loved one (respect and dignity must be afforded to the patient's relatives and the patient's body at all times). It must be remembered that nurses may not be permitted to carry out this procedure, as identified earlier, on religious and cultural grounds.

When turning the body over to wash the back, air that is trapped may be expelled. Some nurses find it easier to speak to the body as they did when the patient was alive. The patient's mouth should be cleaned using a foam stick to remove any dry secretions or debris. If the patient has a wound, the nurse should remove the soiled dressing and replace it with a clean one.

Dress the patient in a disposable shroud or his or her own clothes, depending on the policy of the hospital or relatives' requests.

Jewellery should be removed from the body unless otherwise stated by the family. This should be documented on a 'Notification of Death' form (or as per policy). The patient's valuables should be checked with another nurse, recorded and placed in a sealed envelope and stored according to hospital policy. If the family wishes to view the body before it is removed from the ward, they should be given the opportunity to say their last farewells.

A patient identification bracelet should be placed on the patient's wrist and ankle. A death notification label should be placed on the shroud. The body should be wrapped in a mortuary sheet, ensuring that the head and feet are covered and the legs secured in position by gently tying a tape around the two big toes. The sheet is then secured with Sellotape and the remaining death notification label is placed upside down on the sheet.

The portering staff should be notified to remove the body. However, a nurse must accompany them when they arrive to ensure that the body is removed gently and with respect as this will minimise the effect on the other patients on the ward (Dougherty and Lister, 2008).

Clear away soiled linen and waste in accordance with hospital policy. Remove gloves and apron. The patient's property should be sent to the appropriate administrative office. The bed should be washed thoroughly and disinfected in accordance with hospital policy before being remade. The nurse should also be aware of the needs of the other patients on the ward and be ready to answer their questions without breaching confidentiality.

Cultural and religious beliefs

Dickinson et al. (2000) claim that religion today is a philosophical attitude for many people and not everyone apportions the same relevance to God and the afterlife as in previous generations. It is very important for the nurse to try to find out what the patient fears most, because the patient can communicate more fully with the nurse who empathises with these fears.

Let us consider broadly some of the needs of certain religious groups, remembering that within these groups there are variations about what occurs at the time of death. The only way to be sure and not to offend is to ask (Table 15.1).

Alarm

The fight-or-flight response mirrors a stress reaction and can last for between a few hours and 10 days. It displays itself through restlessness, panic, muscle tension, headaches, loss of appetite, insomnia and emptiness.

Coming to terms with the loss of a loved one is like having to come to terms with enforced change, with the loss of hopes, ambitions and dreams. If the bereaved person's grief is not resolved normally, they may have to be referred to a bereavement counsellor to help them reach the acceptance stage.

Russell (2002) claims that in some studies people's individual experiences of grief may be influenced by culture and social norms. Western societies expect the bereaved to resolve their grief in a short time span; however, for many people, it is a long and painful journey.

Breaking bad news

'Bad news' is any information likely to alter dramatically a patient's view of his or her future. Bad news being conveyed may not be about impending death but could be a diagnosis of diabetes, heart disease or HIV. The patient should be given the opportunity to ask questions, which should be answered sensitively, honestly and with empathy. The patient and family need to be reassured that help will be available if needed and that the nurse understands that they may not have taken all the implications in, and if they wish to make further appointments to ask more questions they must feel free to do so. You cannot soften the impact that bad news can bring because it remains bad news however, regardless of how it is broken, but it can be broken such a way that it conveys caring and support.

Kemp (1999) claims that patients and families frequently grieve for different losses, and that during the dying process they may progress at different speeds. Russell (2002) claims that death may release many different emotions in people; some may be affected greatly and others less so. However, in some instances there may be relief as death means the end of suffering for their loved one.

Murray-Parkes (2000) describes grief as a psychosocial transition in which the bereaved person has to readjust his or her life without the deceased person and has to realise that he or she has to adapt to a new and altered world. However, he claims that each person's experience of grief is unique and states that 'grief is essentially an emotion that draws us towards something or someone that is missing'. Farrell (2002) identifies the ways in which to help the bereaved by:

- Being there
- Listening in a non-judgemental way
- Showing that you have some understanding of what they are going through

Table 15.1 The needs of some religious groups.

Religion	At the time of death	After death occurs
Christianity *Anglican/Church of England*	The hospital chaplain or parish priest may be called to administer Holy Communion if death is imminent. If, however, a chaplain is not available and if prayers are requested, a nurse could say the Lord's Prayer or get another nurse to do so if necessary, or the patient may wish to recite prayers with the family.	Last offices are performed according to hospital practice. A Christian may choose to be buried or cremated. No religious objection to post-mortem.
Free Church, e.g. Baptist, Methodist, Quakers, Salvation Army	A chaplain should be called. Prayers and comfort are available also from their own minister or chaplain who may join the patient and family in informal prayer rather than administer the sacraments.	Last offices are performed according to hospital practice. May choose to be buried or cremated. No religious objection to post-mortem.
Church of Jesus Christ of Latter-Day Saints (The Mormon Church)	There is no specific ritual for the dying; however, spiritual contact is important. The church should be contacted. Mormons may wear a sacred undergarment in death as well as in life.	Last offices are acceptable and burial is preferred. No religious objection to post-mortem.
Roman Catholicism	The sacrament of anointing the sick should be administered to a seriously ill patient who could die. It is important to notify the chaplain at the earliest opportunity. Ward staff should make a record of the sacrament.	Last offices are appropriate and some families may wish to place a crucifix or a rosary with the patient. There is no religious objection to post-mortem. Burial or cremation is acceptable.
Judaism	There is a wide variety of observances within the Jewish faith. However, if possible, open the window to allow the soul departure to heaven. The nurse must always respect the patient's and family's wishes. The patient may wish to recite prayers with the family.	The body should be handled as little as possible and gloves must be worn. The family will usually contact their rabbi. If there is no family, the Hebrew Burial Society or local rabbi should be notified. In some instances, the family will carry out the last offices themselves.

(*Continued*)

Table 15.1 (*Continued*).

Religion	At the time of death	After death occurs
		Jewish people are usually buried within 24 hours of dying, but not on the Sabbath. Post-mortems are usually forbidden unless required by law.
Islam	The *Koran* should be recited by the family or an Imam as the patient faces Mecca. Most hospitals have a Mecca compass, if in doubt contact the local mosque for advice.	Where possible, the patient should not be touched for 30 minutes after death. Non-Muslims should not touch the body. The last offices will be carried out by the family, and if not, nurses must wear gloves and consult the family before washing as they may not want the patient to be washed. In this instance, preparation involves straightening the patient, closing their eyes and mouth and wrapping them in a plain white sheet. Somebody of the same religion and sex should carry out this procedure. Muslims are usually buried within 24 hours of dying. Muslims are opposed to post-mortems unless required by law.
Sikhism	The patient and family may recite passages from the Holy Book.	The family may wish to carry out the last offices themselves; they do not, however, object to others touching the patient. If the patient has taken the vow to abide by the five articles or the five Ks: (1) The *kirpan* means they wear a symbolic sword in a cloth sheath under their clothes (2) The *kara*, an iron, steel or gold wrist band worn on the right wrist

Table 15.1 (*Continued*).

Religion	At the time of death	After death occurs
		(3) The *kach*, cotton shorts (4) The *kesh*, uncut hair (5) The *kangha*, a wooden comb that fixes uncut hair into a bun The turban must remain on, even in death. The nurse should never remove any of these articles or cut the hair. Sikhs are always cremated as soon after death as possible. There is no objection if a post-mortem is required by law.
Hinduism	Hindu patients receive comfort from readings from *Bhagavad Gita*. A side room should be offered for privacy where possible. A Hindu priest should be contacted if the patient or their family wishes to perform certain rituals and blessings. The eldest son should be present. The Ganges water may be administered. Families may wish to burn incense; this may not be possible in certain situations.	The body should be touched only by Hindus. However, if this is not possible then nursing staff must request permission to carry out the last offices, using disposable gloves, as ideally the patient should not be touched by the nurse. No jewellery or sacred objects such as neck and wrist threads should be removed from the patient. All Hindus are cremated. There is no objection to post-mortem if required by law.
Buddhism	There are different sects of Buddhism, so it is important to contact the relatives to establish their wishes. Allow privacy for quiet meditation and chanting by fellow Buddhists may help to relax the patient's state of mind which is very important. At the time of death those around the patient should be calm; this is because Buddhists believe this will influence the character of rebirth.	Before undertaking last offices, check with the family. The body should not be removed if a monk or nun is to attend. The monk or nun may wish to be present during the procedure. Most Buddhists are cremated and their ashes are buried. There is usually no objection to post-mortem; however, some Buddhists from certain countries may object.

Source: Adapted from Green and Green (2006), Neuberger (2004) and Speck (2003).

- Encouraging them to talk about the deceased
- Accepting silence
- Being aware of your own feelings about loss
- Offering reassurance that their grief is normal
- Not taking any anger personally
- Being aware that your feelings may reflect their own
- Resigning yourself to the fact that you cannot make them feel better

Le Mone and Burke (2008) claim that the assessment of the bereaved person's social support systems is important because it helps in the normal outcome of their grief. However, in some instances, loss of a loved one may lead to social isolation, with feelings of loneliness making the person withdraw from their usual social support systems; this results in the bereaved being in danger of prolonged abnormal grieving. The nurse must be aware of this and ascertain how often the person meets friends and encourage them to continue doing so.

Conclusions

Caring for dying patients and supporting bereaved families is a privilege bestowed upon the nurse it can also be a demanding and sometimes stressful experience. If nurses are to offer the highest quality care, they also need to be aware of their own needs. Loss, grief and bereavement will raise many professional and personal issues for all members of the multi-professional health care team. Each member of the team will need support of the others as well as the patient and the family.

It is important that a ward, community and hospice climate exists in which staff are seen to be sincere, sensitive and supporting because this will allow nurses to discuss their painful experience and use the support available without feeling a loss of professional control.

Glossary

Breaking bad news	Any information likely to alter dramatically a person's view of his or her future
Chaplin	A priest, religious minister, rabbi, imam, or other religious leader attached to an institution
Coroner	A judicial officer responsible for investigating deaths that happen under unusual circumstances and determining the cause of death
Death	Cessation of the body's vital function
Hospice	System of care available to the chronically or terminally ill people and their family
Last offices	The care given to a deceased patient, which is focused on fulfilling religious and cultural beliefs as well as health and safety and legal requirements
Palliative care	An approach that improves the quality of life of patients and their families approaching life-limiting illness

Post-mortem	The examination of a body after death; also known as an autopsy
Pathologist	Doctors who specialise in the diagnosis of disease and the identification of the cause of death

Post-chapter quiz

1. List the signs of approaching death
2. Describe the care needed by the dying patient
3. How would you empower the dying patient?
4. Identify three types of support available to the family
5. How has the World Health Organization defined 'palliative care'?
6. What are the three aims identified by the Royal College of Nursing relating to patient dignity?
7. What services might a hospice offer?
8. In what way could a family participate in the care of their dying relative?
9. Discuss the benefits of implementing the Liverpool Care Pathway
10. What procedure is usually undertaken when a patient dies?

References

Beauchamp, T.L. and Childress, J.F. (2001) *Principles of Biomedical Ethics*, 5th edn. Oxford: Oxford University Press.

Bradbury, M. (2000) The good death. In: Dickenson, D., Johnson, H. and Katz, J.S. (eds). *Death, Dying and Bereavement*. London: Sage, pp. 59-63.

Buckman, R. (2000) Communication in patient care. In: Dickenson, D., Johnson, H. and Kratz, J.S. (eds). *Death, Dying and Bereavement*. London: Sage.

Clark, D. (2002) Between hope and acceptance: the medicalisation of dying. *British Medical Journal* 324: 905-907.

Costello, J. (2004) *Nursing the Dying Patient: Caring in Different Contexts*. Basingstoke: Palgrave Macmillan.

Dickinson, D., Johnson, H. and Kratz, J.S. (eds) (2000) *Death, Dying and Bereavement*. London: Sage.

Dimond, B. (2005) *Legal Aspects of Nursing*. 4th ed. Glasgow: Pearson Longman.

Dougherty, L. and Lister, S. (eds) (2008) *The Royal Marsden Hospital Manual of Clinical Nursing Procedures*, 6th ed. Oxford: Blackwell Science.

Ellershaw, J. and Wilkinson, S. (2003) Evaluating the Liverpool Care Pathway for the Dying Patient and future developments. In: Ellershaw, J. and Wilkinson, S. (eds). *Care of the Dying: A Pathway to Excellence*. Oxford: Oxford University Press.

Farrell, M. (2002) Breaking bad news. In: Shaw, T. and Sanders, K. *Foundation of Nursing Studies*. Dissemination Series,Vol. 1. Available at http://www.fons.org/ahcp/completedprojects/pdfs/Diss%20Series%20Vol%201%20No%202.pdf. Accessed 2 July 2009.

Firth, S. (2001) *Wider Horizons: Care of the Dying in a Multicultural Society*. London: The National Council for Hospice and Palliative Care Services.

Fowell, A., Finlay, I.G., Johnstone, R. and Minto, L. (2002) An integrated care pathway for the last two days of life: Wales wide benchmarking in palliative care. *International Journal of Palliative Nursing* 8(12): 566-573.

Freud, S. (1918) *Reflections on War and Death*. New York: Moffat Yard.
Green, J. and Green, M. (2006) *Dealing with Death: A Handbook of Practices, Procedures and Law*, 2nd ed. Suffolk: Jessica Kingsley.
Health and Safety Executive (2007) *Advisory Committee on Dangerous Pathogens*. London: Health and Safety Executive.
Henderson, V. (1996) *The Nature of Nursing*. New York: Macmillan.
Jung, C.G. (1959) *The Archetypes and the Collective Unconscious*. Princeton: Princeton University Press.
Kemp, E. (1999) *Terminal Illness: A Guide to Nursing Care*, 2nd edn. New York: Lippincott.
Kubler-Ross, E. (1969) *On Death and Dying*. New York: Macmillan.
Le Mone, P. and Burke, K.M. (2008) *Medical/Surgical Nursing: Critical Thinking on Client Care*. New Jersey: Pearson International edition.
Murray-Parkes, C.M. (2000) Bereavement as a psychosocial transition, process of adaptation to change. In: Dickinson, D., Johnson, M. and Katz, J.S. (eds). *Death, Dying and Bereavement*. London: Sage, pp. 325–331.
National Health Service (2007) Post-mortem. Available at http://www.nhs.uk/conditions/Post-mortem/Pages/Introduction.aspx?url=Pages/what-i. Accessed 26 January 2009.
National Institute for Health and Clinical Excellence (2004) *Improving Supportive and Palliative Care for Adults with Cancer*. London: NICE.
Neuberger, J. (2004) *Caring for Dying People of Different Faiths*. Abingdon: Radcliff Medical Press.
Nursing and Midwifery Council (2008) *The Code: Standards of Conduct, Performance and Ethics for Nurses and Midwives*. London: NMC.
Russell, P. (2002) Social behaviour and professional interactions. In: Hogston, R. and Simpson, P.M. (eds). *Foundations of Nursing Practice: Making the Difference*, 2nd ed. Basingstoke: Palgrave Macmillan, pp. 343–370.
Speck, P. (2003) Spirituality/religious issues in care of the dying. In: Ellershaw, J. and Wilkingson, S. (eds). *Care of the Dying: A pathway to Excellence*. Oxford: Oxford University Press.
Taylor, C. (2004) Reviewing nursing support in cancer care. *Cancer Nursing Practice* 3(3): 26–31.
The Department of Health (2000) *The National Health Service Plan*. London: DH.
The Royal College of Nursing (2008) *Dignity at the Heart of Everything We Do*. London: RCN.
The World Health Organization (2007) *Cancer Control, Knowledge into Action. WHO Guide for Effective Palliative Care*. Geneva: WHO.
Thayre, K. and Peate, I. (2003) Coping with expected and sudden death. In: Hinchliff, S.M., Norman, S.E. and Schober, J.E. (eds). *Nursing Practice and Health Care*, 4th ed. London: Edward Arnold, Chapter 13, pp. 291–314.
Wilson, V. (2004) Supporting family carers in the community setting. *Nursing Standard* 18(29): 47–53.

Appendix: Normal values

The values given below are representative of the average reference range for adults in:

- Blood
- Cerebrospinal fluid
- Urine

The ranges shown should only be used as a guide. Reference ranges between laboratories will vary; there are many reasons for this, for example the type of analytical equipment used and the temperature used, and you should always consult the ranges used in your own laboratory.

Blood (haematology)

Test	Reference range
Activated partial thromboplastin time (APTT)	30–40 seconds
Erythrocyte sedimentation rate (ESR)	
Women	3–15 mm/hour
Men	1–10 mm/hour
Fibrinogen	1.5–4.0 g/L
Folate (serum)	4–18 μg/L
Haemoglobin (Hb)	
Women	11.5–16.5 g/dL
Men	13–18 g/dL
Haptoglobins	0.3–2.0 g/L
Mean cell haemoglobin (MCH)	27–32 pg
Mean cell haemoglobin concentrate (MCHC)	30–35 g/dL
Mean cell volume (MCV)	78–95 fl
Packed cell volume (PCV or haematocrit)	
Women	0.35–0.47 (35–47%)
Men	0.4–0.54 (40–54%)
Platelets (thrombocytes)	$(150\text{–}400) \times 10^9$/L
Prothrombin time	12–16 seconds
Red cells (erythrocytes)	
Women	$(3.8\text{–}5.3) \times 10^{12}$/L
Men	$(4.5\text{–}6.5) \times 10^{12}$/L
Reticulocytes	$(25\text{–}85) \times 10^9$/L
White cells total (leucocytes)	$(4.0\text{–}11.0) \times 10^9$/L

Blood venous (unless stated) plasma (biochemistry)

Test	Reference range
Alanine aminotransferase (ALT)	10–40 U/L
Albumin	36–47 g/L
Alkaline phosphate	40–125 U/L
Amylase	90–300 U/L
Aspartate aminotransferase (AST)	10–35 U/l
Bicarbonate (arterial)	22–28 mmols/L
Bilirubin (total)	2–17 μmol/L
Calcium	2.1–2.6 mmol/L
Chloride	95–105 mmol/L
Cholesterol (total)	below 5.2 mmol/L
HDL cholesterol	
Women	0.6–1.9 mmol/L
Men	0.5–1.6 mmol/L
$Paco_2$ (arterial)	44.1–6.1 kPa
Copper	13–24 μmol/L
Cortisol (at 0800 hours)	160–565 nmol/L
Creatine kinase (total)	
Women	30–150 U/L
Men	30–200 U/L
Creatinine	50–150 μmol/L
Gamma-glutamyl transferase	
Women	5–35 U/L
Men	10–55 U/L
Globulins	24–37 g/L
Glucose (venous blood fasting)	3.6–5.8 mmol/L
Glycosylated haemoglobin (HbA_1)	4–6%
Hydrogen ion concentration (arterial)	35–44 nmol/L
Iron	
Men	10–28 μmol/L
Women	14–32 μmol/L
Iron binding capacity total (TIBC)	45–70 μmol/L
Lactate (arterial)	0.3–1.4 mmol/L
Lactate dehydrogenase (total)	230–460 U/L
Lead (whole blood)	<1.7 μmol/L
Magnesium	0.7–1.0 mmol/L
Osmolality	275–290 mmol/kg
Pao_2 (arterial)	12–15 kPa
Oxygen saturation (arterial)	>97%
pH	7.36–7.42
Phosphate (fasting)	0.8–1.4 mmol/L
Potassium (serum)	3.6–5.0 mmol/L
Protein (total)	60–80 g/L
Sodium	136–145 mmol/L
Transferrin	2–4 g/L
Triglycerides (fasting)	0.6–1.8 mmol/L

Test	Reference range
Urate	
Women	0.12-0.36 mmol/L
Men	0.12-0.42 mmol/L
Urea	2.5-6.5 mmol/L
Uric acid	
Women	0.09-0.36 mmol/L
Men	0.1-0.45 mmol/L
Vitamin A	0.7-3.5 μmol/L
Vitamin C	23-57 μmol/L
Zinc	11-22 μmol/L

Cerebrospinal fluid

Test	Reference range
Cells	0-5 mm^3
Chloride	120-170 mmol/L
Glucose	2.5-4.0 mmol/L
Pressure	50-180 mm/H_2O
Protein	100-400 mg/L

Urine

Test	Reference range
Albumin/creatinine ratio	<3.5 mg albumin/mmol creatinine
Calcium (diet dependent)	<12 mmol/24 hours (normal diet)
Copper	0.26-0.6 μmol/24 hours
Cortisol	9-50 μmol/24 hours
Creatinine	9-17 mmol/24 hours
5-Hydroxyindole-3-acetic acid (5H1AA)	10-45 μmol/24 hours
Magnesium	3.3-5.0 mmol/24 hours
Oxalate	
Women	40-320 mmol/24 hours
Men	80-490 mmol/24 hours
pH	4-8
Phosphate	15-50 mmol/24 hours
Porphyrins (total)	90-370 mmol/24 hours
Potassium[a]	25-100 mmol/24 hours
Protein (total)	no more than 0.3g/L
Sodium[a]	100-200 mmol/24 hours
Urea	170-500 mmol/24 hours

[a]Depends on intake.

Index